Interoperability in Healthcare Information Systems:

Standards, Management, and Technology

Miguel-Ángel Sicilia
University of Alcalá, Spain

Pablo Serrano Balazote
Hospital de Fuenlabrada, Spain

A volume in the Advances in Healthcare Information Systems and Administration (AHISA) Book Series

Medical Information Science
REFERENCE
An Imprint of IGI Global

Managing Director: Lindsay Johnston
Production Editor: Jennifer Yoder
Development Editor: Erin O'Dea
Acquisitions Editor: Kayla Wolfe
Typesetter: John Crodian
Cover Design: Jason Mull

Published in the United States of America by
Medical Information Science Reference (an imprint of IGI Global)
701 E. Chocolate Avenue
Hershey PA 17033
Tel: 717-533-8845
Fax: 717-533-8661
E-mail: cust@igi-global.com
Web site: http://www.igi-global.com

Library of Congress Cataloging-in-Publication Data

Interoperability in healthcare information systems : standards, management, and technology / Miguel-Angel Sicilia and Pablo Serrano Balazota, editors.
pages cm
Includes bibliographical references and index.
Summary: "This book provides a comprehensive collection on the overview of electronic health records and health services interoperability and the different aspects representing its outlook in a framework that is useful for practitioners, researchers, and decision-makers"-- Provided by publisher.
ISBN 978-1-4666-3000-0 (hardcover) -- ISBN 978-1-4666-3001-7 (ebook) -- ISBN 978-1-4666-3002-4 (print & perpetual access) 1. Medical records--Management. 2. Information storage and retrieval systems--Medical care--Management. 3. Medical informatics--Management. I. Sicilia, Miguel-Angel, 1973- editor of compilation. II. Balazota, Pablo Serrano, 1964- editor of compilation.
RA976.N497 2013
610.285--dc23
2013012831

This book is published in the IGI Global book series Advances in Healthcare Information Systems and Administration (AHISA) (ISSN: 2328-1243; eISSN: 2328-126X)

British Cataloguing in Publication Data
A Cataloguing in Publication record for this book is available from the British Library.

Advances in Healthcare Information Systems and Administration (AHISA) Book Series

Anastasius Moumtzoglou
Hellenic Society for Quality & Safety in Healthcare and P. & A. Kyriakou Children's Hospital, Greece
Anastasia N. Kastania
Athens University of Economics and Business, Greece

ISSN: 2328-1243
EISSN: 2328-126X

Mission

The **Advances in Healthcare Information Systems and Administration (AHISA) Book Series** aims to provide a channel for international researchers to progress the field of study on technology and its implications on healthcare and health information systems. With the growing focus on healthcare and the importance of enhancing this industry to tend to the expanding population, the book series seeks to accelerate the awareness of technological advancements of health information systems and expand awareness and implementation.

Driven by advancing technologies and their clinical applications, the emerging field of health information systems and informatics is still searching for coherent directing frameworks to advance health care and clinical practices and research. Conducting research in these areas is both promising and challenging due to a host of factors, including rapidly evolving technologies and their application complexity. At the same time, organizational issues, including technology adoption, diffusion and acceptance as well as cost benefits and cost effectiveness of advancing health information systems and informatics applications as innovative forms of investment in healthcare are gaining attention as well. **AHISA** addresses these concepts and critical issues.

Coverage

- Clinical Decision Support Design, Development and Implementation
- E-Health and M-Health
- IT Applications in Physical Therapeutic Treatments
- IT Security and Privacy Issues
- Management of Emerging Health Care Technologies
- Pharmaceutical and Home Healthcare Informatics
- Rehabilitative Technologies
- Role of Informatics Specialists
- Telemedicine
- Virtual Health Technologies

IGI Global is currently accepting manuscripts for publication within this series. To submit a proposal for a volume in this series, please contact our Acquisition Editors at Acquisitions@igi-global.com or visit: http://www.igi-global.com/publish/.

The Advances in Healthcare Information Systems and Administration (AHISA) Book Series (ISSN 2328-1243) is published by IGI Global, 701 E. Chocolate Avenue, Hershey, PA 17033-1240, USA, www.igi-global.com. This series is composed of titles available for purchase individually; each title is edited to be contextually exclusive from any other title within the series. For pricing and ordering information please visit http://www.igi-global.com/book-series/advances-healthcare-information-systems-administration/37156. Postmaster: Send all address changes to above address.

Titles in this Series

For a list of additional titles in this series, please visit: www.igi-global.com

Cloud Computing Applications for Quality Health Care Delivery
Anastasius Moumtzoglou (Hellenic Society for Quality & Safety in Healthcare and P. & A. Kyriakou Children's Hospital, Greece) and Anastasia Kastania (Athens University of Economics and Business, Greece)
Medical Information Science Reference • copyright 2014 • 337pp • H/C (ISBN: 9781466661189) • US $245.00 (our price)

Achieving Effective Integrated E-Care Beyond the Silos
Ingo Meyer (empirica, Germany) Sonja Müller (empirica, Germany) and Lutz Kubitschke (empirica, Germany)
Medical Information Science Reference • copyright 2014 • 332pp • H/C (ISBN: 9781466661387) • US $245.00 (our price)

Social Media and Mobile Technologies for Healthcare
Mowafa Househ (College of Public Health and Health Informatics, King Saud Bin Abdulaziz University for Health Sciences, Saudi Arabia) Elizabeth Borycki (University of Victoria, Canada) and Andre Kushniruk (University of Victoria, Canada)
Medical Information Science Reference • copyright 2014 • 308pp • H/C (ISBN: 9781466661509) • US $245.00 (our price)

Advancing Medical Practice through Technology Applications for Healthcare Delivery, Management, and Quality
Joel J.P.C. Rodrigues (Instituto de Telecomunicações, University of Beira Interior, Portugal)
Medical Information Science Reference • copyright 2014 • 361pp • H/C (ISBN: 9781466646193) • US $245.00 (our price)

Handbook of Research on Patient Safety and Quality Care through Health Informatics
Vaughan Michell (University of Reading, UK) Deborah J. Rosenorn-Lanng (Royal Berkshire Hospital Foundation Trust Reading, UK) Stephen R. Gulliver (University of Reading, UK) and Wendy Currie (Audencia, Ecole de Management, Nantes, France)
Medical Information Science Reference • copyright 2014 • 486pp • H/C (ISBN: 9781466645462) • US $365.00 (our price)

Research Perspectives on the Role of Informatics in Health Policy and Management
Christo El Morr (York University, Canada)
Medical Information Science Reference • copyright 2014 • 323pp • H/C (ISBN: 9781466643215) • US $245.00 (our price)

Table of Contents

Detailed Table of Contents

The current healthcare delivery paradigm is defined by integrative care delivery across disparate providers and services. Therefore the ability to deliver efficient and effective healthcare services is dependent on designing and implementing interoperable systems. However, the notion of interoperability is multifaceted and complex. Although the exchange of data is often described as analogous with interoperability it must be remembered that healthcare is a process oriented domain and clinical, management, organizational and other processes must be considered as part of interoperability. This chapter discusses healthcare delivery and the role interoperability plays in supporting its delivery. First, the chapter provides a background on healthcare interoperability from multiple perspectives. Then it presents a case study of collaborative care delivery and uses it to outline specific interoperability requirements. The chapter then uses these requirements to develop a multi-tiered framework of healthcare interoperability, concluding with a discussion of the implications of the framework for interoperability research and for systems design to support integrated healthcare delivery.

The standardization of clinical data represents a major step in the development of information and organizational knowledge of health services. The evolution of information systems from a model of different database owners to a different open software based model is a major challenge. For this reason it is essential to adopt models of metadata based on archetypes to improve the development of information systems and simultaneously integrate all applications. The adoption of clinical terminology that can translate existing knowledge and enhance its growth is a necessary goal. Accessibility, ubiquity, completeness, consistency and durability of the clinical data are essential objectives for efficiency and effectiveness gains in organizations. This chapter presents the concepts and technologies needed to implement a model of EHR (Electronic Health Record) based on a standard, open architecture. It also presents some concepts of decision support systems and business processes that can be integrated with the EHR.

Normalization of data is a prerequisite to achieve semantic interoperability in any domain. This is even more important in the healthcare sector due to the special sensitivity of medical data: data exchange must be done in a meaningful way, avoiding all possibility of misunderstanding or misinterpretation. In this chapter, we present the LinkEHR system for clinical data standardization and exchange. The LinkEHR platform provides tools that simplify meaningful sharing of electronic health records between different systems and organizations. Key contributions of LinkEHR are the development of a powerful medical concept, expressed in the form of archetypes, editing framework based on formal semantics capable of handling multiple electronic health record architectures, the definition of high-level non-procedural mappings to describe the relationship between archetype and legacy clinical data and the semi-automatic generation of XQuery scripts that transform legacy data into XML documents compliant with the underlying electronic health record data architecture and at the same time satisfy the constraints imposed by the archetype.

The semantic interoperability of electronic healthcare record systems is a major issue given that it would increase the quality of healthcare and patient safety. In this chapter, different solutions based on the use of semantic models for representing clinical knowledge are presented. The aim of the research presented here is to contribute to the achievement of semantic interoperability by making explicit the meaning of the exchanged data and knowledge items. In particular, this work is focused on dual model-based electronic healthcare records standards and presents methods and tools for the representation and transformation of clinical archetypes and for the automatic generation of standardized applications.

This chapter presents an approach to translate definitions expressed in openEHR Archetype Definition Language (ADL) to a formal representation using ontology languages. The approach is implemented in the ArchOnt framework, which is also described. The integration of those formal representations with clinical rules is then studied, providing an approach to reuse reasoning on concrete instances of clinical data. Sharing the knowledge expressed in the form of rules is coherent with the philosophy of open sharing underlying clinical archetypes, and it also extends reuse to propositions of declarative knowledge as those encoded for example in clinical guidelines. Thus, this chapter describes the techniques to map archetypes to formal ontologies and how rules can be attached to the resulting representation. In addition, the translation allows specifying logical bindings to equivalent clinical concepts from other knowledge sources. Such bindings encourage reuse as well as ontology reasoning and navigability across different ontologies. Another significant contribution of the chapter is the application of the presented approach as part of two research projects in collaboration with teaching hospitals in Madrid. Examples taken from those cases, such as the development of alerting systems aimed at improving patient safety, are explained. Besides the direct applications described, the automatic translation of archetypes to an ontology language fosters a wide range of semantic and reasoning activities to be designed and implemented on top of a common representation instead of taking an ad-hoc approach.

Semantic interoperability facilitates Health Care and Life Sciences (HCLS) systems in connecting stakeholders at various levels as well as ensuring seamless use of healthcare resources. Their scope ranges from local to regional, national and cross-border. The use of semantics in delivering interoperable solution for HCLS systems is weakened by fact that an Ontology Based Information System (OBIS) has restrictions in modeling, aggregating, and interpreting global knowledge in conjunction with local information (e.g., policy, profiles). This chapter presents an example-scenario that shows such limitations and recognizes that enabling two key features, namely the type and scope of knowledge, within a knowledge base could enhance the overall effectiveness of an OBIS. This chapter provides the idea of separating knowledge bases in types with scope (e.g., global or local) of applicability. Then, it proposes two concrete solutions on this general notion. Finally, the chapter describes open research issues that may be of interest to knowledge system developers and broader research community.

A Wireless Sensor Network (WSN) can be deployed to monitor the health of patients suffering from critical diseases. A wireless network consisting of biomedical sensors can also be implanted into the patient's body and can monitor the patients' conditions. These sensor devices, apart from having an enormous capability of collecting data from their physical surroundings, are also resource constraint in nature with a limited processing and communication ability. Therefore, it is necessary to integrate them with the Grid technology in order to process and store the collected data by the sensor nodes. This chapter proposes the SEnsor Grid Enhancement Data Management system, called SEGEDMA, ensuring the integration of different network technologies and the continuous data access to system users. The main contribution of this work is to achieve the interoperability of both technologies through a novel network architecture ensuring also the interoperability of Open Geospatial Consortium (OGC) and HL7 standards. According to the results SEGEDMA can be applied successfully in a decentralized healthcare environment.

Healthcare is an increasingly collaborative enterprise involving many individuals and organizations that coordinate their efforts toward promoting quality and efficient delivery of healthcare through the use of interoperable healthcare information systems (HIS). Service-oriented architecture (SOA) provides a cost-effective solution to implementing interoperability between heterogeneous HIS which have resulted from extensive investments that most healthcare organizations have made in system resources over the course of many years. However, issues of semantic interoperability still remain unresolved while new challenges arise regarding web service interoperability. This chapter presents a mediator-based approach for achieving data and service interoperability among disparate and geographically dispersed HIS. The proposed system architecture provides a uniform interface to the underlying HIS, thus enabling decoupling of the client applications and the server-side implementations while it ensures security in all transactions. It is a distributed system architecture based on the agent paradigm for both healthcare process management and management of interactions among the participating systems. The healthcare processes and all interactions involved in each process are described according to the workflow metaphor. Thus, robustness, high flexibility and fault tolerance are provided in an environment as dynamic and heterogeneous as healthcare.

Healthcare services are naturally distributed, both from a geographical and an organisational point of view; they include various national and local authorities, as well as different actors ranging from general hospitals to individual physicians. One of the main items on the eHealth agenda of the European Union is the establishment of electronic patient summaries as an instrument to facilitate the pervasive delivery of healthcare and to guarantee its continuity across national boundaries. This chapter analyses several existing large-scale eHealth systems, chosen among the most prominent and established ones in Europe, and analyses their ability to cope with the high heterogeneity challenges of a Europe-wide solution. It then introduces triplespaces, a new-generation middleware based on the concept of semantic spaces, and presents a possible realisation of a European Patient Summary based on a triplespace infrastructure. The chapter shows that this solution can cope with the decentralisation, asynchronicity, subsidiarity, and security requirements arising in the European Patient Summary setting.

Preface

Interoperability is a concern in many domains of Information Technology, and healthcare is no exception for that. On the contrary, the nature of health information calls for advanced interoperability for the benefits of the individual patients, a better management of health institutions, organizations and centres, and also in general for the benefit of clinical practice and science in general, as the ability to combine data opens new avenues for gaining scientific insights.

That was the motivation for compiling this book, since the field of interoperability in health systems is now subject to intense development and research but at the same time is struggling with the practical impediments of deploying interoperable systems that achieve higher levels of integration at the local, regional, national and transnational levels.

In this preface, I try to provide a motivation for the necessity of the book together with an overview of its contents.

MOTIVATION

Interoperability is about sharing information across organizations, administrative domains or countries. And it is about transferring that information in the most effective and efficient form beyond particular micro-integration cases. This entails the alignment of protocols, configurations and data models between computer systems, along with aligning the authorizations, regulation and processes between the organizations sharing the information. And this is thus a complex problem for which there are no easy solutions or "silver bullets", given its inherent complexity.

The domain of healthcare represents a particularly complex case for interoperability still looking for solutions at the macro-scale (Woolman, 2011). This is not only due to the fact that the systems supporting healthcare information are heterogeneous (which is something that occurs in many other domains), but also due to the privacy and security issues surrounding the medical record (Gritzalis, 1998) and also the inherent complexity of representing healthcare-related information (Plsek & Greenhalgh, 2001). This latter aspect is in many cases overlooked in approaches to healthcare interoperability. However, it is an intrinsic, essential characteristic of the domain. Scientific progress and innovation in the healthcare domain are continuous, and the data models required for recording associated information needs to be adaptable in a quick way. In consequence, it is in practice unrealistic to attempt to build comprehensive models for the healthcare domain, and this complicates interoperability. A different approach is needed that accounts for change in its core foundation.

In recent years, this fact has been acknowledged explicitly in the approach to interoperability known as "two-level modelling", of which the OpenEHR initiative represents the most prominent example (Kalra, Beale & Heard, 2005). In this approach, the definition of the models is purposely left open via the provision of a domain-specific language that allows a community-approach to develop new micro-models of clinical information. In OpenEHR, these model fragments are called "archetypes". An archetype may represent known and old measurement concepts as "blood pressure" or "smoking habit" for which conventions exists. But they can be used also to represent new forms of evaluation or measurement instruments that will exist only in the future. In this way, the collection of archetypes openly available can evolve seamlessly in time. Moreover, the provision of a domain specific language enables non-computer professionals to develop archetypes (of course with the appropriate user-friendly tools). This allows the healthcare professionals to drive the development of the models, if needed as a community process with all the practitioners and researchers involved.

In addition to the abovementioned specificities, healthcare information requires the understanding and consistent use of the vocabularies of the different healthcare domains. There is a long, established tradition of using ontologies in the biomedical domain, and the OBO Foundry site provides a good example of them (Smith et al., 2007). Currently, SNOMED CT is arguably the more widely adopted terminology for the clinical domain (Stearns et al., 2001), providing a backbone for achieving a degree of semantic interoperability. However, no current terminology or ontology is perfect for every domain and there is also a lack of guidance and best practice distillation in how to associate terms with information models as archetypes.

The areas within healthcare which benefit most from semantic interoperability can be categorized as follows:

- **Patient care:** The benefits in this area include medical staff saving time, gaining efficiency and improving safety and clinical outcomes through better access to patient information across disciplines, care settings and countries. These influence patient safety, dissemination of good practice, integration of education and care, connecting multiple locations for collaborative care delivery and empowerment of citizens, among others.
- **Public health:** Benefits are also associated to being able to use richer clinical detail, leading to improvement and greater confidence in information used for audit, planning and performance management. These influence international statistics, comparative outcome assessment, pharmacovigilance, coordination of risk assessment, management and surveillance of large-scale adverse health events and population health research, among others.
- **Research and translational medicine:** Semantic interoperability achievement can also lead to the development of multi-centre studies and trials, health data repositories, bio- and tissue-banks and personalised medicine based on genetic and genomic analyses, among others.
- **Support for diverse markets:** Semantic interoperability provides means for the identification of solutions with superior benefit/cost ratios, enabling plug and play best of breed, encouraging industry involvement, stimulating innovations by health service providers and involving clinicians and harmonising legal and regulatory frameworks.

Semantic interoperability not only offers means for new methods and services in the health domain but also contributes to maximise all the benefits from the relation between medicine/healthcare and information technology, given the constraints in resources.

It should be noted that the benefits listed above can be achieved to a greater or lesser extent depending on the degree of level of interoperability achieved. The definition of such levels has evolved from a general perspective oriented to any kind of information system (Sheth, 1999) to a more specific definition in accordance to the requirements of a particular domain. In this manner, Garde et al. (2007) provided three levels adapted to the healthcare environment. Two years later, the levels of IOp established by the SemanticHEALTH report (Stroetmann et al., 2009) were the following:

- **Level 0:** No interoperability at all.
- **Level 1:** Technical and syntactical interoperability (no semantic interoperability)
- **Level 2:** Two orthogonal levels of partial semantic interoperability
  - **Level 2a:** Unidirectional semantic interoperability
  - **Level 2b:** Bidirectional semantic interoperability of meaningful fragments
- **Level 3:** Full semantic interoperability, sharable context, seamless co-operability, that will allow gaining the benefits of computerized support for reminders, alerts, decision support, workflow management and evidence based healthcare, i.e. to improve effectiveness and reduce clinical risks.

In Level 3 the use of an EHR reference model, a rich library of clinical data structures, and the definitions of terminology bindings to value lists for each element of the data structures have all to be agreed within a record sharing community.

However, reaching high levels of interoperability is a resource intensive task while nowadays it is difficult to associate the benefits of interoperability with those who pay for it. Therefore, one of the objectives of this research is to provide a convincing demonstration of the benefit of migration from ad-hoc to interoperable systems.

Another dimension of the interoperability puzzle is that of guidelines and workflows. Typically, guidelines provide procedural knowledge that has been collected through the careful compilation and study of available evidence for a particular health problem. The application of workflows to supporting guideline-based care processes seems straightforward. However, in spite of having a number of available workflow models for the healthcare domain (Lenz & Reichert, 2007), in practice they are not consistently used, and professionals may consider challenging introducing them in their current information systems.

To complicate things even further, security and cross-national boundaries create barriers that need technology, procedures and attention to privacy. While initiatives as the European epSOS project[1] provide the necessary architectural elements and framework for solving them, again practice lags behind theory, and they are far from being widely deployed nowadays.

The multifaceted and complex context of interoperability just briefly portrayed evidences the importance on investing in healthcare interoperability and associated standardization efforts. The technologies and models have been with us for years, but there are still unclear areas and possibilities to go higher in the level of semantics transferred when moving healthcare data across organizations of countries. We hope that the contents of the chapters in this book contribute to give an additional step in that direction.

OVERVIEW AND CONTENTS OF THE BOOK

This book has resulted from a process of selection of chapters with an open call. Initial proposals were screened in a first phase for scope with the topics of the book. Then, selected proposals were developed by their authors and submitted in full form. The chapters passed through a process of peer review for technical adequacy and then authors of accepted chapters developed the final versions integrating the suggestions and recommendations for improvement for the reviewers.

The process has resulted in a selection of nine chapters that cover a broad range of topics and perspectives. An additional introductory chapter covers the broad scope of interoperability to provide the context and outlook in which the contributions should be framed.

In Chapter 1, Kuziemsky discussed healthcare delivery and interoperability from multiple perspectives. A case study of collaborative care delivery is described, together with a multi-tiered framework of healthcare interoperability devised to address the needs of the case.

In Chapter 2, Costa and Isaias present the elements needed to implement a model of Electronic Health Record based on a standard, open architecture.

Elements from decision support systems and business processes that can be integrated with the system are discussed in that context.

Then, Chapter 3 by Maldonado et al. describes LinkEHR, a software framework for interoperability in Health Information Systems that uses the concept of clinical archetype as the central data mode. Archetypes are used to decouple data representations at different systems while making them interoperable through a reference model. The software framework demonstrates how a global interoperability system can be deployed using archetypes as data mapping mechanism.

Chapter 4 by Martínez-Costa et al. presents different solutions based on the use of semantic models for representing clinical knowledge. Concretely, the chapter deals with an archetype-based dual model-based and presents methods and tools for the representation and transformation of clinical archetypes and for the automatic generation of standardized applications.

Lezcano goes a step further in Chapter 5 by introducing the way to use rule-base models together with semantic representations generated from archetype models. This brings an additional dimension in the kinds of clinical knowledge that can be integrated in these systems, and opens the possibilities for new types of reasoning that are not directly supported in other base ontology languages like that of the different OWL variants.

In Chapter 6, Sahay et al. present a case motivating current limitations of ontology based systems in the domain of this book and identify two key features, namely the type and scope of knowledge, within a knowledge base could enhance the overall effectiveness. The idea of separating knowledge bases in types (e.g., general or constraint knowledge) with scope (e.g., global or local) of applicability is discussed as a central concern in this domain.

Chapter 7 by Preve discusses the role of Wireless Sensor Networks (WSN) deployed to monitor the health of patients suffering from critical diseases are presented. This is combined with the needs to standardize internetworked infrastructures according to standards as the Open Geospatial Consortium (OGC) and Health Level (HL7).

Chapter 8 by Koufi et al. brings a new dimension to the scenario of interoperability presented in previous chapters by introducing workflow and agent technologies as supporting machinery for achieving interoperation goals.

Chapter 9 by Carenini et al. analyse several existing large-scale eHealth systems and analyse their ability to cope with the high heterogeneity challenges of a Europe-wide solution. The concept of triplespaces as a semantics-based middleware is described as a key infrastructural element for solving cross-national needs for interoperability.

Chapter 10 by Lezcano et al. deals with a case integrating interoperability and data mining in the context of a concrete pathology. It serves as a prototypical example of dealing with the complexity of data representations and the different kinds of knowledge that needs to be tackled with in real contexts.

CONTRIBUTIONS

This volume contributes to the field of interoperability and healthcare by providing an overview of current research and development in the context of integrating healthcare information. The book includes topics that are related to how advanced techniques as computational semantics can be applied in that context, and also cases and overview information portraying the field of health interoperability nowadays.

Miguel-Ángel Sicilia
University of Alcalá, Spain

REFERENCES

Garde, S., Knaup, P., Hovenga, E. J. S., & Heard, S. (2007). Towards semantic interoperability for electronic health records: Domain knowledge governance for openEHR archetypes. *Methods of Information in Medicine*, *46*(3), 332–343. PMID:17492120

Gritzalis, D. A. (1998). Enhancing security and improving interoperability in healthcare information systems. *Informatics for Health & Social Care*, *23*(4), 309–323. doi:10.3109/14639239809025367 PMID:9922951

Kalra, D., Beale, T., & Heard, S. (2005). The openEHR Foundation. *Studies in Health Technology and Informatics*, *115*, 153–173. PMID:16160223

Lenz, R., & Reichert, M. (2007). IT support for healthcare processes – Premises, challenges, perspectives. *Data & Knowledge Engineering*, *61*(1), 39–58. doi:10.1016/j.datak.2006.04.007

Plsek, P., & Greenhalgh, T. (2001). The challenge of complexity in health care. *BMJ (Clinical Research Ed.)*, *323*, 625–628. doi:10.1136/bmj.323.7313.625 PMID:11557716

Sheth, A. P. (1999). Changing focus on interoperability in information systems: From system, syntax, structure to semantics. In M. Goodchild, M. J. Egenhofer, R. Fegeas, & C. Kottman (Eds.), *Interoperating geographic information systems* (pp. 5–29). Norwell, MA: Kluwer. doi:10.1007/978-1-4615-5189-8_2

Smith, B. et al. (2007). The OBO foundry: Coordinated evolution of ontologies to support biomedical data integration. *Nature Biotechnology*, *25*, 1251–1255. doi:10.1038/nbt1346 PMID:17989687

Stearns, M. Q., Price, C., & Spackman, K. A. et al. (2001). SNOMED clinical terms: Overview of the development process and project status. *In Proc AMIA Symp, 2001*, 662–666. PMID:11825268

Stroetmann, V. N., Kalra, D., Lewalle, P., Rodrigues, J. M., Stroetmann, K. A., & Surjan, G. et al. (2009). *Semantic interoperability for better health and safer healthcare (Project report)*. Luxembourg: Office for Official Publications of the European Communities: European Commission.

Woolman, P. S. (2011). Challenges of managing interoperability in regional healthcare organisations. In *Proceedings of the First International Workshop on Managing Interoperability and Complexity in Health Systems (MIXHS '11)* (pp. 1-2). New York: ACM.

Chapter 1
A Multi-Tiered Perspective on Healthcare Interoperability

Craig Kuziemsky
Telfer School of Management, University of Ottawa, Canada

ABSTRACT

The current healthcare delivery paradigm is defined by integrative care delivery across disparate providers and services. Therefore the ability to deliver efficient and effective healthcare services is dependent on designing and implementing interoperable systems. However, the notion of interoperability is multifaceted and complex. Although the exchange of data is often described as analogous with interoperability it must be remembered that healthcare is a process oriented domain and clinical, management, organizational and other processes must be considered as part of interoperability. This chapter discusses healthcare delivery and the role interoperability plays in supporting its delivery. First, the chapter provides a background on healthcare interoperability from multiple perspectives. Then it presents a case study of collaborative care delivery and uses it to outline specific interoperability requirements. The chapter then uses these requirements to develop a multi-tiered framework of healthcare interoperability, concluding with a discussion of the implications of the framework for interoperability research and for systems design to support integrated healthcare delivery.

INTRODUCTION

The ability to deliver efficient and effective healthcare services is dependent on designing and implementing interoperable health information systems. As healthcare delivery becomes distributed across multiple providers and settings it is interoperability that will allow clinical data and processes to be accessible in these different settings. However, the notion of interoperability is multifaceted and complex. Although the exchange of data is often analogous with interoperability we need to remember that healthcare is a process oriented domain and therefore clinical, management, organizational and healthcare system processes must be considered as part of interoperability.

DOI: 10.4018/978-1-4666-3000-0.ch001

One of the difficulties with interoperability is that it is sometimes discussed as an abstract concept. At basic level, interoperability is the means of connecting two or more computer systems. However, those systems are used by people to conduct healthcare processes and therefore we need to take into consideration the actual processes that we are trying to make interoperable. We suggest that interoperability is not the ends but rather it is the means of supporting healthcare delivery. The 2001 study from the Institute of Medicine 'Crossing the Quality Chasm: A New Healthcare System for the 21st Century' described the quality of care delivery as inadequate and that to improve care delivery would require a commitment to an agenda of efficient, effective, timely, safe, and equitable patient centered care (Institute of Medicine, 2001). Interoperability is the means for achieving those objectives and the true test of interoperability will be how well it helps us achieve them.

This chapter discusses healthcare delivery and the role interoperability plays in it. In particular we emphasize the need to consider interoperability at the process level. In the chapter we first provide a background on healthcare interoperability that looks at it from multiple perspectives. We then present a case study of collaborative care delivery and use it to outline specific interoperability requirements. We then use these requirements to develop a multi-tiered framework of healthcare interoperability. We conclude with a discussion of the implications of the chapter for future interoperability research and for systems design to support healthcare delivery.

BACKGROUND

Types of Interoperability

Interoperability can be formally defined as the 'ability of two or more systems or components to exchange information and to use the information that has been exchanged.' (IEEE, 1990). However, all interoperability is not the same but rather different types of interoperability exist. Benson (2010) describes technical, semantic and process interoperability as three types of interoperability.

Technical interoperability is the ability to move data from computer system A to system B (Benson, 2010). Technical interoperability comprises machine-readable aspects of data representation and addresses the problem of connecting distributed systems on a network. Solutions for technical interoperability have focused on distributed computing and includes Java, proprietary solutions such as the Object Management Group's CORBA (Common Object Request Broker Architecture) and Microsoft's DCOM (Distributed Component Object Model), and XML, web services and service oriented architectures (SOA) (Sartipi and Yarmand, 2008). Technical interoperability connects two or more computer systems without consideration of the meaning of what is exchanged.

Semantic interoperability goes one step further and addresses the need for interoperability of the concepts and vocabulary that is exchanged across computer systems so these systems can interpret and understand the data. Clinical terminologies, defined as "standardized terms and their synonyms which record patient findings, circumstances, events, and interventions with sufficient detail to support clinical care, decision support, outcomes research, and quality improvement; and can be efficiently mapped to broader classifications for administrative, regulatory, oversight and fiscal requirements"(Chute, 2000), are a key provider of semantic interoperability. Clinical terminologies include nomenclature and classification languages such as SNOMED-CT as well as reference models for representing aggregates of domain information into class diagrams such as the HL7 Reference Information Model (RIM).

Process interoperability refers to interoperability of the work processes and people who interact with the technology (Benson, 2010). Simply having the ability to exchange data via standards does not guarantee that it will lead to better healthcare delivery if we do not understand the underlying context of where and how the exchanged data is being used. Even if computers are able to exchange and understand data it does not mean the people using the systems are interoperable. Prinejad et al. point out the need to make a distinction between *interoperable systems* and *interoperable people* (Prinejad et al., 2008). Other interoperability frameworks such as the SemanticHEALTH roadmap (Stroetmann et al., 2009) have similarly pointed out that technical standardization are no longer the most prominent interoperability issues but rather they have been surpassed by political, institutional, organizational and legal issues.

Much of the research on standardization and interoperability have focused on formal or structured types of communication, often facilitated through electronic health records (EHRs). For example the OpenEHR project consists of a reference information model and a set of archetypes (Garde et al., 2007). The archetypes constrain instances of the information model to express a valid structure, data type, and value, which provides technical and semantic interoperability respectively (Garde et al., 2007). However, the extent to which OpenEHR archetypes can support process interoperability is unknown. Ad-hoc communication can be supported if it is communicating archetype data, but that could be problematic given the diverse communication needs of healthcare. We cannot assume that communication and other process interoperability needs will be supported. Before we can develop solutions to support process interoperability we need to understand its needs.

Role of Interoperability in Healthcare Delivery

To understand the role and importance of interoperability we need to look at it in the context of the objectives our healthcare system wants to achieve. Although it is common to define healthcare systems objectives such as a sustainable, effective, efficient, collaborative and safe healthcare system, the challenge is we need the means of operationalizing those objectives. We suggest that interoperability of data and healthcare processes is the means of implementing those objectives.

To better articulate the role of interoperability in healthcare delivery we will discuss it from the perspective of sustainability, patient centered care, team based care delivery, and patient safety.

- Successful organizations must be sustainable, meaning they have the necessary resources to meet their objectives today and also have the ability to adapt to future needs (Coiera and Hovenga, 2007). Healthcare, particularly the way we currently deliver it, is not sustainable in the long term because we have increasing needs and limited or even decreasing resources (Coiera and Hovenga, 2007). As our population ages and people live longer periods with chronic illness we will need to change how healthcare services are resourced and delivered. A sustainable healthcare system is necessary to meet demand and provide access to quality health services to the nation's entire population (Coiera and Hovenga, 2007). Interoperability is a key aspect of sustainability. To foster sustainability we need to integrate patient data across illness, providers and settings, support an educated population and trained workforce through evidence based medicine, and have the ability to evaluate system performance so changes can be made where necessary.

- Patient centered care refers to the need for healthcare delivery to be tailored to the unique needs of each individual patient, as opposed to 'cookie cutter' delivery. Despite all the complexities in healthcare delivery we need to remember that it is still about providing quality care for the patient. Standardization precedes any computer based exchange and is the basis for interoperability (Van Bemmel and Musen, 1997). However a patient centered approach presents a challenge as care delivery that is tailored for each unique patient goes against the notion of standardization. As we standardize data exchanges and other processes to support interoperability we risk limiting our ability to achieve true patient centeredness.
- The need for the development and delivery of patient care by high performing healthcare teams is a common recommendation for healthcare delivery (Institute of Medicine, 2001). A healthcare system supported by collaborative team based healthcare delivery is challenging as our current healthcare system is not designed to support it. Teamwork requires the integration of data and processes across different settings. To date healthcare delivery has largely been single provider and patient oriented and thus interoperability was less important. However, the need for interoperability to facilitate team based care delivery will grow as the benefits of team based care delivery and the prevalence of chronic illness both increase.
- Finally, we can consider patient safety. The 1999 Institute of Medicine (IOM) report: "To err is Human" reported that 45,000 to 98,000 Americans die each year because of preventable medical errors (IOM, 1999). In Canada the "Canadian Adverse Events Study" showed that 7.5% of annual hospital admissions (approx 185,000/year) suffer some type of adverse event and that approximately 70,000 (38%) of those events are preventable (Ross Baker et al., 2004). Poor interoperability leading to fragmentation of the healthcare system and poor data exchange and communication is a significant cause of medical errors (Institute of Medicine, 1999).

Overall, we can see that the desired objectives of the healthcare system can all be viewed from the perspective of interoperability. Health information technology (HIT) will be a key driver of an interoperable healthcare system through integrated electronic health records (EHRs), electronic support for team based care delivery across multiple providers and locations, and real time delivery of medical evidence to ensure healthcare delivery is safe, personalized and evidence based.

Interoperability Outside of Healthcare

A substantial body of research exists on interoperability outside of healthcare. The financial industry and supply chain management are two good examples. The development of interoperable financial systems has been a key driver of economic sustainability (Arduini and Morabito, 2010). I can travel across the world and using my bank card and personal identifier I am able to access my banking information and conduct banking processes (i.e. withdrawal, transfers, bill payment) on my accounts. Yet in Canada I cannot travel across the country and have a physician access my medical data across the various Canadian provinces.

Interoperability is also the basis of supply chain management (SCM), a detailed set of processes that represent the acquisition of raw materials, development of a product and shipment of the product to the customer. SCM is similar to healthcare in that it is increasingly using computerization to automate SCM processes (Zhu et al., 2004). As computerized SCM systems evolved, some believed information technology (IT) was being implemented without understanding the relevant SCM processes (Van Donk, 2008). A disconnect existed between SCM processes and the IT solutions that were being developed to support those processes. SCM overcame that disconnect by first understanding the specific SCM processes, such as how human decision makers interact, and then designing IT that supported these processes (Van Donk, 2008).

It has been recognized that the complexity of healthcare delivery and the processes within it precludes the direct transfer of interoperability research from other domains (Avison and Young, 2007). While that point is true we do suggest that there are some aspects of interoperability research from other domains that is transferable. Foremost is the need to understand interoperability at the processes level. Regardless of whether we are discussing financial, manufacturing or supply chain systems, a key message from business interoperability success is the need for processes to be the driver of interoperability.

Towards New Perspectives and Frameworks for Healthcare Interoperability

The importance of interoperability as a driver of healthcare delivery can be seen through the fact that the development of e-Health strategies and interoperability architectures has become a government priority in several countries. Canada has developed Canada Health Infoway in order to develop an integrated electronic health record system and national strategy for data exchange (Canada Health Infoway, 2010). Australia has a national e-Health strategy for electronically collecting and exchanging health information in order to improve the delivery of healthcare services (Australia 2010; Hovenga, 2008). The United Kingdom formed the Connecting for Health strategy in 2005 with the purpose of delivering a national program for healthcare IT (United Kindgom, 2010). The United States has developed the Healthcare Information Technology Standards Panel to develop interoperability standards for local, regional and national health information networks (United States, 2010).

However, it is interesting to note that many of those national e-Health strategies are struggling to achieve their mandates. In the United Kingdom the Connecting for Health (CFH) strategy has been plagued by criticism, delays and cost overruns. The CFH strategy is currently four years behind schedule (Hazzard, 2008). Similarly in Canada, the initial goal of Canada Health Infoway was for 50% of Canadians to have an electronic health record by 2010. The achievement of that goal will also be delayed.

The message we have delivered so far is that to develop meaningful interoperability solutions we need to ensure they help us achieve the desired objectives of the healthcare system. Further, these solutions have to focus on understanding and developing solutions that support process interoperability. Although HIT will become a key driver of future healthcare delivery, to date widespread HIT implementation has been challenging. The design and implementation of HIT has resulted in large numbers of HIT projects being designated as failures (Avison and Young, 2007). The predominate reason for the failures was we implemented HIT without understanding the underlying complexity of healthcare delivery. To address that issue we need to focus on understanding and supporting process interoperability. Campbell et al. (2006) and Ash et al. (2007) showed that the key to understanding computer physician order entry (CPOE) systems was to understand the underling work processes and interactions of people who used the CPOE systems. The importance of process interoperability has similarly been stated by Shortliffe and Blois who said the key to understanding the complexity with computer based medical records is to understand the *processes* associated with the creation and use of such records (Shortliffe and Blois, 2006). They also suggest the computer-based medical record is not an object, or a product, 'but rather a set of processes that an organization must put into place, supported by technology' (Shortlife and Blois, 2006, p. 6).

As discussed above, we believe the biggest challenge to interoperability is that it is often discussed purely from a data or 'product' perspective. Although many technological and terminological solutions for interoperability exist, we need to recognize that interoperability is more than integrating data across disparate systems. Rather, interoperability needs to integrate people and processes. Interoperability also needs to be done with specific objectives such as efficiency, patient centeredness, and team based care delivery in mind.

We summarize the existing research with a new perspective on healthcare interoperability in the form of with a multi-tiered framework of healthcare interoperability. The framework is based on a case study of collaborative care delivery in hospice palliative care. The framework provides an empirical perspective on many of the interoperability challenges we have already discussed and emphasizes the importance of process interoperability.

CASE STUDY

A case study of collaborative healthcare delivery is the basis for our interoperability framework. Our case study takes place in the domain of hospice palliative care (HPC). HPC is care provided to patients when curative therapies are no longer an option. HPC requires a substantial amount of collaborative healthcare delivery that takes place across different settings and providers making it an ideal domain to study interoperability needs. The case study provides an empirical perspective to integrate the healthcare system objectives and interoperability perspectives we have discussed so far in the chapter.

Setting

We studied collaborative care delivery over a six month period (February to July 2008) at an urban, 9 bed in-patient teaching hospice. At the hospice, healthcare was delivered by a collaborative team consisting of nurses, physicians, medical residents, coordinating administrative staff, personal support workers, and volunteers trained in palliative care. The hospice team generally worked asynchronously. Each patient had a family physician that would coordinate the patient's care. However the family physician's office was external to the hospice and as a result the physician was not at the hospice very frequently. While a nursing staff member was always present on the ward, other members of the healthcare team, including physicians, were intermittently present. Data exchange and communication was a mixture of electronic and paper based tools. Communication between the staff on the ward and the external providers was mainly asynchronous.

Family physicians managed their patient cases remotely and through periodic visits to the hospice. However because family physicians are not palliative care specialists they would sometimes require assistance with complex cases from a palliative care specialist. That assistance could be provided through consultation with a palliative care specialist or through access to medical evidence.

Data Sources

We collected field notes through 90 hours of non-participant observations. A trained qualitative research assistant collected field notes through 90 hours of non-participant observations. The observations were collected by following the care providers during care provision and taking detailed notes of the care activities. The observational data included a wide range of routine day-to-day collaborative processes and tasks, including team activities (such as team rounds, patient admissions and discharges, and managerial meetings) and individual activities that had collaborative implications (such as patient charting and other data entry activities, medication order creation, and communication exchange activities). Observations were conducted at different times of the day and on different days of the week in order to maximize the breadth of ICC activities included in the data.

We also conducted 30 semi-structured interviews with various healthcare team members including 8 nurses, 6 physicians, 6 medical residents, 3 team coordinators (e.g. nursing coordinator), 2 personal support workers and 5 volunteers. Interviews ranged between 30-90 minutes in length. In total 91 members of the hospice's healthcare team participated in the study.

Data Analysis

Grounded theory (GT) methodology was used for data analysis. GT is a research method that uses a systematic set of procedures to develop an inductively derived grounded theory about a phenomenon (Strauss and Corbin, 1994). A GT study does not begin with a preconceived hypothesis or theory that needs to be proven. Instead, a theory emerges from the data. The hallmark of GT is three coding cycles:

open, axial and selective coding (Strauss and Corbin, 1994). Data is coded in open coding into concepts and categories that are refined and interconnected in axial coding. Selective coding establishes the final concepts and categories. GT was chosen for data analysis as it ties theory to data which provides a means of rigor to the analysis.

Multi-Tiered Interoperability Framework

As the data was analyzed we first identified in open coding that there were several interoperability needs. As the codes were refined and interconnected in axial coding it became apparent that the interoperability needs could be grouped within several categories. Those categories were formalized as a multi-tiered framework for healthcare interoperability (Figure 1). The framework has three parts to it. The top part of the framework is data interoperability as obviously data is a key driver of healthcare delivery. We then expand on interoperability by introducing three specific types of process interoperability (knowledge, clinical, and collaborative). Finally, we look at several contextual factors that impact interoperability.

Data Interoperability

Data interoperability is important as data needs to be accessible and sharable across different settings and providers. Indeed, in our case study a recurring issue was the need to integrate several from several sources. One of the benefits of collaborative care delivery is the breadth of providers involved in care delivery. At the hospice in our study nurses, personal support workers, physicians and volunteers all provide care and record patient data. The perspectives of the different care providers are a key part of understanding the overall picture of the patient. However a challenge that arises from that overall picture is that patient data may be in multiple documents and all the data has to be pieced together to obtain the entire picture of the patient. The challenge of reconciling multiple data source sources is particularly significant for family physicians as they are not on the unit as frequently as other providers and thus it is difficult for them to know what individual pieces of data are needed to obtain the entire picture of their patient. In interviews physicians described how they want to be able to come into the hospice and get an overall understanding of

Figure 1. Multi-tiered framework for healthcare interoperability

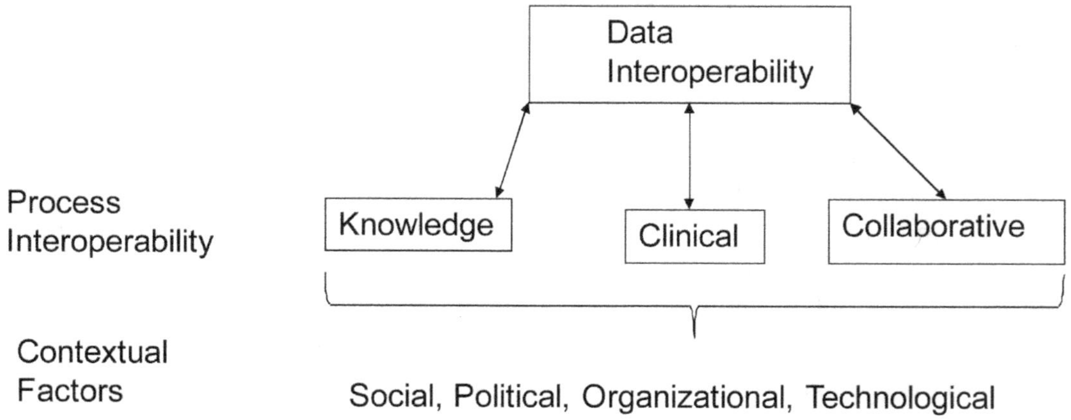

how their patient is doing without having to read through multiple documents.

The data level is the most developed level of the interoperability framework. Existing research has developed technical solutions for data exchange (i.e. XML, Web Services), architectures for data transmission such as the OpenEHR archetypes (Garde et al., 2007) and clinical terminologies to integrate data including SNOMED-CT and HL7.

Process Interoperability

We go back to the earlier statement that just because two computer systems are interoperable does not mean the people using them are interoperable. Thus we need to look at the data interoperability part of the framework in the context of the processes that will use the data. From our data analysis we identified three specific types of process interoperability: knowledge, clinical and collaboration.

Process Interoperability: Knowledge

Knowledge interoperability refers to the use of research evidence by all healthcare actors including clinicians, patients and administrators. Evidence-based medicine (EBM) has been described as "the conscientious, explicit, and judicious use of current best evidence in making medical decisions" (Sackett et al., 1996). Earlier we described how the prevalence of medical errors has prompted the use of research evidence to facilitate safe care delivery. Although it is widely accepted that EBM is a necessary component of health care delivery, it is difficult to implement in day to day healthcare delivery. It is estimated that approximately 30,000 scientific articles are published annually (Choi, 2005) and thus the access and filtering of evidence requires significant time and effort on behalf of the user.

In our case study one of the issues was that although the family physicians wanted to care for their patients they were not formally trained in palliative care. Having access to clinical evidence is one way to increase their comfort level. The ability to access medical evidence has been shown to have a positive impact on physician decision making, mortality rates and cost effectiveness (Westbrook, Gosling and Coiera, 2005). Clinical practice guidelines (CPGs) are one way of incorporating evidence into clinical practice to support healthcare delivery (Sonnenberg and Hagerty, 2006). However, there are many factors complicating effective retrieval of evidence to allow it to be used in a CPG at bedside. These factors include a lack of standardized formatting among libraries and simplistic query mechanisms that are ineffective given the volume of information available (O'Sullivan et al., 2010).

Process Interoperability: Clinical

The clinical level refers to interoperability of the front line care processes. Many of the challenges in implementing HIT have been because of a lack of process interoperability at the clinical level. Earlier we described how Campbell et al. (2006) and Ash et al. (2007) evaluated CPOE systems and discovered numerous clinical process issues caused by the CPOE. It is essential to point out that the CPOE systems functioned as required, meaning they facilitated order entry, and thus were successful from a technical and functional perspective. However the CPOE systems were not interoperable with people and failed from a clinical process perspective. Workflow and communication issues and changes in power structures were some of the process issues caused by the CPOE system (Ash et al, 2007).

Data entry is a common process interoperability issue at the clinical level. Getting clinicians to use structured data entry, which is a significant change from current free text approach, is a particular challenge. There are two key issues with structured data entry. First, although the clinical terminologies discussed in the data interoperability level can assist with structured data entry, there are numerous issues associated with clinical terminologies. Clinical terminologies may not be robust enough to represent complex domains of healthcare. Lau et al. mapped a homecare minimum dataset to SNOMED-CT and were only able to achieve between 68-89% mappings of the terms depending on how the mapping was done (Lau et al., 2008). Other studies have shown similar discrepancies between clinical data needs and terminology standards (Hägglund, 2009). A second issue with standard data entry is reconciling multiple clinical vocabularies into one standard terminology. In our case study the different providers such as physicians, nurses, therapists etc. all use profession specific vocabularies. We observed several examples where a provider would chart patient data in their profession specific language and it would not be understandable by other providers because of the profession specific semantics of the data. In some cases these understandability issues had significant impacts such as delaying a patient's discharge. As clinical terminologies are standardized and electronic charting systems are designed we need to ensure that the terminologies used in these systems are acceptable and understandable by all providers. Therefore, data interoperability takes on a new level of complexity in collaborative care delivery.

Another clinical interoperability issue is the need to recognize that healthcare teams support patient care over the entire continuum of care that includes multiple processes such as assessment, diagnosis, order entry and re-evaluation. In our case study we observed that when a physician would do a diagnosis they would very commonly need to order or change a patient's medication and then provide follow-up on the changed order. Therefore decision support and order entry systems need to be interoperable. We commonly refer to clinical information systems by a particular process such as an electronic health record, decision support or order entry system. However, in reality, care delivery is integrated and not several disparate clinical processes. A 2005 systematic review identified context, computerized access, supporting information, and adaptation with workflow as the factors most needed for a computer decision support system (CDSS) to be successful (Kawamota, 2005). From that perspective although decision support is the objective of the system it is as much about the interoperability of the CDSS to other clinical processes and workflow that will determine its success.

Process Interoperability: Collaboration

The move towards team based healthcare delivery is one of the key changes to our healthcare system. Collaboration is challenging enough when care providers are in the same room. It is substantially more challenging when it takes place asynchronously. Although EHR frameworks and architectures exist a shortcoming is that they have been shown to support individual physician practices rather than facilitating collaborative care activities (Dorr, et al. 2007). Therefore we need to develop frameworks that support collaboration interoperability for team based healthcare delivery.

In our case study the most significant collaboration issue we observed was the need to support collaborative processes asynchronously. One such process was decision making. A specific issue was the need for back and forth dialogue as part of collaborative problem solving. The benefit of collaborative care delivery is that multiple providers contribute to patient decision making and care delivery. However, collaboration is challenging when providers come and go at different times. Participants indicated that achieving the ideal level of collaborative deliberation and information sharing can be difficult, particularly where providers come and go asynchronously. Of all the professions involved in patient care delivery in this setting, physicians spent the least amount of time on the unit and they commonly described being frustrated with not being aware of how problems were being solved. True collaboration must allow multiple providers to be able to brainstorm and problem solve in a collaborative way. Collaborative Health 2.0 tools such as Wikis or blogs could allow multiple providers to asynchronously brainstorm through a problem, interact with each other during the brainstorming, and eventually come to a collaborative solution to the problem.

Another issue was the need to covey the rationale or justification for a treatment or medication decision. In our case study during one observation session a physician ordered a medication for a patient that was an unusual order given the patient's situation. The order was questioned by the nursing staff as they weren't sure whether it was recorded correctly or if it was a prescription error. When the nursing staff finally called the prescribing physician to inquire about the order they were informed that the patient's situation was very unique and thus the medication was both necessary and appropriate. In cases like that a data symbol is needed to indicate that the order is correct and to explain the rationale for the unusual order.

Contextual Factors

Independent of the interoperability needs described above is a number of contextual factors under which interoperability needs to work. Social, political, organizational and technological are some of the contexts under which interoperability needs to occur.

Social contexts refer to the need to remember that the design of HIT is a sociotechnical process. In that context we need to ensure that our move towards e-Health does not limit people's ability to access healthcare services. Although much of society is becoming comfortable with technology we cannot assume that all people will have the willingness or the means to enter data, access medical evidence, or communicate with their care provider electronically. We must ensure that technology does widen the gap between those who have access to healthcare services and those who do not.

Political contexts include the need for e-Health systems to be designed in congruence with national mandates and architectures that are driving e-Health initiatives. These include the national e-Health architectures described earlier. Detailed privacy and security legislations exist in many countries and those legislations must be also incorporated into any e-Health framework. Our case study took place in Canada, where the applicable privacy legislation is the federal Personal Information Protection and Electronic Documents (PIPEDA) act (PIPEDA, 2010). As we design computer based tools to support care delivery in the hospice we will need to ensure that all electronic exchange of clinical data follows the policies and procedures of PIPEDA.

Organizational contexts include the need to consider the rules, regulations and codes of conduct that are maintained in each particular healthcare facility. The setting in our case study was a hospice and one of the policies was that patients could not be admitted if they were undergoing acute interventions such as chemotherapy or radiation. Another policy was that medications requiring intravenous administration were not allowed, which impacted order entry for medications. Also, the hospice did not have an in-house pharmacy and therefore there were medico-legal procedures for obtaining, storing and administering opioid medications. Processes such as patient admission and medication order entry needed to be conducted in consideration of the above policies to prevent delays in having patients admitted or delays in obtaining or administering medications for patients.

Technological contexts include to the need to consider the numerous modalities of how clinical processes take place. Healthcare providers are becoming increasingly mobile and thus we need to factor that mobility into HIT design. The providers in our study liked the potential to receive electronic alerts on a patient but they did not like the fact that alerts would come to a stationary computer as that did not fit with their clinical workflow. One of the primary reasons that providers like the paper based chart is because of its mobility and adaptability. They can take the chart with them from room to room and chart patient data in whatever room they happen to be in. They can also put sticky notes on certain pages to flag key data. HIT needs to provide the same mobility and adaptability as the paper based system.

DISCUSSION

A health informatics saying is that we must model something before we can automate it (Berg and Touissant, 2003). From that perspective it is essential that we understand and model the characteristics of healthcare interoperability before we can build technical solutions to facilitate it. Existing interoperability models and frameworks have largely focused on data interoperability. There is a need for models of process interoperability and the formal and informal contexts that influence interoperability.

This chapter provided a perspective of healthcare interoperability that emphasizes the processes that take place as part of healthcare delivery. We used a case study of collaborative care delivery in hospice palliative care to illustrate of the complexity of process interoperability. We also provided a multi-tiered framework for healthcare interoperability that emphasized process interoperability and the contextual factors that impact interoperability. The key take away message is that interoperability is complex and although there has been extensive research on healthcare interoperability much of it has focused on data interoperability. While data interoperability is important, data by itself cannot facilitate healthcare delivery. We also need to consider the processes that act upon the data, the providers who conduct the processes and contextual issues such as modalities of technology and the policies and procedures of the healthcare setting where the processes are conducted.

Our case study identified several interoperability issues. Table 1 summarizes what we believe are the key issues from the case study around data, process and contextual interoperability, potential solutions to the issues, and ongoing challenges.

The range of issues and challenges from table 1 highlights what is perhaps the most significant challenge the healthcare system faces in trying to establish interoperability - the paradox of wanting standardized data and processes as well as a healthcare system that provides safe, collaborative, team based healthcare delivery to support patient centered care. As we design a healthcare system that is fully standardized we face the risk of moving further away from a patient centered system that is tailored to individual needs. Standardization also makes it harder to support collaborative healthcare delivery because collaboration is not static but rather it is dynamic and evolves in response to each unique circumstance. In our case study we showed the breadth of processes that exist as part of collaborative care delivery and the challenges that exist in making these processes interoperable. We also described how data interoperability can be more complex than initially perceived when considered in the context of collaborative care delivery (row 1 of table 1). Simply exchanging data across two systems is relatively easy. Exchanging data to support specific processes such as collaborative decision making with multiple professions, or providing medical evidence tailored for a specific patient case is far more challenging.

Table 1. Interoperability challenges for collaborative healthcare delivery

Interoperability Type	Issue from Case Study	Potential Solution	Ongoing Challenges
Data	Need for data integration across multiple settings and systems	Common information models such as HL7 RIM and data standards such as SNOMED-CT	Data reconciliation for multiple providers in collaborative healthcare delivery - i.e "data is not one size fits all"; multiple clinical terminologies may have to be reconciled
Process	Collaborative communication	Communication facilitation by Archetypes such as described by Garde et al. (2007)	Communication needs must be prospectively identified and mapped to archetypes
Process	Collaborative decision making	Collaborative technologies such as Health 2.0 offer potential for implementing collaborative process support such as decision making and brainstorming through a problem	We need to design healthcare IT to play an active role as a communication and process facilitator and not just an integrator and transmitter of data
Contextual	Context of where interoperability occurs must be considered	Behavioural and organizational research to understand sociotechnical aspects of interoperability	Need for better integration of "hard" (i.e.technical and syntactical) and "soft" (i.e. social, organizational and political) aspects of interoperability by combining technical and behavioural research

An increased focus on process interoperability could help us with the implementation of HIT such as EHR systems. As described earlier, our struggles at implementing HIT have largely been at the process level because we fail to consider workflow, communication, and the other clinical processes where HIT is used. One of the difficulties with e-Health architectures is that they are developed independent of any specific context of care delivery. Earlier we described how EHR design and implementation is a part of the national e-Health architecture in numerous countries including the United Kingdom, Canada, the United States and Denmark. However we also described earlier how many countries are struggling with their EHR mandates. Many of these struggles are due to resistance from the users of EHR systems because of process interoperability issues (Ford et al., 2009). Often these process interoperability issues are not brought to light until the systems are implemented in real healthcare settings where they are used as part of clinical care processes. Increased attention to process interoperability may help mitigate resistance against EHRs and other types of HIT systems.

The International Standards Association defines the EHR as "a repository of information regarding the health of a subject of care in computer processable form, stored and transmitted securely, and accessible by multiple authorised users. It has a commonly agreed logical information model which is independent of EHR systems. Its primary purpose is the support of continuing, efficient and quality integrated health care and it contains information which is retrospective, concurrent and prospective" (ISO, 2005). Garde et al. add to that definition by stating the EHR needs to be patient centered, longitudinal, comprehensive for all providers and settings, and prospective (Garde et al., 2007). Therefore an EHR is not just a repository of data, or a tool to exchange data, but also a provider of plans, goals and evaluations of healthcare delivery. However the reality is that the current version of the EHR is a long way from that ideal vision. Successful design and implementing of the EHR will require less attention to the product and more attention to the underlying processes and people who will use the EHR.

The case study and interoperability framework presented in this paper highlighted the prevalence and range of process interoperability needs to support collaborative care delivery. The findings from this chapter provide insight to assist in the design and evaluation of formalized interoperability applications such as the OpenEHR archetypes and formal terminologies and information models such as SNOMED-CT and the HL7 RIM. For example it is not just clinical data that needs to be modeled and conveyed but also process data such as an acknowledgement that a task was done or an explanation for a usual medication order as was described in our case study. Those process elements are part of communication to support collaborative care deliver and they need to influence the ad-hoc communication supported by OpenEHR archetypes. The development of communication archetypes to complement the data archetypes is one possibility. Finally, as we develop applications such as EHRs to standardize communication we also need to consider the contextual factors described in our framework. EHRs and other clinical systems do not work in a vacuum. Political, organizational and social contexts will influence how data is acquired and used in a healthcare setting.

The interoperability framework extends also existing work on interoperability such as the SemanticHEALTH roadmap proposed by the by the SemanticHEALTH project. That project described how interoperability challenges are not just technical but rather how political, institutional, organisational, legal and market issues also play a significant role (Stroetmann et al., 2009). Our framework and its emphasis on process interoperability complements the SemanticHEALTH roadmap by providing detailed insight on interoperability issues to support specific aspects of collaborative care delivery. Future research could look at incorporation of our framework into the SemanticHEALTH roadmap.

Overall, this chapter illustrated the importance and complexity of process interoperability. It has provided some insight to assist us in our global desire to build a sustainable healthcare system that can provide the necessary services to all who need them. Shortcomings of this chapter are that case study of collaborative care delivery and multi-tiered framework was based on a single healthcare setting. Other process interoperability needs and contextual factors will arise in other settings. However the framework and method by which it was developed has illustrated the importance of process interoperability and they provide a meta-model to act as a starting point for understanding process interoperability and the contexts that impact it in other healthcare settings.

ACKNOWLEDGMENT

The author acknowledges funding support from the Natural Sciences and Engineering Research Council of Canada.

REFERENCES

Arduini, F., & Morabito, V. (2010). Business continuity and the banking industry. *Communications of the ACM*, *53*(3), 121–125. doi:10.1145/1666420.1666452

Ash, J. S., Sittig, D. F., Poon, E. G., Guappone, K., Campbell, E., & Dykstra, R. H. (2007). The extent and importance of unintended consequences related to computerized provider order entry. *Journal of the American Medical Informatics Association*, *14*, 415–423. doi:10.1197/jamia.M2373 PMID:17460127

Australia National E-Health Transition Authority. (2010). Retrieved June 20, 2010, from http://www.nehta.gov.au/

Avison, D., & Young, T. (2007). Time to rethink health care and ICT? *Communications of the ACM*, *50*(6), 69–74. doi:10.1145/1247001.1247008

Benson, T. (2010). Why interoperability is hard. In *Principles of health interoperability HL7 and SNOMED* (pp. 25–34). London: Springer-Verlag London Ltd. doi:10.1007/978-1-84882-803-2_2

Berg, M., & Toussaint, P. (2003). The mantra of modeling and the forgotten powers of paper: A sociotechnical view on the development of process-oriented ICT in health care. *International Journal of Medical Informatics*, *69*, 223–234. doi:10.1016/S1386-5056(02)00178-8 PMID:12810126

Campbell, E. M., Sittig, D. F., Ash, J. S., Guappone, K. P., & Dykstra, R. H. (2006). Types of unintended consequences related to computerized provider order entry. *Journal of the American Medical Informatics Association, 13*, 547–556. doi:10.1197/jamia.M2042 PMID:16799128

Canada Health Infoway. (2010) Retrieved June 27, 2010, from http://www.infoway-inforoute.ca/lang-en/

Choi, B. C. K. (2005). Understanding the basic principles of knowledge translation. *Journal of Epidemiology and Community Health, 59*(2), 93. PMID:15650137

Chute, C. G. (2000). Clinical classification and terminology: Some history and current observations. *Journal of the American Medical Informatics Association, 7*, 298–303. doi:10.1136/jamia.2000.0070298 PMID:10833167

Coiera, E., & Hovenga, E. J. S. (2007). Building a sustainable health system. *IMIA: Yearbook Medical Informatics, 2*(1), 11–18. PMID:17700898

Dorr, D. A., Jones, S. S., & Wilcox, A. (2007). A framework for information system usage in collaborative care. *Journal of Biomedical Informatics, 40*, 282–287. doi:10.1016/j.jbi.2006.10.001 PMID:17097927

Ford, E. W., Menachemi, N., Peterson, L. T., & Huerta, T. R. (2009). Resistance is futile: But it is slowing the pace of EHR adoption nonetheless. *Journal of the American Medical Informatics Association, 16*, 274–281. doi:10.1197/jamia.M3042 PMID:19261931

Garde, S., Knaup, P., Hovenga, E. J. S., & Heard, S. (2007). Towards semantic interoperability for electronic health records. *Methods of Information in Medicine, 46*, 332–343. PMID:17492120

Hägglund, M. (2009). Sharing is caring: Integrating health information systems to support patient-centred shared homecare. *International Journal of Integrated Care, 9*, e11.

Hazzard. (2008, October 28). UK - Another government IT scheme in trouble. *Telegraph*. Retrieved on June 27, 2010, from http://www.telegraph.co.uk/comment/ telegraph-view/3563090/Another-Government-IT-scheme-introuble. html

Hovenga, E. J. S. (2008). Importance of achieving semantic interoperability for national health information systems. *Texto Contexto Enferm. Florianópolis, 17*(1), 158–167.

IEEE. 1990. IEEE standard computer dictionary: A compilation of IEEE standard computer glossaries. New York: 1990.

Institute of Medicine. (1999). *To err is human: Building a safer health care system*. Washington, DC: National Academies Press.

Institute of Medicine. (2001). *Crossing the quality chasm: A new health system for the twenty-first century*. Washington, DC: National Academies Press.

ISO TR 20514:2005. (2005). *Health informatics - Electronic health record definition, scope and context standard.* International Organization for Standardization (ISO), Geneva, Switzerland.

Kawamoto, K., Houlihan, C. A., Balas, E. A., & Lobach, D. F. (2005). Improving clinical practice using clinical decision support systems: A systematic review of trials to identify features critical to success. *BMJ (Clinical Research Ed.)*, *330*(7494), 765–772. doi:10.1136/bmj.38398.500764.8F PMID:15767266

Lau, F., Yang, J., & Brox, G. (2008). Initial experience in mapping minimum data set home care to SNOMED CT. *Electronic Healthcare*, online.

O'Sullivan, D. M., Wilk, S. A., Michalowski, W. J., & Farion, K. J. (2010). Automatic indexing and retrieval of encounter-specific evidence for point-of-care support. *Journal of Biomedical Informatics*, *43*(4), 623–631. doi:10.1016/j.jbi.2010.03.003 PMID:20230908

Park, H. A., & Hardiker, N. (2009). Clinical terminologies: A Solution for Semantic Interoperability. *J Kor Soc Med Informatics*, *15*(1), 1–11. doi:10.4258/jksmi.2009.15.1.1

PIPEDA. (2010). *Canada's Personal Information Protection and Electronic Documents Act.* Government of Canada. Retrieved on June 29, 2010, from http://www.priv.gc.ca/information/guide_e.cfm

Pirnejad, H., Niazkhani, Z., Berg, M., & Bal, R. (2008). Intra-organizational communication in healthcare. *Methods of Information in Medicine*, *47*(4), 336–345. PMID:18690367

Ross Baker, G., Norton, P. G., & Flintoft, V. et al. (2004). The Canadian adverse events study: The incidence of adverse events among hospital patients in Canada. *Canadian Medical Association Journal*, *170*(11), 1678–1686. doi:10.1503/cmaj.1040498 PMID:15159366

Sackett, D. L., Rosenberg, W. M., Muir Gray, J. A., Haynes, B. R., & Richardson, W. S. (1996). Evidence based medicine: What it is and what it isn't. *BMJ (Clinical Research Ed.)*, *312*, 71–72. doi:10.1136/bmj.312.7023.71 PMID:8555924

Sartipi, K., & Mohammad, H. Y. (2008). Standard-based data and service interoperability in eHealth systems. *In Proceedings of the* International Conference on Software Maintenance (pp. 187 – 196). IEEE pres.,

Shortliffe, E. H., & Blois, M. A. (2006). The computer meets medicine and biology: Emergence of a discipline. In E. H. Shortliffe & J. J. Cimino (Eds.), *Medical informatics: Computer applications in healthcare and biomedicine (3rd Ed.),* Springer Press.

Sonnenberg, F. A., & Hagerty, C. G. (2006). Computer-interpretable clinical practice guidelines – Where we are and where we are going? *AMIA Yearbook*, *11*, 45–158.

Strauss, A., & Corbin, J. (1994). Grounded theory methodology: An overview. In N. K. Denzin, & Y. S. Lincoln (Eds.), *Handbook of qualitative research* (pp. 273–285). Thousand Oaks, CA: Sage.

Stroetmann, V. N. (Ed.). Kalra, D., Lewalle, P., Rector, A., Rodrigues, J.M., Stroetmann, K.A., Surjan, G., Ustun, B., Virtanen, M., & Zanstra, P.E. (2009). Semantic interoperability for better health and safer healthcare. SemanticHEALTH Report. ISBN-13: 978-92-79-11139-6, DOI: doi:10.2759/38514

United Kingdom. (2010). Retrieved on June 26, 2010, from http://www.connectingforhealth.nhs.uk/

United States. (2010). *Healthcare Information Technology Standards Panel*. Retrieved on June 26, 2010, from http://www.ansi.org/standards_activities/standards_boards_panels/hisb/hitsp.aspx?menuid=3

Van Bemmel, J. H., & Musen, M. (1997). *Handbook of medical informatics* (1st ed.). Houten, The Netherlands: Bohen Stafeu Van Loghum.

Van Donk, P. (2008). Challenges in relating supply chain management and information and communication technology. An introduction. *International Journal of Operations & Production Management*, *28*(4), 308–312. doi:10.1108/01443570810861534

Westbrook, J. I., Gosling, A. S., & Coiera, E. (2005). Do online information retrieval systems help experienced clinicians answer clinical questions? *Journal of the American Medical Informatics Association*, *12*(3), 113–120. doi:10.1197/jamia.M1717 PMID:15561783

Zhu, K., Kraemer, K., Xu, S., & Dedrick, J. (2004). Information technology payoff in e-business environments: An international perspective on value creation of e-business in the financial services industry. *Journal of Management Information Systems*, *21*(1), 17–54.

Chapter 2
Standards Related to Interoperability in EHR & HS

Mário Macedo
Instituto Politécnico de Tomar, Portugal

Pedro Isaías
Universidade Aberta, Portugal

ABSTRACT

The standardization of clinical data represents a major step in the development of information and organizational knowledge of health services. The evolution of information systems from a model of different database owners to a different open software based model is a major challenge. For this reason it is essential to adopt models of metadata based on archetypes to improve the development of information systems and simultaneously integrate all applications. The adoption of clinical terminology that can translate existing knowledge and enhance its growth is a necessary goal. Accessibility, ubiquity, completeness, consistency and durability of the clinical data are essential objectives for efficiency and effectiveness gains in organizations. This chapter presents the concepts and technologies needed to implement a model of EHR (Electronic Health Record) based on a standard, open architecture. It also presents some concepts of decision support systems and business processes that can be integrated with the EHR.

INTRODUCTION

A knowledge of Information Systems in healthcare leads to an increase in the wealth of societies and an improvement in the quality of life.

"Health" according to the Merriam-Webster Dictionary (n. d.) is "the condition of being sound in body, mind, or spirit ; especially **:** freedom from physical disease or pain." The WHO (World Health Organization, n. d.) defines "Health" as a "state of complete physical, mental, and social well-being and not merely the absence of disease, or infirmity."

The use of ICTs (Information and Communication Technologies) in the areas of health has been slow as a result of two factors:

DOI: 10.4018/978-1-4666-3000-0.ch002

- Some conservatism;
- Great complexity of healthcare associated with its constant evolution.

It is common to hear doctors note, for example, that their profession is a mix of science and art. Actually the number of variables to consider in the provision of healthcare is enormous and difficult to integrate. For this reason the automation of workflows, the definition of data models and development of knowledge databases are complex and difficult to construct. Another issue is that until now it has not been possible to develop systems entirely appropriate to the requirements of this area. According to Downing (2007), healthcare must be safe, effective, patient focused, timely, efficient and equitable. Patterson (2004) states that we are moving towards a knowledge network society.

The main advantage of Information Systems concerning digitized clinical data is the fact that Health professionals are not interested in looking at data but in building up knowledge from it. Many available systems on the market just transform the previous paper records into electronic records.

Another concept emerges from these issues: the concept of e-Health. According to the WHO, e-Health "is a new term used to describe the combined use of electronic communication and information technology in the health sector or is the use, in the health sector, of digital data-transmitted, stored and retrieved electronically-for clinical, educational and administrative purposes, both at the local site and at a distance."

The ICTs and the creation of knowledge from them are the engine of modern society.

According to Langley and Carol (2007) information systems can improve the quality of Health services in the following dimensions:

- Improving existing resources management;
- Supporting diagnosis and care through additional information being made available in databases;
- Increasing accessibility to clinical data;
- Automation of care processes;
- Increasing communication with the user/patient.

Improving Existing Resources Management

Improving existing resources management will allow better planning of needs in terms of capacity, use and supply. Information systems can also create knowledge based on historical data and support future planning avoiding flaws in answering requests.

Supporting Diagnosis and Care Through More Information Made Available in Databases

One of the great difficulties for doctors is accessing, assimilating and contextualizing the huge amount of information that is produced daily about improvements in medicine. According to Patterson (2004), the fragmentation and simultaneous explosion of knowledge in healthcare systems are not compatible with traditional care methods.

With the advent of the information society, it is possible to develop systems that search, in a permanent, automatic way, available databases on the internet, (called crawlers), and generate local knowledge through the use of data mining. These systems are foundations of knowledge which may be associated with neural networks and they can integrate expert systems to support the decision making process. According to Bergman (2008), the information available on the Web and not accessed by ordinary search engines is between four hundred to five hundred times greater. There are also about one hundred thousand sites in the area of the "Deep Web" that are not searched.

Increasing Accessibility to Clinical Data

ICTs allow the integration and digital processing of all the data that was traditionally produced in other media. In order to integrate and transmit clinical data, several protocols were developed, such as HL7 (Health Level Seven), version 3, that is the most widely used today.

One of the advantages of electronic data is the standardization of clinical terms in the field of clinical diagnosis, equipment and procedures. This standardization also decreases the variability of services among Healthcare Organizations. Patterson (2004) stated that it is common in hospitals, for example, for the expression "*heart attack*" to be used simultaneously along with "*myocardial infarction*."

Another advantage of electronic clinical data is the automation of communication of infectious disease cases to public Health agencies that study epidemiology, for example. Increased access to clinical data translates into an increase in the efficiency of provided services and it influences a crucial element of treatment, time.

Automation of Care Processes

The automation of care processes allows us to optimize the management of resources, reduce human error and improve the overall quality of services. Due to the capacity of information systems, workflows check some data automatically and are able to generate alerts when certain conditions exceed standards or rules. In this way, it is possible to increase the efficiency of healthcare.

Increasing Communication with the User/Patient

Nowadays, portals for user support are an important communication tool. These portals also provide advice and information. They are also an important means of communication between the citizen and the healthcare technician enabling the prevention of health problems and patient personal care. This is the (CRM) Custom Relationship Management domain, which customizes the citizen healthcare needs and citizen relationship management.

With the concept of Web 2.0 and collaborative work, the concept of Health 2.0 arose. Web 2.0 provides dynamic, social, collaborative platforms, with different integrated services without the use of static pages. We are in the field of rich Internet applications, that is, the applications in which the user is both consumer and producer of content. The keyword is interactivity with the environment.

The concept of Health 2.0 appears associated with Web 2.0 but it is focused on healthcare.

According to Shreeve (n.d.), Health 2.0 is a new concept in healthcare in which all stakeholders (i.e. patients, doctors, suppliers and donors), collaboratively contribute to the services provided and their costs using the means available to improve safety, efficiency and quality of care. Also according to this author, Health 2.0 implies observation of the principles of standardization and connectivity in the cooperation, exchange of information and knowledge transfer platforms. The main vector of this concept is value added services and allowing free choice and assessment of the value delivered to the user.

Within healthcare organizations there are, however, great difficulties in integrating systems. Due to technological advances and the advent of information systems integrated with medical equipment, developed by each manufacturer, there is a state of lack of integration and redundancy of data. However, this integration is possible provided that there are interfaces and protocols appropriate for each computer application. Some of the most important advances in this area are object oriented languages and the protocols of standard messages for communication between systems in the field of healthcare. The protocols of standard messages still have the characteristic of being flexible in their structure and include different types of clinical data, for example, images of medical examinations.

In conclusion, according to Patterson (2004), the new paradigms of healthcare are:

- Transition of hierarchical systems to network systems;
- Transition of systems guided by functions to systems oriented by proceedings;
- Systems with rigid structures of medical records change into flexible records, focused on tasks.

The needs of permanently increasing knowledge of clinical data have enhanced the use of Data Mining tools in healthcare. According to Kraft et al. (2003), the Decision Support Systems in healthcare supported by neural networks have been used in several cases, such as in estimating a need for blood for transfusions, myocardial strokes, needs of medicine supplies and prediction of risk of coronary heart disease. The neural networks are used to solve complex problems that cannot be described by algorithms. For data classification, Baysean models, associations in clusters and fuzzy networks have also been used.

BACKGROUND

Healthcare can be analyzed from the perspective of persons, groups of persons or populations.

Information systems applied to healthcare services improve the services delivered to each patient and also improve the quality of life. Information systems can also enhance the provision of care simultaneously to groups of individuals or populations thus increasing the efficiency of Health services.

The new paradigm of information systems applied to healthcare is moving towards the concept called EBM (Evidence Based Medicine). This new paradigm enables the implementation of systems to support clinical decisions as well as providing data relevant to management.

According to the AHRQ (Agency of Healthcare Research and Quality), Electronic Health Records improve quality in primary care settings and healthcare knowledge. There are two types of analysis that an information system should be able to do in an epidemiological perspective:

- Identify the population clusters that correspond to specific attributes including diseases;

- Examine the state of Health of the population in each cluster.

These studies allow those responsible for public health to act proactively in the development of individual Health plans of a preventive or curative nature.

Increase of efficiency in healthcare delivery can also be achieved by increasing the accessibility, completeness, ubiquity and availability of data needed to provide services.

Accessibility to patients' data is ensured through filters for selecting the desired field of data and a standard interface with the user. The completeness of all data ensures the availability of all their sizes and attributes. Due to differences in working environments and the fact that plans for treatment of certain patients may involve different organizations, it is crucial to ensure data availability, independently of the environment and the place of access.

Reduction of clinical risk with the adoption of medical guidelines along with real time procedures and drug verifications are together a fundamental issue for improving the quality of care provided.

With the adoption of decision support systems in the clinical area, it will be possible to find appropriate guidelines for treating certain diseases and supporting diagnosis definition as well as treatment plans for each patient. One of the great advantages of decision support systems is supporting the doctor in designing the best treatment plan relevant to each diagnosis.

The use of electronic prescriptions can also validate drugs, dosages and doses prescribed according to the established drug protocols. Drugs tracking in all supply chains decreases clinical risk. This tracking should use automatic identification and data capture.

Information systems can also improve communication with the public and contribute to better information on diseases, treatments and healthcare organizations. The creation of virtual communities for advice and information is one of the marketing tools in health care today.

PERSONALIZED MEDICINE

Standardization of clinical data also enables the delivery of personalized healthcare services.

The possibility to include genetic data in electronic records of the clinical data of each patient also adds, according to Shabo (2005), knowledge for decision making in healthcare services.

According to this author, there are three fundamental barriers to full recording of all clinical data of a patient:

- The internal data protection procedures for each hospital determine security policies and how to archive data to enable a hospital to preserve the patient's privacy and keep data confidential. For this reason it is not possible for a patient to receive treatment at different hospitals on different dates and have all the data aggregated.
- Another barrier is the time. Indeed, the average life of an individual is much greater than the deadlines of data storage. Thus, if a person lives 70 years, it is not likely that the hospital keeps a record that long.
- Another barrier is the fact that even if the clinical terminology is the same, for different healthcare organizations, it would be very difficult to ensure

semantics compatibility over several years, especially since their own terminologies are in permanent evolution.

Along with these 3 barriers there is the problem of genetic data that has evolved in structure and complexity as science also evolves.

Despite these barriers, the need to include genetic data in electronic registration of clinical data becomes evident. The SNOMED (Systematized Nomenclature of Medicine) standard according to IHTSDO (International Health Terminology Standards) now includes genetic terminology, which will enhance the creation of archetypes of genetic data.

For the HL7 standard, a working group developed a model restricted to storing data from chromosomes. This data is referenced by a set of metadata stored in a RIM platform (Reference Information Model). This model is strictly used to communicate data between hospitals and the pharmaceutical industry.

The Open EHR works in this area but there is a defined genotype. Two questions arise:

- Should the clinical data be kept for a long time and reflect all the genetic data, diseases and individual's care?
- Who should have the storage infrastructure?

Some authors argue that it should be distributed through different databases, whilst others argue that it should be a centralized clinical data bank. The concept of FEHR (Federation Health Electronic Record) is now being used. It is increasingly present in the creation of models for integrating data among different hospitals.

THE STANDARDIZATION OF CLINICAL SEMANTICS

There are many components for establishing a standard for HER involving clinical data. One component of great importance is clinical terminology. It is essential that all records are referenced to a single syntax and semantic. Due to knowledge developments, different cultures and the different services provided, there are different classifications for the same type of diseases, procedures, epidemiological data, demographic data, etymological data, equipment, chemical substances pharmaceuticals, etc.

Terminology standardization could establish communication between different care agents and allow data sharing.

The type, range and possible aggregations among data are essential to an EHR architecture (Figure 1). Due to the nature of the data related to models of these types of information systems, the metadata model is flexible and evolutionary. The architecture of archetypes allows the necessary flexibility to the metadata model to monitor the context in which care is provided.

The standardization of medical records allows implementation of Process Management Business models. There are ratings and open standards for information systems

Figure 1. An EHR architecture (author´s proposal)

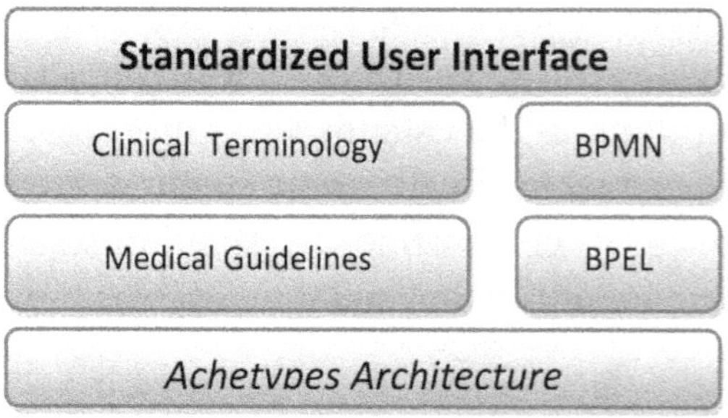

integration from different organizations. The BPMN (Business Process Modeling Notation) and the implementation of workflow engines using the BPEL (Business Process Execution Language) enable the automation of business processes and their integration with various healthcare organizations.

Another important aspect is user interface normalization. The screen layout and the used symbols used should be software independent. The user should not have to learn how to use a software application each time changes are made.

Another very important issue is to have medical guidelines for the chosen terminology. These guidelines would avoid some medical errors and missing information.

Clinical Ontology and Terminology

According to Moore (2001), "in medical informatics, ontology has come to mean a structured list of concepts, typically prepared by an expert or panel of experts."

The domain of concepts properly structured and related to each other has the name of clinical terminology.

One of the main components of an Electronic Health Record model is a standardized database of clinical terminology. There are several clinical terminologies developed by different organizations and with different objectives. The codification of diseases has been improved in successive works and is the origin of some codifications like ICD (International Classification Diseases) and SNOMED, as they are known today.

A standardized terminology should present the features necessary to be implemented by information systems, provide proper syntax and semantics and be able to be reproduced. A standardized terminology consists of a set of concepts, terms and relations. Due to the particularities of regions, cultures, diseases or treatments, it must be flexible and extended in accordance with the needs of each application. The data set that defines the terminology should be integrated into the information system and form a basis of reference of all electronic registration of clinical data.

Thus, the representation of an item in a terminology cannot depend on the interface with the standardized, user settings, place or time. The use of terminology also increases the quality of healthcare services. It allows a better quality of recorded data and enables the use of systems to support clinical decision. In addition, it allows the implementation of audit systems, Workflow Management Systems and condition alerts. Thus, any EHR (Electronic Health Record) system should refer to clinical terminology that relates to the data stored.

ICD-10

The ICD-10 (International Classification Diseases) terminology was developed by the WHO in order to classify mortality and causes of morbidity

This is a codification structured with three characters for each disease and cause of injury. This encryption is divided into 21 chapters beginning in chapter 1 with infectious diseases through to Chapter 21 with the factors that influence health and welfare.

The code is quite accurate with the main specialties (Taylor, 2006, p. 101). The three characters of the classification of a disease can be expanded into others that define its features and the causes of death. A situation can also be described using more than one ICD-10 code. For instance, in Table 1 code A02.2 could be linked with other codes, from other chapters to fully describe a disease.

Table 1. Some codes of Chapter I, ICD-10, (Source: NCHS)

Code	Description	
A02	Other salmonella infections	
	Includes:	infection or foodborne intoxication due to any Salmonella species other than S. typhi and S. paratyphi
A02.0	Salmonella enteritis	
	Salmonellosis	
A02.1	Salmonella septicaemia	
A02.2	Localized salmonella infections	
	Salmonella:	
	· arthritis+ (M01.3*)	
	· meningitis+ (G01*)	
	· osteomyelitis+ (M90.2*)	
	· pneumonia+ (J17.0*)	
	· renal tubulo-interstitial disease+ (N16.0*)	
A02.8	Other specified salmonella infections	
A02.9	Salmonella infection, unspecified	

The ICD-10 code provides a strong hierarchy of concepts. In some situations there are several codes to identify a disease with different anatomical or morphological parts.

Another criticism that is made of ICD-10 is that it is not possible to extend the codification to specificy fields needs of each organization.

Finally, the ICD-10 codifies diseases but not medical devices, procedures, drugs or additional means of diagnosis and treatment.

ICD-10 can neither develop terminology in accordance with local practices, cultural or religious values nor set up a table of cross-tables to allow linking codes of different terminologies. However, ICD-10 is widely used because it allows simple adequate codification of hospital production and standardization of healthcare costs.

SNOMED-CT

One of the best known organizations in Europe is the IHTSDO (International Health Terminology Standards Development Organization) based in Denmark. This organization is responsible for the development of the SNOMED-CT (Systematized Nomenclature of Medicine-Clinical Terms) Standard. The SNOMED-CT standard was created by the CAP (College of American Pathologists) and continues to be maintained and developed by this organization under contract with the IHTSDO.

Meanwhile the NLM (National Library of Medicine), an organization of North American standards and a member of the IHTSDO, joined SNOMED-CT in a standard model of EHR that was developed in the USA and is called the Unified Medical Language System.

Meanwhile, Europe and Australia followed a different path through an organization called Open EHR. Archetype's architecture, a different approach discussed in this chapter, was developed and was the essence of some case studies in the United Kingdom, Denmark, Finland, Sweden and Australia. The NLM model is based on a server that can be accessed with different technologies, Web, API (Application Programmer Interface) and XML (Extensible Markup Language). This server has a database called metathesaurus which owns the codification of all the terminology, a database of relationships and a semantic lexicographic analyzer. Software providers are encouraged to develop applications using the NLM online service for codification of all terms related to healthcare services.

The SNOMED-CT Terminology is used by two information systems: OpenEHR and NLM.

According to the IHTSDO the scope of the current SNOMED-CT embraces:

- Clinical findings, including disorders;
- Medical procedures;
- All kind of entities, (eg: labs, exams, conditions and so forth);
- Anatomy, morphology and body structures;
- Chemicals and drugs;
- Organisms relevant to Health and healthcare;
- Etiology of diseases;
- Function and activities;
- Social content relevant to Health;
- Types of clinical records, documents and certificates;
- Staging, scales, classifications and all kinds of health information;
- Variables and values necessary to organize and structure the terminology.

The SNOMED-CT terminology is based on three fundamental components:

- Concepts;
- Descriptions;
- Relationships.

The concepts are atomic entities with clinical significance and identified by a unique code. The concepts involved in hierarchies may have different levels of detail and may belong simultaneously to more than one hierarchy. Therefore, main concepts are aggregated and are divided into more specific concepts.

The SNOMED-CT terminology also permits a desegregation of the codes in more atomic concepts according with health service practices and different cultures.

Each concept has a full description called FSN (Fully Specified Name) and may have several abbreviated descriptions and synonyms. Relationship is what links concepts and establishes semantic meanings between them. There are different types of relationships between concepts:

- Definition;
- Qualification;
- Historical;

Each of these types of relationships has variables that create the various semantic contents of the standard.

Figure 2 illustrates an example of how it is possible to specify a condition. Each of these concepts, in turn can be subdivided into others as well as the relationship "FINDING SITE", which belongs to the Clinical Finding type which have other attributes such as

Figure 2. Adapted from SNOMED CT User Guide, illustrating pneumonia finding site lung structure

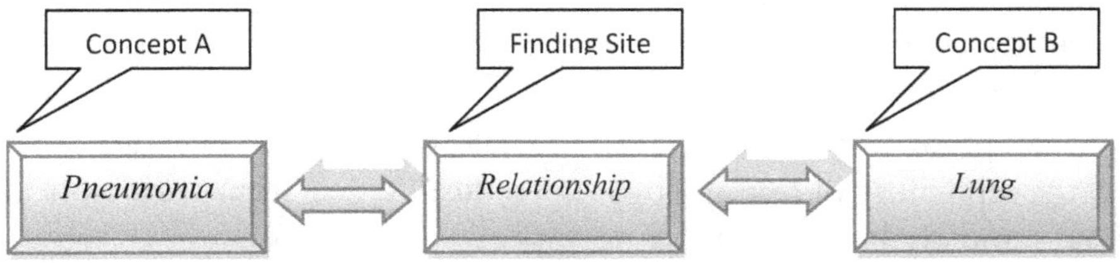

supplementary morphology, associations with agents, causes, disease, gravity or episode.

The SNOMED-CT terminology uses cross tables to establish equivalence with one single or multiple codes of other terminologies.

The United States National Library of Medicine

The NLM (National Library of Medicine) developed a multilingual metathesaurus with translation into several languages to support various activities related to health care. This thesaurus covers several areas of terminology related to health care and includes several classifications which emphasize pathological, medical devices, as well as pharmaceutical laboratory, demographic, social and billing aspects.

The metathesaurus codifications include vocabularies from different sources. These codifications include not only the concepts but also their inter-relationship to enable an accurate transcript of the semantics linked to healthcare. According to the NLM, the metathesaurus is not only a model of clinical ontology, but a different set of ontologies to observe and relate healthcare according to different perspectives resulting from each culture.

The metathesaurus has a set of concepts, attributes and validation rules to establish the inter-related entities. It is possible to have more than one codification for the same concept. This situation is always given in the codification terminology. The main objective of the metathesaurus is the creation of standardized data that can be communicated and understood by different healthcare services and used by Decision Support Systems.

Another advantage of using the metathesaurus is that the repository of terminology can be accessed remotely by the systems of each healthcare organization, which ensures data alignment between all systems and full compatibility.

There is an exception; when a healthcare organization wants to develop its own extensions to the known standard extensions, which are known as "subsets". This implies that only the standard codes can be used to communicate between different organizations as each one has its own extensions.

The Metathesaurus can be accessed remotely through an API (Application Program Interface) available in NLM or by direct access to a database installed locally. In the latter case, one will get higher speed access but it is critical to ensure an ongoing review of the same.

Standardization of Electronic Medical Records

According to the European Standards Committee, an EHR model should comprise the following aspects:

- Record clinical data so that the record is communicable to all systems;
- The data should be complete;
- The data should be useful;
- The data should be ethico-legal.

The EHR model of the Open EHR organization was the result of huge investigations carried out under the GEHR (Good European Health Record) project.The working group called the GEHR had two sources. A Belgian oncologist, Dr. Alain Maskens, who was interested in recording data in order to identify the causes of cancer. The system built allows storage of structured data created and consolidated from various healthcare units.

His team, which was created in the 80s, was perhaps the first EHR system.

In the UK, a general medical practitioner, Dr. Sam Heard, with his team of work colleagues from London, wanted a system for medical records in one of the major London hospitals, St Bartholomew's. Dr. Alain Maskens' project received the name of HealthOne and proved to be effective.

The GEHR group was founded in the early 90s with the aim of creating a structure for sharing clinical information between different departments, organizations, regions, countries and creating historical archives of simple and complex data. The project involved GEHR doctors and researchers from around twenty different organizations in eight countries. Twenty-three volumes of documentation were produced over four years.

The GEHR project was completed in 1995. The case studies now known as the result of this research project are Synapses, EHCR Support Action (EHCR SupA) and SynEx.

According to Dr Peter Schloeffel, Dr Sam Heard, Mr Tom Beale and Dr David Rowed, in June 1999, these were contributions made by the GEHR:

- A clear statement of requirements;
- A description of the architecture;
- A formal expression of the architecture as a compliable source code;
- A generated CASE (diagrammatic) expression of the model;
- Various exchange specifications (IDL, XML, etc.);
- An application programmer's interface (API);
- A GEHR term set;
- A provisional set of archetypes;
- Development guidelines.

The architecture is designed according to the Open EHR ISO model for distributed processing, RM-ODP (Reference Model - Open Distributed Processing).

According to Vallecillo (n. d.) the main objective of the RM-ODP model for information systems is to provide the following characteristics:

- The main functionalities should be implemented;
- The systems should be flexible in line with the evolution of the organization and should be flexible to integrate heterogeneous systems;
- There should be a clear, appropriate terminology for the activity semantics that permits communication between people and organizations;
- The information systems should be scalable in relation to the size of the organizations;
- It should be possible to integrate different technologies and systems manufacturers.

The ISO (International Standards Organization) and ITU-T (International Telecommunication Union) formed a working group to define the ODP model that includes distributed processing.

The reference model called RM (Reference Model), is a framework designed to enable interoperability of distribution and processing.

The OpenEHR model is an architecture based on a modular structure. The OpenEHR model consists of three main components:

- RM (Reference Model);
- SM (Service Model);
- AM (Archetype Model).

The RM and SM correspond to the ISO model RM / ODP and serve to ensure distributed processing (Figure 3).

The AM model liaises with the clinical ontologies. The concept of archetype was defined by the Dipark Kalra EurRec Conference in 2006 (Kalra, 2006):

An archetype defines a data structure, including optionally and multiplicity, data value constraints, and relevant bindings to natural language and terminology systems.

An archetype might define or constrain relationships between data values within a data structure, expressed as algorithms, formulas or rules.

An archetype may locally include other archetypes, and may be a specialization of another archetype.

The concept of archetype is thus very broad and includes all clinical ontologies at different levels of granularity. It also allows the location of concepts with the creation of specific derivatives of archetypes defined within the terminology in use and the management of different versions of clinical terminology. This way the archetypes model creates a middleware that virtualizes the physical data models and the computational infrastructure behind it.

Figure 3. Open EHR model architecture (adapted from open EHR architecture overview)

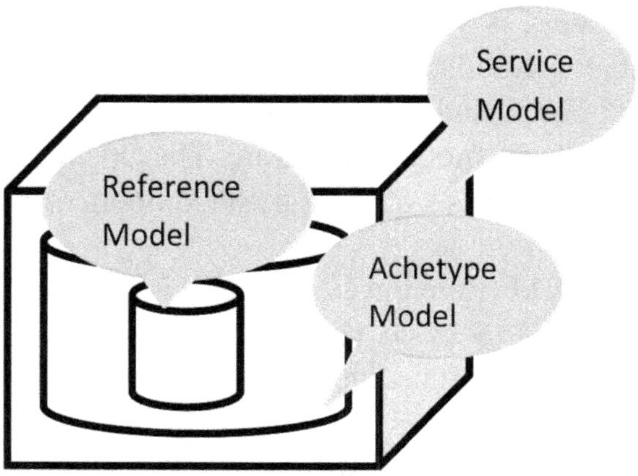

The concept of archetypes is intended to overcome the limitations of traditional metadata models. The archetypes have a similarity with the concept of object-oriented databases with the characteristics of inheritance, encapsulation, inherence and polymorphism.

Access and maintenance of terminologies, search for related knowledge and establishment of medical guidelines, are also still part of the archetype functions modules. These medical guidelines are fundamental to the procedure workflows for the patients' treatment. Some systems also allow the creation of medical guidelines on the archetypes.

In an archetype model, the data structure, the semantic content and the software are independent of each other. Another significant advantage of this model is that it allows the creation of new concepts and the update of their templates with control over all the versions.

This data model will be recorded on the RM-ODP model, according to the terminology and the archetypes defined. The archetypes give semantic meaning to data as a function of the selected terminology.

To define archetypes there is still a language called ADL (Archetype Model / Definition Language). This language allows a description of the whole structure of archetypes. The definition of an archetype may have clauses, returns of attributes and validations of clauses to guarantee the data validity.

The SM model incorporates definitions of services that are provided by the Open EHR model. This model has an interface that allows access to repositories of archetypes, terminology and clinical data through an API

(Application Programming Interface), which can also be used by any software.

An electronic registry of clinical standard data can be created. This standard should be evolutionary and available to any system to support clinical decision or management. This model also allows the integration of heterogeneous systems in the same healthcare unit or in different units.

Finally, one can also provide data for epidemiological studies or other types of research. A very important aspect of the OpenEHR model is privacy, confidentiality and data security. Thus, clinical information sharing identifying the patients should be made with patients' consent. This issue is very problematic. For example, a patient may wish to limit the data sharing that identifies certain diseases such as AIDS. However, through analysis of different data chunks, confidential diseases can be inferred. On the other hand, it is very important to have data about previous treatments and correlated data to avoid treatment-induced or an erroneous diagnosis; in other words, to avoid clinical error. So, the problem of privacy, confidentiality and security of clinical data is much more than a technological problem: it is primarily an ethical issue.

In some cases, a doctor responsible for a patient could have access to all data about that patient but the question is: who would have permission to set access levels for other health professionals?

This question is made worse by patient mobility. But, in fact, data sharing between healthcare organizations and the use of information technology to prescribe medication and to schedule exams at external laboratories are responsible for the complexity of this problem. A possible solution is to allow data access only to healthcare professionals related to the clinical episode in question. However the doctor who is making the diagnosis may need to continue to have access to the patient's clinical history. On the other hand, there is a risk in the implementation of systems managed by processes that hide the identification of the patient because they can cause errors of a technical or procedural nature.

Keeping the above in mind, it can be concluded that there is no single recipe for the implementation of a security system. The model must be selected and adapted to each case.

According to the OpenEHR Achitecture Overview, the OpenEHR model of archetypes provides the following features:

- Inability to physically eliminate records;
- Enabling the audit of all the introductions, changes and access to identification of date and time, user, reason and with digital signature;
- Possibility of providing access data on each patient;
- The model by default allows records with restrictions of access;
- Permission can be given by patients;
- Control of hits with a login possibility of entry logs;
- Whenever a data error is detected, it is possible to determine all the related records to identify possible diagnosis errors, mistakes in treatment plans or in communications with other entities.
- Possibility of establishing a correlation between records to identify more than one entity for the same patient. For example, if there is an error in the identification of a patient and two different entities are created for the same individual, the model should detect this situation;

- Limitation of time to access each clinical data episode. Data is accessed with the permission of the staff. The connection between these areas can be established outside the EHR model or within the model. Also the access can be parameterized to be permanent or the data can be accessed only once.

There is w wide variety of security policies that can be implemented.

EN13606 - a Standard for EHR System Communication within the CEN standard provides some of these policies.

"THE MODEL DRIVER ARCHITECTURE" AS A NEW APPROACH TO MODELING INFORMATION SYSTEMS

The modeling of architectures with archetypes also known as MDA (Model Driver Architecture) has a symbolic and semantic structure similar to the UML (Unified Modeling Language) with some added features. Among these features is a language for defining attribute domains called OCL (Object Constraint Language).

The OCL language is much more than a grammar for defining possible types and ranges for numerical variables. It is possible to set all kinds of variable types used in programming languages.

It is also possible to define the OCL types of language associations and restrictions of consistency between classes of objects.

The OCL language also has a syntax like JAVA to describe business rules that will be part of the model. Functions and procedures can be created to be part of the model semantics.

These rules are part of the business logic and they will be included in the MDA model independently of the software application.

The major innovation of this approach is that it enables modeling of the organization as a whole and establishes the architecture of information systems that integrates and standardizes all sorts of different data in clinical and administrative areas as well as human resources, stocks, property, financial and strategic management.

MDA is a methodology that reinforces improvement in the quality of global information systems. This methodology defines a different approach: instead of being composed of individual applications software without an overall overview, there is a macroscopic analysis of correctness and consistency among all the applications. Along with the terminology, these archetypes can also be called business objects. The OMG archetypes standardize delivery and offer maintenance and modeling tools for business processes.

According to the OMG, a model is a formal specification of the structure, functions and behavior of a system. According to the OMG the characteristics of this model are:

- Independence from the technology platform;
- Ability to generate machine executable codes for different platforms.

The use of models, that can be independent of technology, is very important because it allows a completely independent technological option and the ability to integrate systems from different vendors. The modeling tool should provide the following advantages:

- Creation of a metadata model in XML Metadata Interchange;

- Ability to create instances of variables in functions;
- Definition of business objects with characteristics of isomorphism and homomorphism.

The MDA model also includes specific definitions for the transformation of the abstract model called PIM (Platform Independent Model) into the physical model PSM (Platform Specific Platform). These processing definitions are directly related to the technology chosen and to specific platforms. These settings may still be characterized by some private aspects of the physical model such as whether a subject belongs to a physical or abstract platform and if the conversion is for one or more platforms. The main types of transformation are:

- Manual, in which each option is specified by the user at the time of transformation;
- Using the profile of a file that defines the actions to be taken;
- According to predefined templates;
- Automatic.

There are many tools to create models. Among the various available products, some of those most commonly used are Arcstyler of Interactive Objects, and PowerDesigner of Sybase.

In healthcare information systems there is a main electronic data record that is a general pointer to all the data for each patient. As far as data protection is concerned, it is imperative that the clinical data is separated from the names of each individual.

The Master Index database is thus the component that ensures the privacy and confidentiality of data and it helps to establish the relationships required when it is necessary to access the patients' private information.

One problem that arises in the migration between systems is data alignment with this Master Index. That is, if the same patient data is recorded in two Master Index databases, it can be perceived as two different patients when in fact it is only one patient.

There are several technologies based on fuzzy networks to analyze the databases to identify individuals and to determine if the data belong to the same individual or not.

Some companies like IBM are developing EAS (Entity Analytic Resolution) software. These systems are called Entity Analytic Resolution Systems and have the following features:

- Storage of all relevant data for the identification of persons in a database. The more information available, the easier it is to identify the individual reliably;
- Multiple views on resolution of the identity of each individual. Different views will make it easier to identify the person (for example, a person can be searched by name and address or name and date of birth);
- Person identification in real time. Whenever new data is recorded, it is compared with the existing data to check if identification is pending. If the data confirms the identification a new record is created;
- Resolution of identity is independent of the order in which data is recorded;
- All attributes are searchable;
- Relations between individuals are created and maintained dynamically.

Bilgic et. al. (2006) presented a new method to identify social networks and the relationships between persons. According to these authors this method and the software tool called D-Dupe, "is an interactive tool that combines data mining algorithms for entity resolution with a task-specific network visualization."

The use of these software tools can be extremely useful not only to prevent duplication in databases and improve data quality and for clinical decision support, but also for epidemiological studies because it is possible to establish socio-cultural, marital, genealogical, and other links among patients.

THE UTILIZATION OF BUSINESS PROCESS MANAGEMENT IN HEALTHCARE SERVICES

This methodology enables description of activities, conditions and events. It is possible to create groups of activities. The BPM (Business Process Management) model is a structural approach for all the activities of an organization and the interfaces between each layer with reference to different functions.

The BPM models can be implemented with different technologies and meet all the process requirements to develop and implement dynamic models. According to Perkonigg, (2006) the main steps are:

- Model creation;
- Development of a technology platform;
- Workflow implementation;
- Monitoring;
- Optimization.

The creation of the model represents one of the fundamental steps of the process and has the following aspects to be considered: activity definition, their relationships, operating conditions, variables and their relevant fields.

There are several tools for BPM modeling. Many are open source and others are commercial. All these tools provide a model in a standardized format that could be interpreted by different workflow engines.

The development of a platform, its implementation, monitoring and optimization technologies depend on the chosen technology. Some organizations have promoted efforts to standardize tools for BPM. Among these organizations, there is BPMI (Business Process Management Initiative) belonging to the OMG (Object Management Group). According to OMG this organization was founded in 1989 with the aim of defining norms and standards to enable interoperability, portability and integration of software developed on distributed, heterogeneous platforms.

BPMI was established in August 2000. The first syntax for creating models was published in 2002. For a description of the model, BPMI published in May 2004, a set of recommendations called 1.0 BPMN (Business Process Management Notation). The first objective was to present a syntax for managers, analysts, software engineers and end users.

According to the BPMI this organization joined OMG in June, 2005, with the objective of defining a standard for the modeling of business processes. This standard is based on the following concepts:

- Actors;
- Activities;
- Events;
- States.

With these four concepts the whole process can be defined. The main objective of BPMN syntax is to enable the automatic generation of executable code from the business model. For example, one can set the stage for a chart that describes graphically the business process model.

The business model is described in BPMN notation and converted into a language capable of being understood by a BPM engine. This language is known as BPEL (Business Process Execution Language). These languages have an XML format and are based on Web Services as described by the WSDL (Web Service Description Language) of the W3C. One of the best known is BPEL4WS created by BEA, nowadays linked with Oracle, IBM and Microsoft. Integration between different organizations is a must. Therefore, the development, implementation and evaluation of a BPM system within an organization becomes necessary to integrate the business process with other organizations. Thus, it is necessary to publish and orchestrate different services provided by BPM models. The systems that perform these tasks are called BPMS (Business Process Management Systems).

BPMS thus provide an integrated set of services with workflows for different organizations in the e-business field. An instance of the BPM model is called a workflow. According to Hollingsworth(1995), the definition of workflow is as follows:

The computerised facilitation or automation of a business process, in whole or part.

The workflow establishes which documents, information or tasks are passed from one participant to another according to activity sequence and rules.

The Workflow Management Coalition (n. d.) also offers the following definition of a Workflow Management System:

A system that completely defines, manages and executes "workflows" through the execution of software whose order of execution is driven by a computer representation of the workflow logic.

Healthcare workflows are very diverse: examinations, diagnosis, treatment plans and administrative procedures, logistical and operational decision-making and strategic management, among others. The workflows may also vary according to each organization and, in some cases, they can integrate more than one healthcare organization.

Dazzi et al. (n.d.) developed a model called PW(f)MS (Patient Workflow for Management System), based on Petri Nets to automate patient treatment activities. This model has been implemented in an Extranet and Intranet and aimed at pediatric patients with acute myeloid leukemia. The system's main components were a medical guidelines publisher that described the ontologies, a translation feature of the guidelines for the type of workflow engine and the workflow itself.

Clinical ontologies were described with a model known as The EON Model of Intervention Protocols and Guidelines. This model has a syntax to describe the activities, their connections and the conditions related to them. The workflows applied to healthcare issues are a new approach to Health Services based on evidence consisting of standardized data. The systems-based workflows can still implement policies to secure access to data and monitor the various activities.

In environments of shared care it is still possible to implement workflows with collaborative data sharing. The patients' identification and their demographics should be stored in a shared database. This is of utmost importance in healthcare not only because of the need to share resources between departments in healthcare organizations but also because in most cases the same patient suffers from several diseases and the treatment plans and guidelines differ.

In other cases the treatment plans cannot be established in advance. These situations are derived from three types of factors: uncertainties in the diagnosis, rare diseases or new therapies. In this context the workflows enable the use of non-deterministic models. The workflows still have some of the healthcare features such as the impossibility of carrying out rollback activities, that is, to go backwards as a result of activities undertaken. The workflows are not fully deterministic due to the uncertainty that always exists in the outcome of medical activities; they are complex in the number of variables in their relationships to each other. Each player also has his/her own ideas and perceptions as to whether or not it is appropriate to authorize treatment offers.

The model proposed by Browne (2005, p. 30) defines the architecture of the Clinical Information System with the following components:

- Knowledge stored by guidelines algorithms;
- Data stored as an EHR model;
- Workflow processes stored like metadata.

After all, the most important components of the Clinical Information System are the clinical terminology and archetypes. The terminology might include several clinical taggings and should comprise the semantic content of medical guidelines and the data stored in EHR. The archetypes, in turn, will define the structure of all the clinical data.

Several standards and technologies for the implementation of a workflow must be considered.

The different implementations and languages depend on one single, conceptual model called cross BPM (Figure 4).

Figure 4. BPM models (authors' proposal)

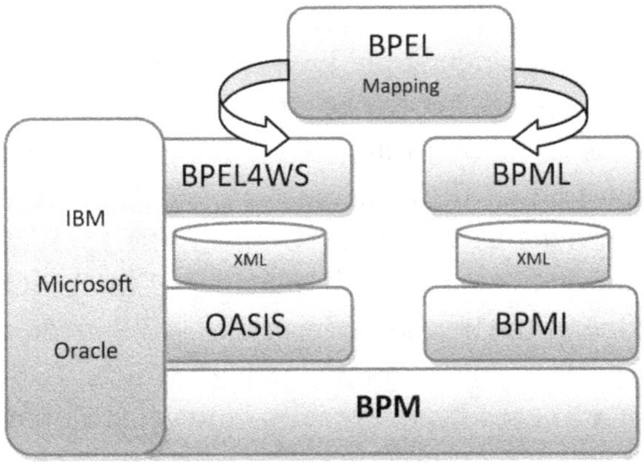

IBM, Microsoft and Oracle have developed a technology based on XML web services that allows this interoperability. This language was given the name BPE4LWS (Business Process Execution Language for Web Services). The BPEL4WS is supported by an organization called OASIS created by various manufacturers. A process in BPEL is physically in two types of files:

- Definition Language, web service files that describe the interfaces with the web services;
- BPEL files that define the processes, activities, links, events and variables.

When the WSDL (Web Services Definition Language) and BPEL files are put together, a process is obtained that can communicate with other processes or external sites. Many companies in 2000 like BEA which was bought by Oracle as well as BM, SAP, Peoplesoft and others created an organization called BPMI (Business Process Modeling Initiative), to promote the standard BPM. This organization is in turn a member of the W3C, OASIS, OMG and WfMC.

The main specifications focus on the following action lines:

- BPMN (Business Process Modeling Notation) which is a graphical language to develop models;
- BPML (Business Process Modeling Language) which is an XML language to transcribe the model chart in a syntax that can be run by an engine.

Other specifications are:

- BPQL (Business Process Query Language) which is a query language for procedures aimed at monitoring.
- BPSM (Business Process Semantic Model) which is a semantic appropriate for business.
- BPXL (Business Process Execution Layers) which is a BPEL standard for commercial transactions.

The WS-CDL (Web Services Choreography Description Language) is a language developed by W3C. The main goals of this language are to solve models of a collaborative nature in which there are interactions between different actors and data sharing.

The main distinction between the model described in standard WS-DL and WS-CDL is that, while the former implies a centralized management, the latter includes several models, each with its own management but with relationships and dependencies between them.

The characteristics of the standard WS-CDL are the interaction between the business processes of different BPMs, the possibility of channels of communication and setting interaction permission levels between processes.

THE DEVELOPMENT OF MEDICAL GUIDELINES

The CDA language (Clinical Document Architecture) was developed for the standard HL7 version 3 and it is intended to describe clinical ontologies. This language is based on the XML standard. Beyond text, it also includes sound, image and all kinds of known file types.

The document written in the language structure, CDA, presents a header with demographic data and information of the episode, a body that may be made of free text or structured in sections and each section with structured items and a digital signature.

The possible use of free text is very important for the standard because it enables not only covering all possible situations but also, in an implementation phase of this standard, and a gradual progressing.

There are several types of document associated with each activity and each episode of a document can be read with a simple text editor because it is in XML.

The reason for not having used exclusively the XML standard as defined by W3C, and creating a specific language, is due to the need to create objects of different types and rules to validate the structure of the messages.

According to HL7 Clinical Document Architecture, Release 2.0 the main features of a document in CDA are:

- Persistence;
- Possibility to be read by any browser;
- Security of access and authenticity guaranteed by digital signatures;
- Link to clinical terminology;

The types of documents that exist in CDA are:

- Financial;
- Clinical Observation;
- Diagnostics;
- Laboratory exams;
- Reports to public health.

The implementation of the HL7 protocol with the CDA language makes possible independent messages from each other, as well as completeness and consistency which can be implemented gradually within an organization.

The terminologies to be used may be different but the most commonly used are ICD10 and SNOMED-CT.These terminologies are available through the NLM (National Library of Medicine).

According to the HL7- EHR System Functional Model: A Major Development Towards Consensus on Electronic Health Record System Functionality (2004), the technical requisites for the development of this standard were:

- The architecture must be compatible with XML;
- The architecture specifies the schemas required for exchange;
- The architecture should impose minimal constraints or requirements on a document structure and content required for exchange;
- The architecture must be scalable to accommodate fine-grained highly structured markup such as text and coded data;
- Document specifications based on this architecture should accommodate such constraints and requirements according to appropriate professional, commercial, and regulatory agencies;
- Document specifications for document creation and processing, if intended for exchange, should map to this exchange architecture;
- CDA documents must be human-readable using widely available and commonly-deployed XML aware browsers and print drivers and a generic CDA style sheet written in a standard style sheet language;
- Use of open standards.

Another very important aspect of this standard is that it may include, in the same message, terminology of different rules.

A tag named codeSystemName may have the terminology identification. This possibility is of utmost importance for the ease of integration between different systems and cultures.

KEY ISSUES TO IMPLEMENT AN ELECTRONIC OPEN HEALTH RECORD SYSTEM

There are some issues that should be addressed to develop an EHR System. There are two different normalized approaches:

- HL7
- OpenEHR

Both of them have their basis in archetypes patterns. An archetype pattern is a library of stereotypes of object classes. There are different types of stereotypes. According to Robert et. Al. (2006), for instance HL7 uses six different domains of stereotypes: act, participation, entity, role, actRelationship and rolelink).

Physically a stereotype is a XML metadata class that defines a data structure.The OpenEHR association developed an archetype library like HL7. These two models are very similar. The main difference is perhaps the metamodel arquitecture. The HL7 uses a RIM, (Reference Information Model) and Open EHR uses an Archetype Model Architecture.

A description of OpenEHR gateways to HL7 versions and other protocols is available on OpenEHR Achitecture Overview, (2007).

All these models are documented, described and available to download in each association sites.The user can prune some classes or select some optional attributes and classes. It is not allowed to change structures that modify the consistency, coherency and well formed data definition classes.

The syntactic reference database is a very important piece of the EHR system. The most used terminology is SNOMED. Joining the archetype system, database terminology and a database data repository, an EHR system will be achieved.

The EHR system is a middleware and data repository to support the hospital Information system and hospital communication system. The communication system should communicate with other hospitals using an authentication and encryption protocol.

The EHR system is the repository of all data. To integrate with other software applications there are different technologies mainly Webservices, BPM, As1 and As2. The proprietary databases of each software should be substituted by the EHR repository system.

FUTURE RESEARCH DIRECTIONS

The normalization and standardization of clinical data are a current objective to be achieved.

The main drivers are the healthcare delivery 100% focused on the patient, improving care quality, increasing the efficiency and effectiveness of healthcare units and lowering medical risk.

Other drivers are related to the high mobility of people in an increasingly globalized society. It can be said that people are increasingly citizens of the world rather than just a region. That statement implies a large interoperability between the age of Information Systems and healthcare organizations in different regions, countries and continents.

The new paradigm of Evidence-based medicine also involves an increase in the type and quantity of clinical data originating from various sources: emergency services, outpatient and inpatient care, continuing care, palliative care, laboratories, additional methodologies of diagnosis and treatment, pharmacies and also the patient himself. In this model, the patient is active in the production of clinical data. There are still some barriers for which there is no complete solution:

- How to ensure a unique identification of the patient anywhere in the health-care network?
- Where should clinical data be stored?
- How to ensure complete privacy and confidentiality of clinical data?
- Clinical data is aligned with clinical terminology. How to ensure data interpretation throughout the patient's life, bearing in mind that the terminology is evolving?
- And yet, if the average lifespan of a citizen may be more than 70 years, how to ensure data availability over this period?

Single patient identification is an aspect of great importance. Many concepts have been identified to set a single key. This issue remains unresolved and the question is how to identify citizens of different countries. The current trend is to have a DNA key identification for patients. This would be the only valid guarantee of unique identification.

Clinical data storage is a very pertinent question because there is the problem of moving towards large volumes of data distributed by various organizations. The topology of storage with guarantees of access, length of time available and integration of data is very important and still unresolved.

How to guarantee privacy and data confidentiality is another very important aspect. It is possible to set policies to access data within a hospital, but how can the access by collaborative systems between different hospitals? How to avoid the individual's identification through datamining tools and cross-checking? (despite some systems having no permission to access the patients' identity). If, on the one hand, we must use Business Intelligence tools, how can use set levels of access that prevent the construction of undue or illegal knowledge about the clinical data?

The development of clinical terminology is a fact . Also its location and suitability for religious values (E.g.: a blood transfusion cannot be made without the patient's consent. Some religions do not allow people to have blood transfusions.) and practices of each hospital are objectives to be achieved. But how to ensure alignment of semantics over the life of a patient if the terms are dynamic and evolving?

Records on paper last for a long time and do not depend on technology to be interpreted. Moreover paper records do not need an appropriate technology to be read. Any technology in the field of ITs lasts only for a short time. The question again is how to ensure access to the data of an individual over his/her entire life.

These issues will be the subject of discussions, research and future developments because they are barriers to the development of models of medical records.

CONCLUSION

This matter is complex with contours that touch on several areas including clinical ontologies and cybernetics.

The models developed so far solve some of the existing needs but some major steps must be taken to ensure interoperability between all systems, safety and long life of clinical data.

The certification of information systems is also a very important milestone towards the development of an integration network for clinical data.

However, much work needs to be done especially in information systems governance, normalization and standardization.

Patient healthcare will benefit greatly from these developments as will epidemiology, medical research and the economy in general.

Increasing the quality of life is one of the drivers of the economy in many nations.

REFERENCES

AHRQ. (n. d.). *Agency for Healthcare Research and Quality*. Retrieved December 20, 2009, from http://www.ahrq.gov/.

Arcstyler. (n. d.). *Interactive objects*. Retrieved December 20, 2009 from http://www.interactive-objects.com/

Bergman, M. K. The deep Web: Surfacing hidden value. *Journal of Electronic Publishing*. Retrieved December 8, 2009, from http://www.brightplanet.com/pdf/deepwebwhitepaper.pdf

Bilgic, M., Licamele, L., Getoor, L., & Shneiderman, B. (2006). D-Dupe: an interactive tool for entity resolution in social networks. *Visual Analytics Science and Technology*. Retrieved December 8, 2009 from http://waimea.cs.umd.edu:8080/basilic/web/Publications/2006/bilgic:vast06/

BPMI. (n. d.). *Business Process Management Initiative*. Retrieved December 8, 2009 from http://www.bpmi.org/

Browne, E. D. (2005). *Workflow modelling of coordinated inter. health-provider care plans* (Unpublished doctoral dissertation). School of Computer and Information Science, University of South Australia, Adelaide.

CAP. (n. d.). College of American Pathologists. Retrieved December 8, 2009 from http://www.cap.org/apps/cap.portal

Dazzi, L., Fassino, C., & Saracco, R. Quaglini, S., & Stefanelli, Mario. (n.d.). A patient workflow management system built on guidelines. *Consorzio di Bioingegneria e Informatica Medica, Pavia, Italy*. Retrieved December 8, 2009 from http://www2.amia.org/pubs/symposia/D004083.PDF

Dolin, H. R., Alschudler, L., Boyer, S., Beebe, C., Behlen, M. F., Biron, P.V., & Shabo, Amnon. (2006). HL7 clinical document, release 2. *Journal of American Informatics Association*. Retrieved November 20, 2009 from http://www.jamia.org/cgi/content/abstract/13/1/30

Downing, G. (2007). Improving health and accelerating personalized health care through health information technology and genetic information in population-and community-based health care delivery systems. *Personalized Medicine Coalition*. Retrieved December 8, 2009 from http://www.personalizedmedicinecoalition.org/PMC_Response_to_HHS_RFI_on_HIT_final_1_25_071.pdf

EN13606 - a standard for EHR system communication. (n. d.). Retrieved December 8, 2009 from http://www.openehr.org/standards/cen.html

GEHR – Good European Health Record (n.d.). Retrieved December 8, 2009 from http://www.chime.ucl.ac.uk/work-areas/ehrs/GEHR/.

HL7-clinical document architecture release 2.0. (n. d.). Retrieved December 8, 2009 from http://xml.coverpages.org/CDA-20040830v3.pdf

HL7- EHR system functional model: A major development towards consensus on electronic health record system functionality. (2004). Retrieved December 8, 2009, from http://www.providersedge.com/ehdocs/ehr_articles/HL7_EHR_System_Functional_Model-White_Paper.pdf

HealthOne. Retrieved December 8, 2009 from http://www.openehr.org/114-OE.html

Hollingsworth, D. (1995). The workflow reference model. *Workflow Management Coalition*. Retrieved December 8, 2009, from http://www.e-workflow.org/standards/workflow_ref_model.pdf

IBM EAS. (n. d.). Retrieved December 8, 2009 from http://www-01.ibm.com/software/data/ips/products/masterdata/eas/

IHTSDO. (n. d.). *International Health Terminology Standards Development Organization*. Retrieved December 8, 2009 from http://www.ihtsdo.org/

ISO. (n. d.). *International Standard Organization*. Retrieved December 8, 2009 from http://www.iso.org/iso/home.htm

ITU. (n. d.). *International Telecommunication Union*. Retrieved December 8, 2009 from http://www.itu.int/net/home/index.aspx

Kalra, D. (2006). *Archetypes: The missing link*. Retrieved December 8, 2009 from http://www.eurorec.org/eurorec2006/programme.cfm?actief=programme

Kraft, M. R., Desouza, K. C., & Androwich, I. (2002). Data mining in healthcare information systems: Case study of a Veterans' Administration spinal cord injury population. In *Proceedings of the 36th Hawaii International Conference on System Sciences*. Retrieved December 8, 2009 from http://csdl2.computer.org/comp/proceedings/hicss/2003/1874/06/187460159a.pdf

Merriam-Webster Dictionary. (n.d.). Retrieved December 8, 2009 from http://www.merriam-webster.com/dictionary/health.

Moore, G. W. (2001). *What is a medical ontology?* Retrieved December 8, 2009 from http://www.netautopsy.org/whatonto.htm retrieved

NCHS. (n. d.). *Nation Center of Health Statistics*. Retrieved December 8, 2009 from http://www.cdc.gov/nchs/icd9.htm

NLM. (n. d.). *National Library of Medicine*. Retrieved December 8, 2009 from http://www.nlm.nih.gov/healthit.html

OMG. (n. d.). *Business process management with OMG specifications*. Retrieved December 8, 2009 from http://www.bpmroundtable.org/101807_BPM_Fact_Sheet.pdf

OpenEHR. (n. d.). Retrieved December 8, 2009 from http://www.openehr.org

OpenEHR architecture overview. (n. d.). Retrieved December 8, 2009 from http://svn.openehr.org/specification/BRANCHES/Release-1.0.1-candidate/publishing/architecture/overview.pdf

Patterson, N. L. (2004). *The mission of IT in health care: Creating a system that cares in healthcare information system management*. London: Springer. doi:10.1007/978-1-4757-4041-7_1

Perkonigg, F. (2006). *Application of business process management in Web-based education* (Unpublished Master Thesis). Institute for Information Systems and Computer Media (IICM), Graz University of Technology, Austria.

PowerDesigner. (n. d.). *Sybase*. Retrieved December 8, 2009 from http://Sybase.com */products/modelingdevelopment/powerdesigner*.

Samson, W. T., & Musen, M. A. (1996). The EON model of intervention protocols and guidelines. *EON Project at Stanford Medical Informatics*. Retrieved December 8, 2009 from http://www.smi.stanford.edu/projects/eon/96scamc/tu96scamc.html

Schloeffel, P., Heard, S., Beale, T., & Rowed, D. (1999). *Overview of GEHR from an Australian perspective*. Retrieved December 8, 2009 from http://www.omg.org/docs/corbamed/00-01-17.txt

Shabo, A. (2005). The implications of electronic health records for personalized medicine. *Personalized Medicine*. Retrieved on December 8, 2009 from http://www.haifa.ibm.com/projects/software/cgl7/papers/the_implications_of_ehrs_for_perso-nalized_medicine-shabo.pdf

Shreeve, S. (n. d.). The Enabling technologies and reform initiatives for next generation health care. Retrieved December 8, 2009 from http://health20.org/wiki/Shreeve_Health_2.0_Whitepaper.

SNOMED CT style guide. Retrieved December 8, 2009 from http://www.ihtsdo.org/snomed-ct/snomed-ct-publications/

Taylor, P. (2006). *From patient data to medical knowledge*. London: BMJ. doi:10.1002/9780470994702

Vallecillo, A. (n. d.). RM-ODP: *The ISO reference model for open distributed processing*. Retrieved December 8, 2009 from http://www.enterprise-architecture.info/Images/Documents/RM-ODP.pdf

W3C. (n. d.). Retrieved December 8, 2009 from http://www.w3.org

WfMC. (n. d.). *Workflow Management Coalition*. Retrieved December 8, 2009 from http://www.wfmc.org

WHO. (n. d.). *World Health Organization*. Retrieved December 8, 2009 from http://www.who.int/

KEY TERMS AND DEFINITIONS

Archetypes: According to Kalra (2006), an archetype defines a data structure, including optionality and multiplicity, data value constraints, and relevant bindings to natural language and terminology systems.

Business Process Management (BPM): According to OMG (n.d.), BPM is a set of techniques for the continuous, or improvement of all the processes involved in running a business.

Clinical Terminology: According to SNOMED CT, Style Guide (2008, p. 6), a terminology resource consists of concepts, terms and interrelationship between them and is intended to ensure comprehensive coverage of terms that are appropriate and expressive.

E-Health: According to the WHO (n. d.), e-Health is a new term used to describe the combined use of electronic communication and information technology in the health sector or is the use, in the health sector, of digital data-transmitted, stored and retrieved electronically for clinical, educational and administrative purposes, both at the local site and at a distance.

Electronic Health Record (EHR): According to Taylor (2006, p. 28), EHR is the architecture of a model of the generic features necessary [...] for it to be communicable and complete, retain integrity across systems, countries and time, and be a useful and effective ethico-legal record of care.

Personalized Medicine: According to Shabo (2005), personalized medicine relies on the ability to effectively associate personalized genomic data with clinical data to support the clinical decision.

Workflow: It is a component of a Business Process Management. A workflow describes the flows of activities inside an organization. A Business Process Management integrates different workflows across one or several organizations.

Chapter 3
LinkEHR:
A Platform for the Normalization of Legacy Clinical Data Based on Archetypes

José Alberto Maldonado
Instituto ITACA, Universitat Politècnica de València, Spain

Diego Boscá
Instituto ITACA, Universitat Politècnica de València, Spain

David Moner
Instituto ITACA, Universitat Politècnica de València, Spain

Montserrat Robles
Instituto ITACA, Universitat Politècnica de València, Spain

ABSTRACT

Normalization of data is a prerequisite to achieve semantic interoperability in any domain. This is even more important in the healthcare sector due to the special sensitivity of medical data: data exchange must be done in a meaningful way, avoiding any possibility of misunderstanding or misinterpretation. In this chapter, we present the LinkEHR system for clinical data standardization and exchange. The LinkEHR platform provides tools that simplify meaningful sharing of electronic health records between different systems and organizations. Key contributions of LinkEHR are the development of a powerful medical concept, expressed in the form of archetypes, editing framework based on formal semantics capable of handling multiple electronic health record architectures, the definition of high-level non-procedural mappings to describe the relationship between archetype and legacy clinical data and the semi-automatic generation of XQuery scripts that transform legacy data into XML documents compliant with the underlying electronic health record data architecture and at the same time satisfy the constraints imposed by the archetype.

DOI: 10.4018/978-1-4666-3000-0.ch003

1. INTRODUCTION

Nowadays, patient health data is scattered among many information systems. This leads to distributed and heterogeneous data resources creating a large gap between the potential and actual value of the information content of Electronic Health Record (EHR) systems. Closing this gap by making efficient use of the health data held by these systems, could improve significantly patient care, clinical efficiency, patient safety and empower research activities.

To achieve a complete EHR that encompasses all existing health information about a patient independently of where it was generated or where it is stored and maintained crucially depends on a high level of semantic interoperability among EHR systems. Semantic interoperability is the ability of computer-based systems to seamlessly communicate, incorporate and use information generated by external systems. Data standardization (normalization) is a prerequisite to achieve semantic interoperability in any domain. The use of standards enables clear, complete, and efficient communication of data by means of agreements on language and procedures. This is even more important in the health-care sector due to the special sensitivity of medical data. Data exchange must be done in a meaningful way, avoiding all possibility of misunderstanding or misinterpretation. As a consequence any project involving the sharing or communication of EHR must face the challenge of how to model faithfully the data to be communicated. The first and basic requirement is the definition of a common information architecture for communicating EHR extracts. The good news are that considerable effort has been invested over the years on the definition of EHR architectures (Kalra, 2006) and currently a mature body of EHR standards is available.

In this chapter we describe the LinkEHR platform along with some use cases in real settings. LinkEHR is a software platform whose main purpose is the creation a virtual, standardized and federated EHR view from data distributed among heterogeneous and autonomous health information systems. LinkEHR uses archetypes as a means to achieve semantic enrichment and normalization of existing health data. The main objectives of LinkEHR are then twofold. Firstly, in the context of data integration, the use of archetypes as a semantic layer over the data repositories, whose contents need to be integrated, described and exchanged, associating them with formal semantics. Secondly, the use of archetypes for making public existing clinical information in the form of XML EHR extracts compliant with the underlying EHR architecture.

2. DUAL MODEL EHR ARCHITECTURES

During the last decade different organizations have been working on the definition of an EHR architecture for the faithful communication of health data. The Technical Committee 251 (health informatics) of the European Committee for Standardization (CEN/TC251) completed in 2007 a European Standard for the communication of the EHR called EN13606 whose part 1 (reference model) (International Organization for Standardization, 2008a) became an ISO standard in February 2008. One of the main contributions of CEN/ISO 13606 is the utilization of an EHR architecture based on the dual model methodology (Beale, 2002) for the description of the structure and semantics of health data. The dual model methodology distinguishes a reference model and archetypes. In a broad sense, a reference model is an abstract representation of the entities and relationships of a domain which is designed to provide a basis for the development of more concrete models and implementations. The reference model is represented by a stable and small object oriented model that models the generic and stable properties of health record information. The generality of the reference model is complemented by the particularity of archetypes. Archetypes are detailed and domain-specific definitions of clinical concepts (Apgar score, discharge report, primary care EHR, etc.) in the form of structured and constrained combinations of the entities of the reference model. Their principal purpose is to provide a powerful, reusable and interoperable way of managing the creation, description, validation and query of EHRs. From a data point of view, archetypes are a means for providing semantics to data instances that conform to some reference model by assuring that data obey a particular structure and satisfy a set of constraints. The semantic description of domain concepts is achieved by linking the data structures and content to knowledge resources such as terminologies and ontologies (Maldonado et al., 2009).

In this methodology, only the stable reference model is hard-coded in database schemas or software, while the possible numerous and volatile domain concepts (archetypes) are modeled separately by domain specialists and their definitions are maintained in a repository. Since the software is only bound to the reference model it has no direct dependency on domain concepts. Furthermore, when new concepts are introduced or existing ones are altered the system does not need to be changed. Archetypes can be re-used to define new archetypes by different means. They can be composed (i.e., previously defined archetypes can be components of new and more complex archetypes). Archetypes may also be specialized: an archetype is considered a specialization of another archetype if it specifies that archetype as its parent, and only makes changes to its definition such that its constraints are narrower than those of the parent.

2.1 The CEN/ISO 13606 Norm

The CEN/ISO 13606 norm is a five part standard for communication and semantic interoperability of EHR data. The first part of the standard describes a Reference Model (RM) for EHR data. It describes a generic object oriented model for representing any clinical annotation of the EHR. The overall goal is to define a rigorous and stable information architecture for communicating part or all of the EHR of a single subject of care (patient). The reference model imposes a hierarchical structure and organization on EHR data. To do this, the model sub-divides the EHR hierarchy into parts with different levels of granularity ranging from organisational folders all the way down to single data values. It also specifies the data structures for meeting published requirements in order to be faithful to the original clinical context and to preserve meaning when records are communicated. This is to support the interoperability of systems and components that need to communicate EHR data via electronic messages or as distributed objects.

The second part of the standard (International Organization for Standardization, 2008b) defines an Archetype Model (AM) for the description of clinical domain concepts in the form of structured and constrained combinations of the reference model classes. The overall archetype model consists of identifying information, a description (its meta-data), a definition (expressed in terms of constraints on instances of a model model class), and an ontology. Only those classes of the reference model that define logical building blocks of EHRs can be used to construct archetypes, we call them business concepts. CEN/ISO 13606 defines six business concepts, namely: Folder, Composition, Section, Entry, Cluster and Element. Therefore, the root of the constraint structure of an archetype shall always take the form of a constraint on one of these classes. ADL (Archetype Definition Language) is a formal language developed by the openEHR consortium for expressing textually archetypes that has been adopted by CEN/ISO 13606.

3. A INTEGRATION AND NORMALIZATION OF LEGACY HEALTH DATA

3.1 Data Integration

In most health organisations the coexistence of several heterogeneous information sources in terms of platform, structure (data model) and semantics is a common scenario. They were created and are maintained to fulfill the requirements of a particular user, application or hospital service. As a consequence they are suitable for the department they were created for but not for other applications that may also need to use the information held by these systems, i.e. here we face a problem of data integration. Data integration is the problem of combining data residing at different sources and providing the user with a unified view of these data (Lenzerini, 2002). This unified view may be created from a set of existing data repositories in order to facilitate information access through a single information access point or given a certain information need it may be constructed by combining different but complementary repositories in order to satisfy the need.

LinkEHR follows one of most commonly solutions used in data integration: the mediator/wrapper architecture. Wiederhold (1992) defines a mediator as "a software module that exploits encoded knowledge about a certain set or subset of data to create information for a higher layer of applications". A mediator, which can be seen as a read-only virtual database which is introduced between the data sources and the application using them, is capable of answering queries about the underlying data. For this purpose the mediator uses the sources, suitable interfaced by a wrapper which are specialized programs that interface with the sources and hide their technical details, and/or another mediator to answer the queries. The mediator maintains a common data model and relies on schema mapping for integration of the data source usually supported by wrappers, in order to overcome the difficulties that can arise in dealing with the heterogeneity of data sources (relational, XML, object oriented, etc.), mediators use a global conceptualization model, called mediated schema, for the data from all integrated databases which describes the domain entities and their relationship. Data sources are mapped to the mediated schema by defining the entities they contain. Users pose queries on the virtual view and a query engine is in charge of decomposing and translating the query into an equivalent set of local subqueries that are executed against the local data sources, whose results are then combined.

In order to take the maximum advantage of information it is necessary to transform source data to meet the data format of the target applications. This problem is known in the literature as *data exchange*, which is the problem of taking data structures under a source schema and creating an instance of a target schema that reflects the source data as accurately as possible (Fagin, Kolaitis, Miller, & Popa, 2005).

3.2 LinkEHR Integration Engine

LinkEHR integration engine is a data federation system, emphasized in flexibility and quick deployment. Briefly, LinkEHR integration engine is a data integration system that provides a virtual, integrated and global XML (Wiederhold, 1992)view over distributed health data sources. Although a materialized solution is generally more efficient computationally, we prefer virtual approach as it does not involve data replication, which may cause data update and synchronization problems, a significant limitation in an EHR application where up-to-date information is needed. In LinkEHR integration engine, the virtual global view is easily customizable for different user groups whose needs may change over time. In an evolving environment as healthcare, the local databases may change often. The databases are designed and maintained to meet local needs and changes are almost made independently of the integrated global view. LinkEHR integration engine can be classified as a generic middleware that integrates clinical information. LinkEHR integration engine currently supports access to XML and relational sources, web services and access to other LinkEHR integration engines.

3.3 LinkEHR-Ed Archetype Editor

LinkEHR-Ed (www.linkehr.com) (Maldonado et al., 2009, 2011) is a visual tool implemented in Java under the Eclipse platform which allows the edition of archetypes based on different reference models, the specification of mappings between archetypes and data sources and the semi-automatic generation of data conversion scripts which translate unnormalized data into XML documents conforming to the selected RM (in our context the standard chosen to represent the EHR extract) and at the same time satisfy all data constraints imposed by archetypes. We intend to employ archetypes for publication of existing clinical information in the form of standardized EHR extracts. We call them *Integration Archetypes*. Figure 1 shows a usage overview of integration archetypes.

The archetype mapping process is divided into four main steps in LinkEHR-Ed. The first step deals with the import of reference models. A new reference model expressed as a W3C XML Schema can be imported at any time. The second step is the actual archetype editing process, for this purpose a visual editor is provided. Step 3 deals with mapping specification between archetypes and data sources. In step 4, an XQuery expression that encodes the mapping specification is automatically created. The execution of the XQuery expression over a set of data sources yields a XML instance that satisfies the constraints imposed by the archetype and is at the same time compliant with the underlying reference model. Therefore, LinkEHR-Ed helps data engineers to write possibly long and complex programs to standardize data. In summary, LinkEHR-Ed combines the formal representation of knowledge of a health domain expert in the form of archetypes (steps 1 and 2), with mapping information to clinical data sources for the standardization and semantic description of existing information (steps 3 and 4). Four different reference models (target schemas) have been tested successfully, namely CEN/ISO 13606, OpenEHR, HL7-CDA, and CCR. To the authors' knowledge, LinkEHR-Ed is the only editor capable of handling archetypes as a data transformation mechanism.

3.3.1 Archetype Editing

The archetype editing process in LinkEHR-Ed is based on a clear formalization of the archetype model. The formalization is based on types over tree-structured data with labeled nodes (i.e. XML data) and a subsumption relation is used to model the specialization of archetypes and the relationship between archetypes and reference models. For a detailed explanation we refer to (Maldonado et al., 2009).

In LinkEHR-Ed a new reference model expressed as W3C XML Schema can be imported at any time. Users must indicate the set of classes of the reference model that define logical building blocks of EHRs, i.e. the set of business concepts. Obviously, this step only needs to be performed once for each reference model. One of the main features of LinkEHR-Ed is that the set of business concepts are also represented as archetypes, we call them business archetypes. Note that business archetypes are the most general archetypes that can be defined for a reference model and therefore any archetype must be a specialization of one of them.

Business archetypes allow us to apply the same logic either when a new archetype is defined from scratch or when an existing one is specialized to create a more refined medical concept. As consequence, only the rules specified in the archetype model to control the archetype creation need to be directly implemented in the tool. This allows the definition of archetypes based on different standards.

3.3.2 Mapping of Archetype to Data Sources

One of the difficulties in setting up a data integration system is the definition of the semantic mappings between the sources and the federated virtual schemas. It requires both database expertise to express them in a formal language and domain knowledge to understand

Figure 1. Integration archetype usage for data exchange

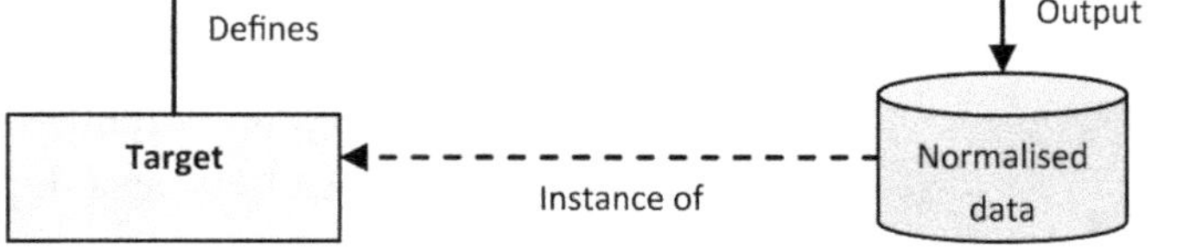

the meaning of the schemas being mapped (Fagin et al., 2005). Mappings between two schemas can be specified either procedurally, i.e. by programs that physically import objects stored in the underlying databases into corresponding objects of the global environment or declaratively, i.e. by defining a set of correspondences between entities from the local and global schemas. Procedural mappings allow dealing with a wide range of data source formats and transformations but they are more difficult to maintain because the mapping is encoded in actual programs. On the other hand, declarative mappings are easier to maintain and can accommodate query optimization but they are less powerful in specifying complex data transformation.

Existing clinical data must be transformed to meet the data structures and constraints defined by reference models and archetypes. Therefore mapping specifications must define how to create archetype instances from the content of the data sources. In LinkEHR-Ed, an archetype with a mapping specification to a data source is called an integration archetype. Data exchange at the schema level requires an explicit representation of how the source schema (legacy data schema) and target schema (archetypes) are related to each other; these explicit representations are called mappings. The effort required to create and manage such mappings is considerable. It involves writing and managing complex data transformations programs. The common case is to write intricate custom and non-reusable software to perform the required transformations. This is even more complex with archetypes, since they are defined to model arbitrary complex domain concepts without any consideration regarding the potential internal architecture or database design of EHR systems. As a consequence, complex and expressive mapping specifications are necessary. It is not only necessary to specify value couplings between atomic entities but also structural mappings, i.e. how the data structures of source and target schemas are related, due to the potential low similarity between archetypes and clinical data sources. In the health care domain very few generic EHR data transformation efforts exist. Many commercial mapping tools are capable of processing XML schemas but they cannot handle archetypes.

LinkEHR-Ed is designed to map hierarchical data; the source schema must be expressed in W3C XML Schema and the target schema (archetypes) in ADL. LinkEHR-Ed can also handle source relational schemas, as long as they are converted in a canonical way into a W3C XML Schema. For this purpose, it comes with a visual tool for handling relational schemas that can also generate a set of Hibernate (Hibernate, 2013) mapping definitions that construct such canonical XML views. During the mapping definition from relational sources users do not have to interact with the canonical XML view, a visual representation in the form of tables and relationships is provided instead.

In ADL only those entities (classes and attributes) of the reference model that are actually constrained need to appear in the archetype definition. This rule poses a difficulty when an archetype is mapped to a data source. It may be necessary to define a mapping for an unconstrained attribute and therefore it is not present in the archetype definition. Thus, for the sake of mapping we are forced to temporally complete the archetype definition with entities from the underlying business archetype. In LinkEHR-Ed, we have defined a merge function that takes an archetype and a business archetype as input and outputs what we call a comprehensive archetype, which contains all the entities defined in the latter but at the same time preserves all the constraints imposed by the former. Put in other words, comprehensive archetypes include all the explicit constraints (those defined by the archetype to be specialized or mapped) and all the implicit ones (those defined by the business archetype) that data instances must satisfy. Figure 2 shows an example of comprehensive archetype. On the left-hand side the original CEN/ISO 13606 archetype is depicted whereas on the right-hand side the corresponding comprehensive archetype is shown. Note that the comprehensive archetype contains all the constraints of the original archetype as well as all the unconstrained entities from the reference model class such as act_status, archetype_id, etc.

LinkEHR-Ed can be considered as a high-level schema mapping tool (Raffio, Braga, Ceri, Papotti, & Hernandez, 2008). Users are responsible of defining a high-level non-procedural mapping specification. This high-level specification is defined by defining correspondences between entities of archetypes and source schemas. Two types of correspondences are supported, namely between atomic entities (leaf nodes) and between complex entities (inner nodes). The former are value correspondences that specify how to calculate atomic values whereas the latter are structural correspondence that may be used to control the generation and grouping of elements in the target.

Value correspondences are defined by a set of pairs, consisting of a transformation function that specifies how to calculate a value in the target from a set of source values, and a filter, indicating the conditions that source data must satisfy to be used in the transformation function. The simplest kind of transformation function is the identity function which copies a single source value into a target value. But quite often it is necessary to specify arbitrary complex functions which transform a set of source values into a target value. To achieve this, a wide range of transformation functions are supported such as type conversion, mathematical, logical, string, date and time, set value, and ontological. When the filter is missing it is supposed that its value is true; hence it will be applied always. For instance, Table 1 contains a simple correspondence transforming gender codes. It transforms the local gender code in the path: /patient/gender of the source XML EHR extract into a normalized code. Note that the order is relevant and only the first applicable function is used, consequently the last filter acts as a 'default' condition. Therefore, this correspondence should be interpreted as:

If (/patient/gender='M' OR /patient/gender='m') then 0
Else if (/patient/gender='W' OR /patient/gender='w') then 1
Else if (/patient/gender=0 OR /patient/gender=1) then /patient/gender
Else 9

Value correspondences are easy to specify but lack expressive power regarding grouping semantics, i.e. when target instances must be grouped and nested inside the same element. LinkEHR-Ed comes with a default groping semantics which is context-aware, in the sense that data with the same context (atomic elements at the upper levels) are grouped together. The context data depends on reference models and it is calculated on the fly for each archetype. For instance, in the case of CEN/ISO 13606 data that share the same committed time, attester, etc. are grouped together.

On the other hand, structural correspondences are defined by a set of source paths

Figure 2. Example of comprehensive archetype

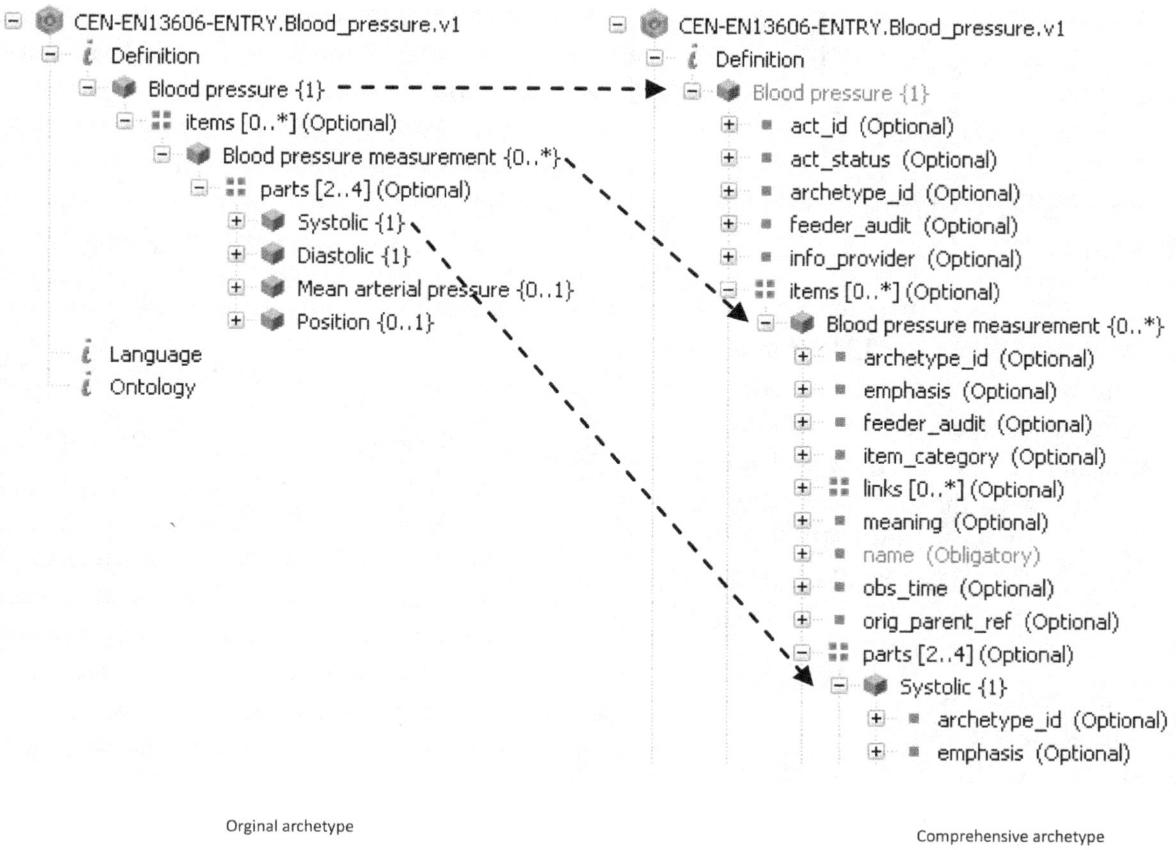

and a filter. They control the creation of target instances, in such a way that a new target instance is constructed for each set of source nodes addressed by the paths that satisfies the filter. It should be note that value correspondences are mandatory, at least one value correspondence must be define for every mandatory attribute in the target whereas structural correspondences are optional, if they are not present default grouping semantics is applied.

The abstract mapping specification is then compiled into an executable transformation script expressed using XQuery. The resulting transformation script takes as input an instance of the source EHR data and generates a XML document that is compliant both with the archetype and the underlying reference model.

LinkEHR-Ed is a visual programming environment for the definition and management of abstract mappings and for the generation and validation against real data of the XQuery transformation scripts.

4. OTHER MODULES

LinkEHR-Ed is just one part of a bigger system called LinkEHR Normalization Platform. This platform allows to create a VFEHR infrastructure, that is, to create a virtual and federated view of the patient's EHR whose data are distributed among heterogeneous HIS. The global architecture of the LinkEHR platform can be seen on Figure 3.

Table 1. An example of value correspondence

Filter	Function
/patient/gender='M' OR /patient/gender='m'	0
/patient/gender='W' OR /patient/gender='w'	1
/patient/gender=0 OR /patient/gender=1	/patient/gender
true	9

- **Extract server**: An EHR extract server must be deployed in each HIS or data source to receive the requests of information, extract data and normalize it by using the transformation scripts generated with LinkEHR-Ed. Then, it builds the extract header and communicates the result to the requester. The requester might be a final system or another extract server. Our Extract server implementation follows part five of the CEN/ISO 13606 norm and is accessible through web services.
- **Detailed Clinical Model repository**: This repository stores common concept definitions as detailed clinical models. Our DCM repository implementation supports the storage and recovering of DCM concepts and their specific definitions in other standards such as HL7 templates, archetype definitions and also integration archetypes. Those definitions can be recovered on demand to be applied to existing data during the normalization process.
- **Demographic server**: This patient information repository does not substitute the master patient index, but normalizes the basic demographic information of patients, health professionals and organisations using CEN/ISO 13606.
- **Terminology server**: This server uses the Common Terminology Services (CTS) specification developed by HL7 and implemented by LexGrid (Pathak, Solbrig, Buntrock, Johnson, & Chute, 2009). Beneath it, SNOMED-CT is available in order to provide semantic descriptions of health data.
- **Clinical information index**: An index of locations of clinical information for each patient. This system avoids unnecessary queries to HIS nodes where do not exist relevant information. This is a fundamental component of any distributed system such as the VFEHR that we define in this work.
- **EHR Viewer (EHR*flex*)**: A web-based generic EHR viewer for standardized clinical information. It is the main user entrance to the VFEHR and permits the automatic generation of interfaces based on archetypes. It also allows the introduction of new data that will be directly stored in a standard format (EHRflex, 2013)
- **Agent-based communication layer**: The distributed EHR infrastructure depends on a flexible and adaptable communication layer. This layer has been implemented with software agent technologies over web services which will provide a high degree of independence and scalability for the complete LinkEHR platform.

All these modules are in different stages of development. Extract server, clinical information index and the EHR viewer are already available. Demographic server, terminology server, DCM repository and agent-based communication are still in development or in a research phase. We must mention a common property of these developments: they are always independent of a particular RM, as is LinkEHR-Ed. This platform can thus

Figure 3. The LinkEHR Standardisation Platform architecture

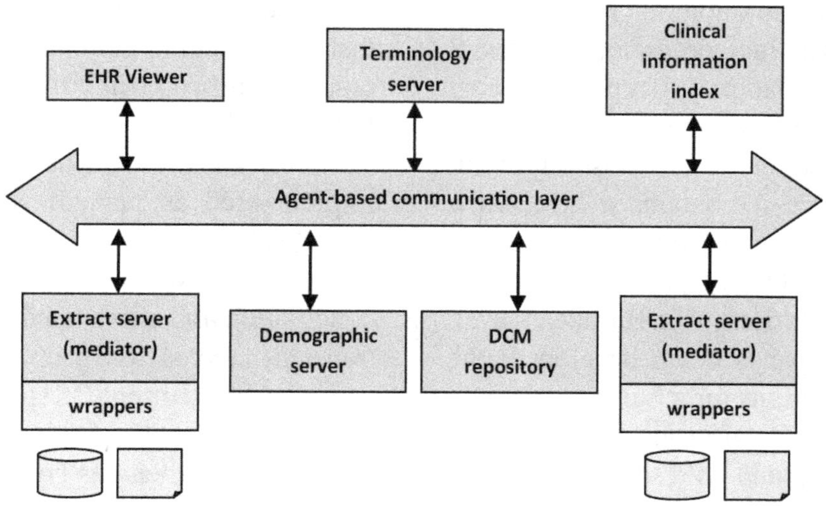

potentially work with any EHR standard that we decide to use.

5. STUDY CASES

The CEN/ISO 13606 norm and archetype based systems are slowly being adopted and tested in several countries. Outstandingly, the Swedish official adoption of this norm as the national standard is the most firm initiative in Europe. The Department of Health for the State of Minas Gerais, in Brazil, is developing a central repository and a message infrastructure, based on CEN/ISO 13606, aiming at the semantic interoperability of the EHR systems. In Germany, the ByMedConnect project develops and demonstrates a communication solution based on the standards "Continuity of Care Record" (CCR) and CEN/ISO 13606 for semantic interoperability. The communication models developed will be tested and evaluated in the region of Ingolstadt (Bayern). In Spain, our experiences and pilot projects that are briefly presented in this section are among the first ones to make use of this norm.

The presented applications and systems have been mainly developed in collaboration with two healthcare institutions: the *Consorcio Hospital General Universitario de Valencia* (CHGUV, a 592-bed hospital with more than 1,000 medical and nursery professionals which serves a population of nearly 350,000 people) and the *Hospital de Fuenlabrada* (HF, 385 beds and 676 medical and nursery professionals serving a population of 220,000 people), in Madrid. The implementations in real clinical organisations have helped to the validation of the CEN/ISO 13606 reference model.

The developed works can be considered as an example of the three main phases of the normalization process of existing EHR systems; namely the definition of data structures and concepts in the form of archetypes, the normalization of existing data and finally the communication of the normalized data among several organisations.

5.1 Definition of Clinical Archetypes

The Spanish Ministry of Health is developing the HCDSNS project in order to gain a national partial access to EHR information from the diverse autonomous regions. This partial EHR will include, among others, a patient summary, laboratory reports, clinical images and outpatient reports. The patient summary will be one of the most important documents, since it contains a brief view over the health state of the patient including solved and current health problems, allergies and active medications. At a European level, a similar initiative is being developed: the epSOS specifications for a European Patient Summary (Smart Open Services for European Patients, 2012a) and ePrescription (Smart Open Services for European Patients, 2012b)

We have defined both Spanish and European specifications in the form of archetypes. The flexibility of the RM and the different constraints that can be expressed in an archetype have made possible to represent the entire requirements faithfully. In fact, our developed epSOS archetypes have been included as the reference implementation in CEN/ISO 13606 of the epSOS project at the final reports (Smart Open Services for European Patients, 2009)

5.2 Normalization of Legacy EHR Systems

At the CHGUV a full standardisation of the information included in their EHR systems is being developed. Currently, all the information is expressed in proprietary formats. The aim of the project was to implement the LinkEHR Normalization Platform over the existing LinkEHR integration engine. Archetypes for each type of document or data structure supported by LinkEHR integration engine have been defined first and then mapped to the original data sources. Those archetypes were based on the European epSOS specification. The result of this work is the availability of standardised views of the existing information that can be securely communicated outside the organisation or used internally by the CHGUV HIS (Angulo et al., 2007)

At the HF different use cases have been implemented as part of several research projects, including the measurement of pressure ulcer risk with the Norton score and the conciliation of active medication between transient patients from primary to specialized care (also based on epSOS specifications). All that information has been normalized with LinkEHR and then has been integrated into the EHR system of the hospital, SELENE from Siemens.

6. EVALUATION AND CONCLUSION

The implementation and use of the CEN/ISO 13606 norm in our pilot projects has not been problem-free, but it has demonstrated to be feasible due to its very flexible nature.

The main problem to face was the lack of previous implementation experiences and implementation support. Other problems were the lack of a well defined archetype definition methodology and CEN/ISO 13606 archetypes. Finally, lessons learned from the implementation experiences could improve the norm itself in a future revision.

Among the benefits of using the norm, we could mention the seamless transition and integration of the norm implementation with the existing systems. The flexibility of the reference model was more than enough to represent all of our data structures. Developed archetypes were easily understood by participant clinicians and were easily adaptable to any required change. In fact, clinicians have been the developers of some of the projects archetypes. As a difference from other clinical documentation standards, CEN/ISO 13606 does not impose technical limitations to the representation of health information, but it adapts to any clinical requirement.

We have presented LinkEHR, a platform that allows the utilization of archetypes for upgrading already deployed systems in order to make them compatible with an EHR standard. The overall objective is to maintain in-production systems and applications without any changes while providing a mean for publication of clinical information in the form of standardised EHR extracts, hiding technical details, location and heterogeneity of data repositories. Therefore, archetypes could be used as a semantic layer over the underlying databases associating them with domain specific concepts and therefore upgrading the semantics of the data they hold. In all presented cases the mapping capabilities of LinkEHR-Ed were enough to generate normalized extracts with the intended semantics in a short period of time. As a performance indicator, we considered the response time for serving a patient summary request. Transformations of source data for a single patient into a CEN/ISO 13606 XML documents using the generated XQuery script took a fraction of a second, which was found to be insignificant with respect to the data-retrieving time.

Future evolution of the platform includes the transformation of the archetype repository into a generic Detailed Clinical Model (DCM) repository, the inclusion of a security layer to apply the patient personal access policies to his EHR data and the connection of the platform with decision support systems.

Finally, as an additional result of our implementation experiences, we found that the community of users and implementers of the CEN/ISO 13606 norm needs a place to share experiences and solve doubts. We have launched an open web site to serve as a place for cooperation and future renewal of the standard (http://www.en13606.org).

ACKNOWLEDGMENT

We would like to thank the collaboration of the *Consorcio Hospital General Universitario de Valencia* and the *Hospital de Fuenlabrada* for they support during the execution of these projects. This work has been partially funded by the Ministerio de Economía y Competitividad and the FEDER programme through grants TIN2010-21388-C01, the *Plan de Calidad para el Sistema Nacional de Salud* of the Spanish Ministry of Health together with the Madrid Regional Government, and by the Health Institute Carlos III through the RETICS Combiomed, RD07/0067/2001.

REFERENCES

Angulo, C., Crespo, P., Maldonado, J. A., Moner, D., Pérez, D., & Abad, I. et al. (2007). Non-invasive lightweight integration engine for building EHR from autonomous distributed systems. *International Journal of Medical Informatics*, *76*(Suppl 3), S417–S424. doi:10.1016/j.ijmedinf.2007.05.002 PMID:17600763

Beale, T. (2002). Archetypes: Constraint-based domain models for future-proof information systems. In OOPSLA 2002 workshop on Behavioural Semantics (pp. 1–18).

EHRflex. (2013). EHRflex project. Retrieved from http://ehrflex.sourceforge.net

Fagin, R., Kolaitis, P. G., Miller, R. J., & Popa, L. (2005). Data exchange: Semantics and query answering. *Theoretical Computer Science*, *336*, 89–124. doi:10.1016/j.tcs.2004.10.033

Hibernate. (2013). Relational Persistence for Java and.NET. Retrieved from http://www.hibernate.org/

International Organization for Standardization. (2008a). Health informatics — Electronic health record communication — Part 1: Reference model.

International Organization for Standardization. (2008b). Health Informatics-Electronic health record communication, Part II: Archetypes.

Kalra, D. (2006). Electronic health record standards. *Yearbook of Medical Informatics*, *45*, 136–144. PMID:17051307

Lenzerini, M. (2002). Data integration: A theoretical perspective. In *Proceedings of the Twenty-First ACM SIGMOD-SIGACT Symposium on Principles of Database Systems* (Vol. 4, pp. 233–246). doi:10.1145/543613.543644

Maldonado, J., Moner, D., Bosca, D., Angulo, C., Marco, L., Reig, E., & Robles, M. (2011). Concept-Based Exchange Of Healthcare Information: The LinkEHR approach. In *2011 IEEE First International Conference on Healthcare Informatics, Imaging and Systems Biology*, 150–157. doi:10.1109/HISB.2011.18

Maldonado, J., Moner, D., Boscá, D., Fernández-Breis, J. T., Angulo, C., & Robles, M. (2009). LinkEHR-Ed: A multi-reference model archetype editor based on formal semantics. *International Journal of Medical Informatics*, *78*(8), 559–570. doi:10.1016/j.ijmedinf.2009.03.006 PMID:19386540

Pathak, J., Solbrig, H. R., Buntrock, J. D., Johnson, T. M., & Chute, C. G. (2009). LexGrid: A framework for representing, storing, and querying biomedical terminologies from simple to sublime. *Journal of the American Medical Informatics Association*, *16*, 305–315. doi:10.1197/jamia.M3006 PMID:19261933

Raffio, A., Braga, D., Ceri, S., Papotti, P., & Hernandez, M. A. (2008). Clip: A visual language for explicit schema mappings. In *2008 IEEE 24th International Conference on Data Engineering*, 30–39. doi:10.1109/ICDE.2008.4497411

Smart Open Services for European Patients. (2009). *D.3.5.2. work package 3.5 - semantic services appendix G - CEN EN13606 technical specifications*. Retrieved from http://www.epsos.eu/uploads/tx_epsosfileshare/D3.5.2_Appendix_G_EN13606_Implementation_01.pdf

Smart Open Services for European Patients. (2012a). *D3.2.2 Final definition of functional service requirements- Patient summary*. Retrieved from http://www.epsos.eu/uploads/tx_epsosfileshare/D3.2.2_Final_Definition_Functional_Service_Req_Patient_Summary.pdf

Smart Open Services for European Patients. (2012b). *D.3.1.2 final definition of functional service requirements - ePrescription*. Retrieved from http://www.epsos.eu/uploads/tx_epsosfileshare/D3.1.2_Final_Definition_of_Functional_Service_Requirements_ePrescription_01.pdf

Wiederhold, G. (1992). Mediators in the architecture of future information systems. *Computer*, *25*, 38–49. doi:10.1109/2.121508

Chapter 4
Interoperability of EHR Systems Based on Semantic Representation and Transformation Models

Catalina Martínez-Costa
Institute of Medical Informatics, Medical University of Graz, Austria & Universidad de Murcia, Spain

Marcos Menárguez-Tortosa
Universidad de Murcia, Spain

Jesualdo Tomás Fernández-Breis
Universidad de Murcia, Spain

ABSTRACT

The semantic interoperability of electronic healthcare record systems is a major issue given that it would increase the quality of healthcare and patient safety. In this chapter, different solutions based on the use of semantic models for representing clinical knowledge are presented. The aim of the research presented here is to contribute to the achievement of semantic interoperability by making explicit the meaning of the exchanged data and knowledge items. In particular, this work is focused on dual model-based electronic healthcare records standards and presents methods and tools for the representation and transformation of clinical archetypes and for the automatic generation of standardized applications.

INTRODUCTION

A healthcare record is the set of non-redundant, ordered, and complete information concerning the relation between an individual and any healthcare centre, and it is a basic tool to achieve quality in healthcare. Healthcare records can be queried in different situations and due to different reasons, and they can play different roles in the healthcare process. However, their main use is to support clinical care. The lifelong clinical information of

DOI: 10.4018/978-1-4666-3000-0.ch004

any person supported by electronic means configures the Electronic Healthcare Record (EHR). An EHR is then a healthcare record digitally stored in one or more information systems. It contains information about one patient although it can contain references to other people. As pointed out in Blobel (2006), EHR systems must support life-long EHR, be technology and data format independent, facilitate sharing of EHRs via interoperability at data and knowledge levels, integrate with any/multiple terminologies, support for clinical data structures and prioritise the patient / clinician interaction.

As a consequence of the technological development, there are currently many different Health Information Systems (HIS) in daily practice in healthcare institutions. Most of these systems are built on different information models, so the exchange of information between clinical information systems has become a major challenge for the last decades. In this context, the adoption of EHR standards will facilitate the achievement of the information exchange goal. In fact, it is more a requirement than a goal given the increasing fragmentation of healthcare and the increasing mobility of citizens around the world, who need effective and quality healthcare.

Nowadays, there are some advanced standards and architectures for representing and communicating electronic healthcare records, among which HL7 (HL7, n.d.), OpenEHR (OpenEHR, n. d.) and ISO EN 13606 (ISO 13606, 2013) should be pointed out given their relevance. So far, the availability of such standards has not solved the problem, because each standard defines its own information models and manages the information in a particular way. However, they play a fundamental role because they are currently the targets of the interoperability methods that are currently being developed by the community. In particular, this chapter will be focused on the interoperability of EHR standards that follow the dual model architecture approach (Beale, 2001).

This architecture is based on the metamodeling of healthcare records, which distinguishes two conceptual levels, information and knowledge. Therefore, our effort will be mainly put on the interoperability at knowledge level. It should be noted that the following three levels of interoperability are usually identified in healthcare:

- **Level 1:** Technical and Syntactical interoperability. Example: Dr Smith is able to receive patient clinical data but he cannot understand them, because they are in French.
- **Level 2:** Partial semantic interoperability. Example: Dr Smith is able to understand some important data because they are codified according to an international coding system. However most of them are in French.
- **Level 3:** Full semantic interoperability. Example: Dr Smith is able to access patient data, to understand them and to integrate them in the hospital information system.

In this chapter, we will describe solutions for representing and transforming knowledge between dual model based EHR systems, and for the automatic generation of applications from clinical knowledge units. All these solutions intend to support the achievement of interoperability level 3 by following the technological recommendations of the Semantic Interoperability for Better Health and Safer Healthcare report (EC Roadmap, 2009), which identifies the use of standards and technologies that will be explained further in this chapter, such as archetypes and ontologies, as key for the semantic interoperability.

Finally, the content of this chapter can be described as follows. First, the main technological concepts needed to understand this work will be explained. Then, our semantic model for representing clinical knowledge for dual based EHR standards will be presented. This constitutes the basis of our technological solutions for transforming archetypes between standards and generating applications, which will be presented then.

BACKGROUND

First, we will present the EHR standards we are working with. Next, the technologies applied to facilitate the interoperability will be described.

Electronic Healthcare Records

The dual model architecture is based on the meta-modeling of healthcare records, which distinguishes two conceptual levels: (1) reference model (information), and (2) archetype model (knowledge). The reference model represents the global features of the annotations of healthcare records, how they are aggregated and the context information required to meet the ethical, legal, etc requirements. This model defines the set of classes that forms the generic building blocks of the electronic healthcare record and it contains the non volatile features of the electronic healthcare record.

On the other hand, an archetype models the common features of types of entities and, therefore, it defines valid information structures in terms of taxonomic ("is a class of") and partonomic ("is a part of") components. Archetypes restrict the business objects, which can be considered descriptors of domain ontological levels, defined in a reference model. Archetypes bridge the generality of business concepts defined in the reference model and the variability of clinical practice, thus becoming a standard tool to represent this issue. The second principle is that the information system is based on the Reference Model, and the valid healthcare records extracts are instances of this reference model. In clinical settings, they refer to clinical concepts. Clinical archetypes are usually built by domain experts, so they are based on clinical knowledge, and they define valid data configurations. In fact, they are an attempt to standardize clinical practice. They can be used to control and validate the data obtained by clinicians and to guide the processing of clinical queries. In summary, their primary purpose is to provide a reusable, interoperable way of managing data creation, validation and querying, by ensuring that data conform to particular structures and semantic constraints. Consequently, archetypes will be the semantic interoperability unit in this chapter.

Archetypes are defined using the Archetype Definition Language (ADL). An ADL archetype has different sections: header, description, definition and ontology. The header includes the name of the archetype, language, specialization information and so on. The description section includes audit information, such as original author, purpose or lifecycle status. The definition section contains the structure and restrictions associated with the particular clinical concept. Finally, the ontology section includes the terminological definitions and bindings associated with the archetype terms.

Figure 1 shows an excerpt of the definition section of the OpenEHR Blood Pressure (BP) archetype. It describes the BP as formed by systolic and diastolic pressure, their mean and

Figure 1. Excerpt of the definition part of the OpenEHR BP archetype

```
OBSERVATION[at0000] matches {  -- Blood pressure
  data matches {
    HISTORY[at0001] occurrences matches {0..1} matches {  History
      events cardinality matches {1..*; unordered} matches {
        EVENT[at0006] occurrences matches {0..*} matches {  any event
          data matches {
            ITEM_LIST[at0003] occurrences matches {0..1} matches {  Blood pressure
              items cardinality matches {0..*; ordered} matches {
                ELEMENT[at0004] occurrences matches {0..1} matches { systolic
                  value matches {
                    C_DV_QUANTITY <
                       property = <[openehr::125]>
                       list = <
                            ["1"] = <
                                  units = <"mm[Hg]">
                                  magnitude = <|0.0..<1000.0|>
                                  precision = <|0|>
                            >>>
                }}
                ELEMENT[at0005] occurrences matches {0..1} matches {...}  diastolic
                ELEMENT[at1006] occurrences matches {0..1} matches {...}  mean
          }
          state matches {
            ITEM_LIST[at0007] occurrences matches {0..1} matches {  state structure
             items cardinality matches {0..*; ordered} matches {
              ELEMENT[at0008] occurrences matches {0..1} matches {  Position
                value matches {
                  DV_CODED_TEXT[at0036] occurrences matches {0..1} matches {
                   defining_code matches {
                    CODE_PHRASE[at1000] occurrences matches {0..1} matches { Standing
                       terminology_id matches {
                         TERMINOLOGY_ID[at0066] occurrences matches {0..1} matches {
                           value matches {"SNOMED-CT"}
                         }}
                       code_string matches {"10904000"}}
                    CODE_PHRASE[at1001] occurrences matches{0..1}matches{...} Sitting
                    CODE_PHRASE[at1002] occurrences matches{0..1}matches{...}Reclining
                    CODE_PHRASE[at1003] occurrences matches{0..1}matches {...} Lying
                  }
          }}}}
}}}}}
```

the position in which it should be measured. The systolic, diastolic and mean pressures are measured in *mmHg* and their value must be between *0* and *1000* for the systolic and diastolic case and between *0* and *750* for the mean pressure case. The position in which it should be measured is encoded using the SNOMED-CT terminology.

As it has been aforementioned, two standards are addressed in this work, ISO EN 13606 and OpenEHR. The ISO EN 13606 specification is proposed by the CEN/TC251, Technical Committee 251 of the Normalization European Committee (TC251, n. d.), and it intends to support the interoperability of systems and components that need to interact with EHR services. On the other hand, the OpenEHR standard is promoted by the OpenEHR Foundation and provides a full specification for the creation, storage, maintenance, and querying of EHRs whereas the ISO EN 13606 standard was developed to exchange EHR extracts, so it does not provide proper methods for version management, workflow management, interfaces to other systems etc. Both standards have a proper reference model, whereas they share the archetype model.

The analysis of both reference models (see Figure 2) reveals that OpenEHR defines more and richer data structures and data types, but they share the main data structure organization. In ISO EN 13606 data are organized in *COMPOSITIONs*, which can be included into an optional *FOLDER* hierarchy. A *COMPOSITION* includes *ENTRYs*, which can be also grouped in *SECTIONs*. Finally, *ENTRYs* include *ELEMENTs*, which can be grouped in *CLUSTERs*. Some differences are found in OpenEHR. First, *ENTRYs* are classified according to their type of information in *ADMIN_ENTRY*, *OBSERVATION*, *INSTRUCTION*, *ACTION*, etc. Second, it also allows for the definition of data structures such as table (*ITEM_TABLE*), tree (*ITEM_TREE*), list (*ITEM_LIST*) and a single *ELEMENT* (*ITEM_SINGLE*). Finally, it provides other structures to represent the *HISTORY* of *EVENTs*.

Semantic Approaches and Interoperability

Semantic technologies offer a working environment that allows for connecting distributed data and describe their content according to particular contexts. Therefore, the use of semantic technologies makes it possible the description of the nature and logical context of the information to exchange, whereas it allows each system to remain independent, which is fundamental for the interoperability of EHR systems and standards.

An advantage of using semantic approaches is that they do not require to replace current integration technologies, databases and ap-

Figure 2. ISO EN 13606 and OpenEHR RMs

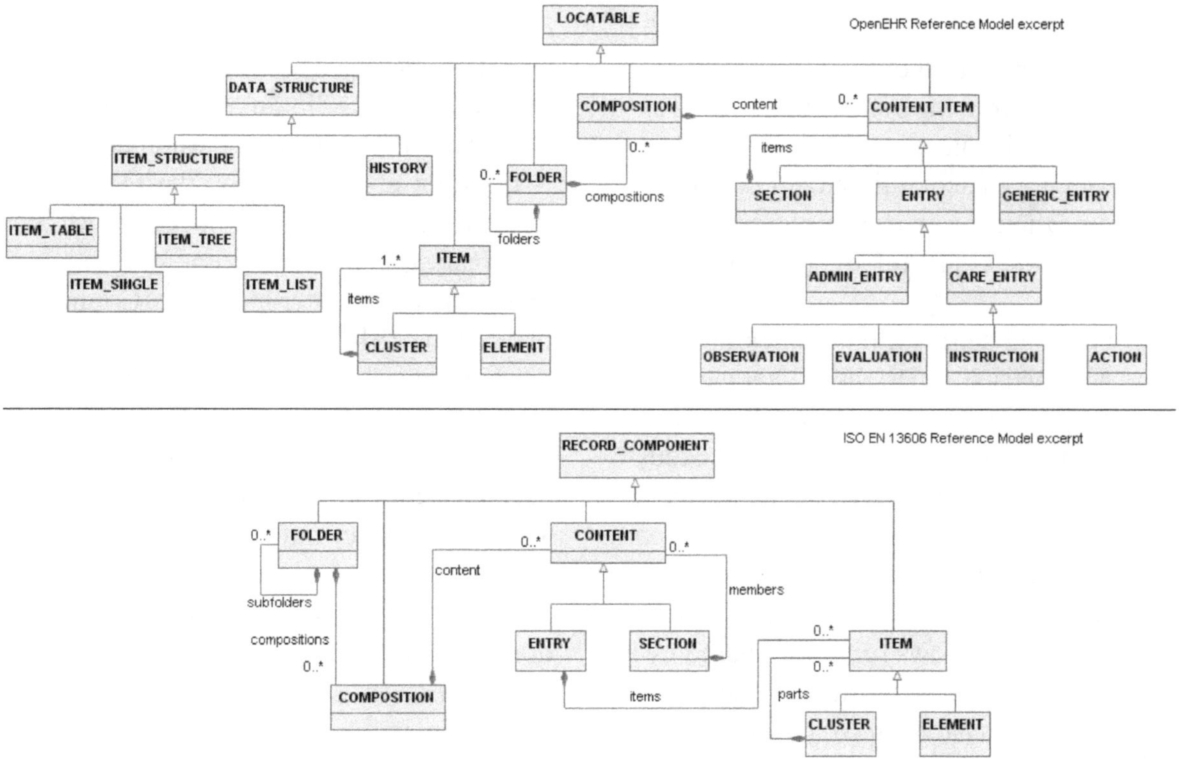

plications, but to add a new layer that takes advantage of the already existing infrastructure (Dogac et al., 2006). Interoperability requires real-time transformations of the information and knowledge that flows between systems. The transformations must take into account the semantic differences between the standards and systems. The most important factors that make it difficult to integrate and obtain interoperability between systems are the semantic and structural heterogeneity, as well as different meaning information has in different systems.

Amongst the different available semantic technologies, ontologies are considered a basic technology to promote semantic interoperability between independent and heterogeneous systems. In literature, multiple definitions for ontology can be found (see for instance (Van Heijst et al., 1997). An ontology represents a common, shareable and reusable view of a particular application domain, and they give meaning to information structures that are exchanged by information systems. An ontology can be seen as a semantic model containing concepts, their properties, interconceptual relations, and axioms related to the previous elements.

In practical settings, ontologies have become widely used due to the advantages they have (see for instance (Brewster & O'Hara, 2007). On the one hand, ontologies are reusable, that is, a same ontology can be reused in different applications, either individually or in combination with other ontologies. On the other hand, ontologies are shareable, that is, their knowledge allows for being shared by a particular community. Therefore, ontologies may help EHR systems to share information and knowledge. They help to fully understand the meaning and context of the information, and this is very important for achieving semantic interoperability, as suggested in EC Roadmap (2009).

In this work, ontologies are proposed to represent clinical information semantics. The ontologies will be modeled by using the Ontology Web Language (OWL) (OWL, 2013), which is the recommendation of the W3C for the exchange of semantic content on the web. In particular, OWL-DL (where DL stands for ''Description Logics") is used, because of its decidability and computability nature. It offers enough expressiveness and the possibility of reasoning over the information that it describes.

Ontologies have also been used in biomedical domains for integration and interoperability. In (Paterson, 2004), ontologies were used to promote integration and interoperability between information systems for three medical communities by combining data with HL7 and terminologies such as UMLS (UMLS, n. d.), MEDCIN (MEDCIN, n. d.) and SNOMED-CT (SNOMED CT, n. d.). Another example is the joint effort made by the ONTOLOG forum (http://ontolog.cim3.net/), the Medical Informatics department of Stanford University and the Semantic Interoperability Community of Practice (SICOP) (http://colab.cim3.net/cgi-bin/wiki.pl?SICoP) to make the Federal Health Architecture and the National Health Information Network interoperable. They defined a three level ontological architecture. The medium level ontologies were FEA-RMO (Federal Enterprise Architecture- Reference Model Ontology) and HL7 RIM, and different domain ontologies were obtained from the Federal Health Architecture. This effort was carried out in the context of HL7, so different EHR models were not targeted as we intend in semantic interoperability environments.

In this chapter, we propose semantic models for representing and transforming clinical archetypes. Given that archetypes are usually represented in ADL, mechanisms for obtaining the semantic, ontological representation of ADL archetypes are required. This means the connection of two different technological spaces, the corresponding ones to ADL archetypes and ontologies. Our technological solution makes use of Model-Driven Engineering (MDE) as an intermediate technological space, which will play the role of bridge between both spaces. MDE is based on the idea of using models at different abstraction levels for developing systems. The Object Management Group (OMG, 2006) defines a four-level meta-modeling architecture (MOF), amongst which two levels are relevant for this work: models (e.g., an ADL archetype) and metamodels (e.g., the ADL language). A model is an instance of a particular metamodel. MDE approaches facilitate the development of formal, maintainable solutions, so they constitute an optimal technological infrastructure for achieving our goals (Stahl, 2006). In MDE, model transformation is the process of converting a model Mx conforming to metamodel MMx into a model My conforming to metamodel MMy. Consequently, archetypes and ontologies will be represented in MDE for facilitating representation and transformation processes. In this work, model transformations will be expressed in RubyTL (Sánchez-Cuadrado et al., 2006).

SEMANTIC REPRESENTATION OF ARCHETYPES

The semantics in archetypes have a double nature, namely, structural and terminological. The structural semantics is provided by the proper structure of the archetype, whereas the terminological one comes from the set of inter-related conceptual clinical entities contained in the archetype, each having a set of links to terms of specific medical terminologies, such as SNOMED-CT.

We have designed a series of ontologies that form an infrastructure for facilitating the interoperability between OpenEHR and ISO EN 13606 systems. These ontologies have been the result of the semantic interpretation of the reference and archetype models. Some conclusions are drawn from the interpretation of both models. First, the representation of the information models is oriented to the transmission via a communication network rather than to representing contents semantically. In fact, the different model diagrams provided in the documentation of both standards have little semantic information; they are similar to UML class diagrams. For instance, there are some references to elements belonging to different classes modelled by string attributes. This representation may make it harder to understand the underlying semantics. Therefore, it would be more appropriate to model this sort of references through a relation between the corresponding classes. In our ontological approach, referential semantics is modelled through semantic relations between the concepts.

This archetype model is common to both ISO EN 13606 and OpenEHR standards. It contains general information such as the auditory details, the archetype description, assertions, translations to other languages, and a set of available terminologies. Furthermore, an archetype contains the definition of a concept (i.e., heart rate pulse), that may be a specialization of another archetype, and it contains a set of archetype terms, which are the domain elements in which the archetype is structured. The ontological section and the constraints are the most important parts since they contain the definition of the archetype terms, which are instances of some specific type of concepts belonging to the respective reference models. However, the archetype model does not structure appropriately or represent formally this information. So, the archetype terms are central in our semantic model.

As a result of the semantic interpretation process some ontologies were designed. The one that represents the archetype model and that is common to both standards (AR) and one specific for each one that defines the reference model aspects (SP). The OpenEHR and ISO13606 ontologies will define the reference model (SP) and will include the archetype model ontology (AR). Thus, the final ontology will combine archetype and reference model concepts. Some of the main classes of ISO EN 13606 ontology are shown in Figure 3. As it can be observed, concepts from the reference and archetype models are put together expressing the archetype structure in a more comprehensible way. For instance, concepts as *archetype*, *archetype description*, *archetype description item*, *occurrences*, *clinical datatype* or *archetype term* exist in the archetype model, but other ones more standard-specific as *folder*, *composition*, *section*, *entry* or *element* belong to the reference model. Thus, this modelling decision captures the common features of both standards, these are the mentioned archetype model concepts, and allows including the specific concepts that exist in each one. In fact, the OpenEHR ontological representation will be similar, except for the concepts as *folder*, *composition*, *section*, etc, that is, those which belong to the respective reference model.

In this chapter, we describe advances in the semantic interoperability between ISO EN 13606 and openEHR, although we aim at applying our results to other standards too. Therefore, the solutions must consider

Figure 3. Fragment of the semantic representation for ISO EN 13606

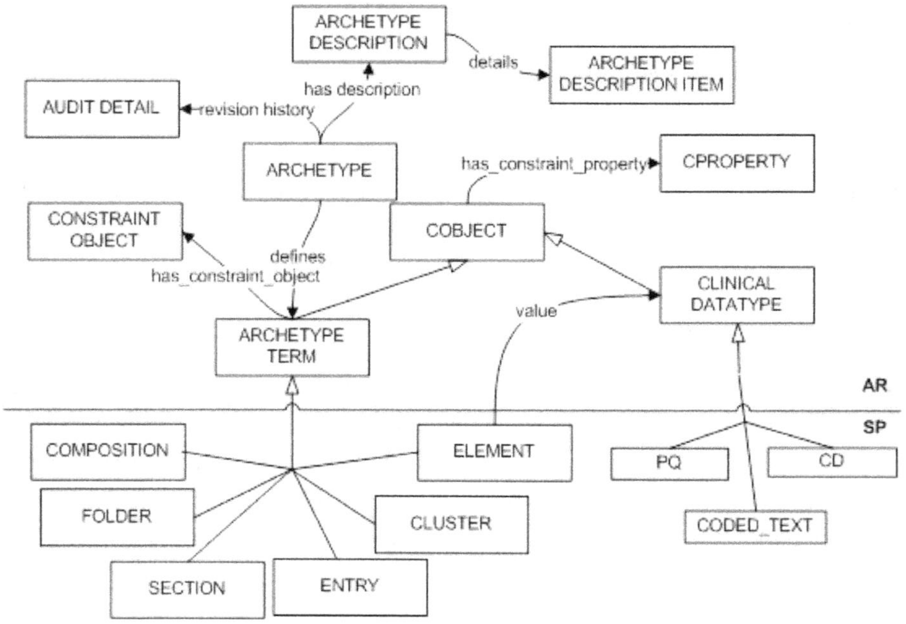

such aim. In Figure 4, part of our semantic interoperability architecture is presented. This figure is oriented to show the relations between the ontologies we have developed. This set includes the ones for the standards, as it has been previously described, plus the common one. The current version of this ontology, called Common ontology, combines ISO EN 13606 and OpenEHR reference models. This ontology was built by identifying the common and disjoint knowledge defined in the ontologies of both standards, so it is not a global EHR ontology at this moment. The Common ontology acts as a mediator in the communication process between standards. This ontology imports the AR ontology and the Common-SP one. All the ontologies are available in a public repository (Poseacle, 2013).

The use of ontologies for representing clinical archetypes offers some benefits against the use of ADL. Ontologies allow performing activities such as comparison, selection, classification and consistency checking in a more generic, easier and efficient way. Moreover, there is very limited work on the implementation of queries on archetypes. The OpenEHR Foundation is developing the Archetype Query Language (AQL) (AQL, n. d.), a declarative query language based on a path syntax that does not offer the possibility of exploiting the semantics of archetypes, since the queries have also a syntactic nature. In this modeling approach, archetypes are considered as individuals of the previously described ontologies, so queries for searching particular archetypes can be defined. We have developed a system (see Figure 5) for guiding the execution of semantic queries on archetype repositories, which can be used without any knowledge of semantic query languages as SPARQL (SPARQL, n. d.). The "Search for" area contains the ontology entities from which the information has to be retrieved. By clicking on "Select Concept" the ontological tree is shown to the user, who makes a choice and that concept is added into the query. The conditions and constraints over the selected

Figure 4. Ontologies relation map

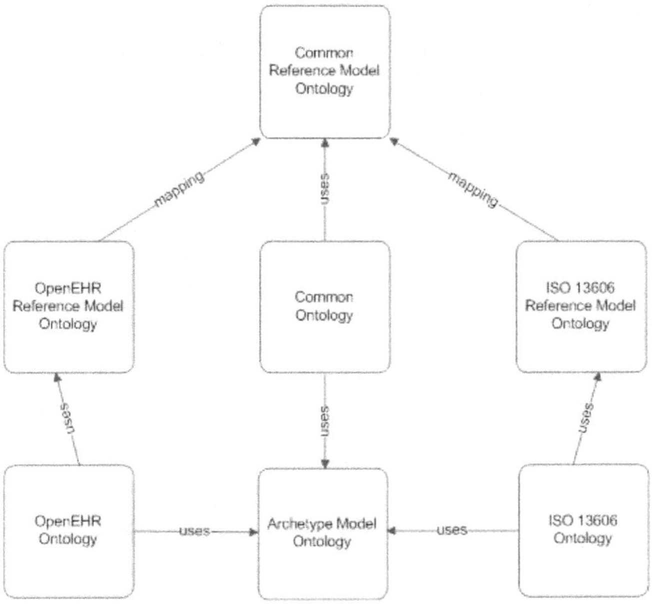

Figure 5. GUI interface for the design of queries

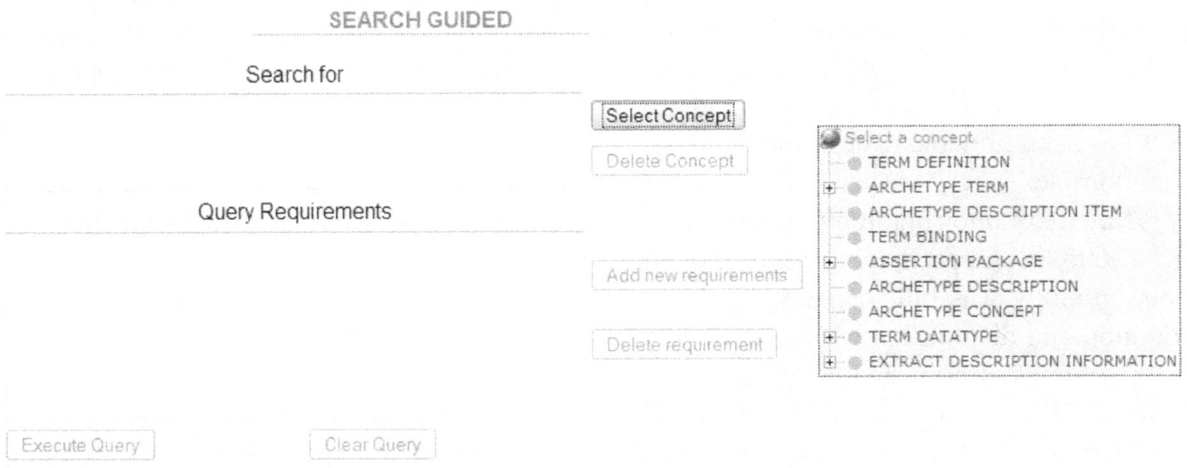

concepts are displayed in "Query Requirements", and can be added by clicking on "Add new requirement". When this occurs, a list of allowed condition clauses is shown. The system will translate this query into the corresponding one in SPARQL.

A possible query might be "finding the unit in which the systolic blood pressure is measured and its allowed values". After the interaction with the GUI interface, three main concepts are required for answering this query (see Figure 6): ELEMENT, which is the category of systolic blood pressure in the reference model, its units and its value, which are a string and a real number respectively. The "Query requirements" defines the properties that must meet the results. The resulting *ELEMENT* must contain "Systolic blood pressure" as *TERM DEFINITION* value. Then, we will retrieve its value, which is a *PHYSICAL QUANTITY* and has the properties *units* and *value_real*.

This query can be then be translated into SPARQL and issued. Figure 7 shows the result of the query. The left hand side shows the units in which the systolic blood pressure is measured: mm[Hg], whereas the right one is the range of allowed values: 0 (lower_bound) and 1000 (upper_bound).

Figure 6. Query: Find the unit in which the systolic blood pressure is measured and its allowed values

```
Search for:
        ELEMENT[0]
        String Type[1]
        Real Type[2]
Query requirements:
        ELEMENT[0]→term_definitions→TERM DEFINITION[3]
        TERM DEFINITION[3] →text→Systolic blood pressure
        ELEMENT[0] →element_value→PHYSICAL QUANTITY[4]
        PHYSICAL QUANTITY[4] →units→CODED SIMPLE VALUE[5]
        CODED SIMPLE VALUE[5] →code_value→String Type[1]
        PHYSICAL QUANTITY[4] →value_real→Real Type[2]
```

Figure 7. Query result

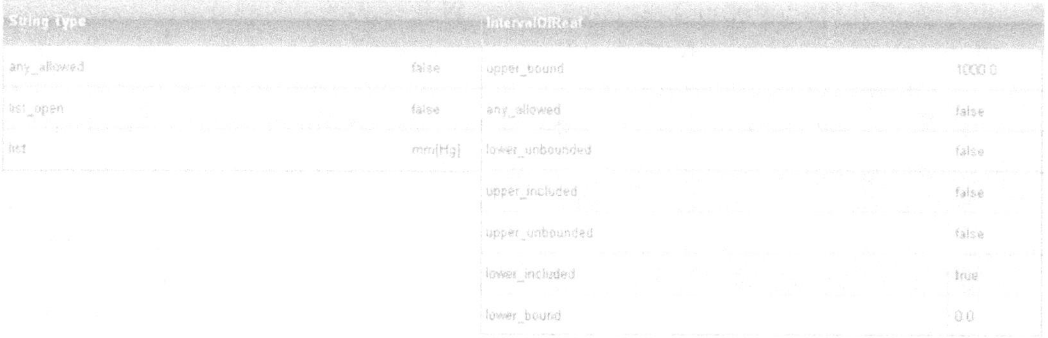

String Type		IntervalOfReal	
any_allowed	false	upper_bound	1000.0
list_open	false	any_allowed	false
list	mm[Hg]	lower_unbounded	false
		upper_included	false
		upper_unbounded	false
		lower_included	true
		lower_bound	0.0

SEMANTIC TRANSFORMATION OF ARCHETYPES

Dual model-based EHR standards are designed to exchange archetyped data, that is, the meaning of data included EHR extracts is given by the archetypes used for data acquisition. Therefore, the goal of semantic interoperability requires EHR systems to be capable of understanding archetypes developed for other standards. The architecture designed for this purpose is shown in Figure 8 and aims to be general enough to deal not only with ISO EN 13606 and OpenEHR, but also with other ones.

The input to this transformation process is an ADL archetype of the source standard (i.e., OpenEHR), which is first transformed into its semantic representation in the MDE technical space. The output of the process is an ADL archetype of the target standard (i.e., ISO EN 13606). Hence, the transformation process includes these four transformation steps can be distinguished in the transformation process:

1. The ADL source archetype is transformed into its MDE representation, which is a model conforming to the metamodel of the source standard (source standard model).
2. The source standard model is transformed into the common archetype representation (Common model).
3. The Common model is transformed into MDE representation of the target model (target standard model).
4. The target standard model is transformed into ADL code (ADL target archetype).

Figure 8. Architecture of the transformation process

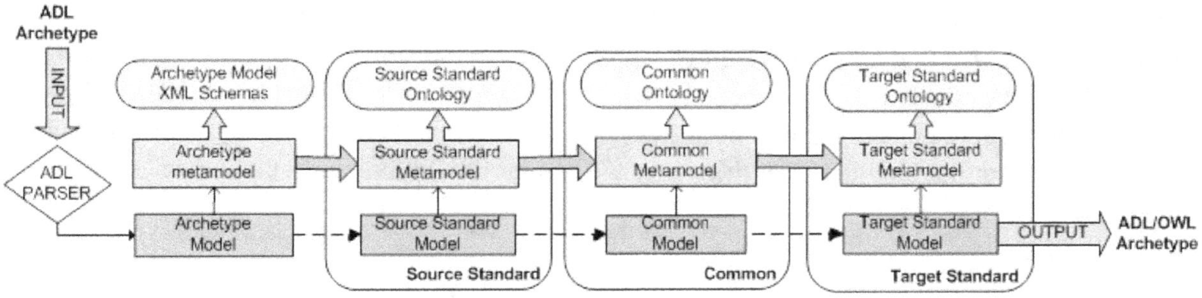

This transformation approach is based on the availability of bidirectional mappings between the common semantic representation and the semantic representation for a particular EHR standard. In our work, we define the mappings at metamodel level due to the availability and maturity of tools provided by MDE. These mappings have been conceptually defined at concept and property levels and implemented using the model transformation language RubyTL by means of rule definition. In order to get the target ADL archetype, model to text rules have been defined in MOFScript (MOFScript, n. d.) and applied to the target model. The last phase of the workflow can be configured to produce an OWL archetype.

We have currently addressed the interoperability of ISO EN 13606 and OpenEHR archetypes. Both information models share the main structure organization having every ISO EN 13606 entity a similar one defined in the OpenEHR standard, but not the opposite. For instance, in OpenEHR an *ENTRY* is an abstract entity that defines different subtypes such as *OBSERVATION*, *EVALUATION*, etc. However, there is an only *ENTRY* concept in ISO EN 13606 and it is a concrete class. Each subtype will be represented in ISO EN 13606 as an *ENTRY* entity and its multiple relation items will contain *CLUSTERs* and *ELEMENTs*. Also, OpenEHR defines an Item structure hierarchy (*ITEM LIST, ITEM TABLE, ITEM TREE and ITEM SINGLE*) that does not have any direct mapping in ISO 13606. They can be represented in this standard by means of *CLUSTER* and *ELEMENT* entities, what makes the transformation between both standards possible. Therefore, from the above it can be deduced that OpenEHR entities that do not have any direct correspondence in ISO EN 13606 are mapped to more general entities such as *CLUSTER*, *ELEMENT* or *ENTRY*.

With regards to data types, some of them are also common to both standards but other ones are defined in a different way or with different granularity. This may provoke some information loss in the transformation process. The mappings defined between these standards are available at (http://miuras.inf.um.es/~researchehr/ISO13606-OpenEHR-Mappings.html). Finally, the result of transforming the archetype shown in Figure 1 to ISO EN 13606 is displayed in Figure 9.

The Poseacle Converter

We have developed a software tool that implements the archetype transformation architecture. This tool is called Poseacle converter and is accessible at http://miuras.inf.um.es/PoseacleConverter). The Poseacle Converter (see Figure 10) implements three different workflows:

- The transformation of ADL ISO13606 or OpenEHR archetypes into OWL
- The transformation of ADL OpenEHR archetypes into ADL ISO EN 13606
- The transformation of ADL ISO EN 13606 archetypes into ADL OpenEHR

The Poseacle Converter has been tested using the archetypes available at the OpenEHR repository (OpenEHR-repository, n. d.) and some archetypes available for ISO EN 13606. The transformed archetypes are available in our repository (Poseacle, 2013). Using the converter is very easy. The user only has to input the ADL archetype by browsing the lo-

Figure 9. Extract of the definition part of the ISO EN 13606 blood pressure archetype

```
ENTRY[at0000] occurrences matches {1..1} matches {  Blood pressure
  items matches {
    CLUSTER[at0001] occurrences matches {1..1} matches { history
        meaning cardinality matches {1..*; ordered; unique} matches {
         CV[at0032] occurrences matches {1..1} matches {
           codeValue matches {"http://miuras.inf.um.es/~researchehr/ontologies/OpenEHR-SP-v2.1.owl#HISTORY"}
        }}
        parts cardinality matches {1..*; ordered; unique} matches {
         CLUSTER[at0006] occurrences matches {0..*} matches {  any event
           meaning cardinality matches {1..*; ordered; unique} matches {
            CV[at0032] occurrences matches {1..1} matches {
              codeValue matches {" http:// miuras.inf.um.es/~researchehr/ontologies/OpenEHR-SP-v2.1.owl#EVENT"}
            }}
           parts matches {
             CLUSTER[at0003] occurrences matches {1..1} matches { blood pressure
               meaning cardinality matches {1..*; ordered; unique} matches {
                 CV[at0032] occurrences matches {1..1} matches {
                   codeValue matches{"http://miuras.inf.um.es/~researchehr/ontologies/OpenEHR-SP-v2.1.owl#data"}
                 }}
               structure_type cardinality matches {0..*; ordered} matches {
                 CS[at0023] occurrences matches {1..1} matches {
                  codeValue matches{"http://miuras.inf.um.es/~researchehr/ontologies/OpenEHR-SP-
                                                                                       v2.1.owl#ITEM_LIST"}
               }}
               parts cardinality matches {0..*; ordered} matches {
                 ELEMENT[at0004] occurrences matches {0..1} matches {  systolic
                   value matches {
                     PQ[at0047] occurrences matches {0..1} matches {
                       value matches {|0.0..<1000.0|}
                       property matches {[openehr::125]}
                       units matches {
                         CS[at0063] occurrences matches {0..1} matches {
                           codeValue matches {"mm[Hg]"}}}}}}
                 ELEMENT[at0005] occurrences matches {0..1} matches {...}diastolic
                 ELEMENT[at1006] occurrences matches {0..1} matches {...} mean
             }}
            CLUSTER[at0007] occurrences matches {1..1} matches {  state structure
               meaning cardinality matches {1..*; ordered; unique} matches {
                 CV[at0032] occurrences matches {1..1} matches {
                   codeValue matches {"http://miuras.inf.um.es/~researchehr/ontologies/OpenEHR-SP-
                                                                                       v2.1.owl#state"}
               }}
               structure_type cardinality matches {0..*; ordered} matches {
                 CS[at0023] occurrences matches {1..1} matches {
                  codeValue matches {"http://miuras.inf.um.es/~researchehr/ontologies/OpenEHR-SP-
                                                                                       v2.1.owl#ITEM_LIST"}
               }}
               parts cardinality matches {0..*; ordered} matches {
                 ELEMENT[at0008] occurrences matches {0..1} matches { Position
                   value matches {
                      CODED_TEXT[at0036] occurrences matches {1..1} matches {
                         codedValue matches {
                            CD[at1000] occurrences matches {0..1} matches { Standing
                              codingSchemeName matches {"SNOMED-CT"}
                              codeValue matches {"10904000"}}
                             CD[at1001] occurrences matches {0..1} matches {...} Sitting
                            CD[at1002] occurrences matches {0..1} matches{...} Reclining
                            CD[at1003] occurrences matches {0..1} matches {...} Lying
                 }}}...}}
}}}}}}
```

cal file system or entering its URL, to select the source and target EHR standard (ISO EN 13606 / OpenEHR) and to choose the target representation format (ADL/OWL). Finally, the result is obtained by pressing the convert button.

AUTOMATIC APPLICATIONS FROM SEMANTIC ARCHETYPES

In previous sections, we have described how archetypes of EHR standards can be represented semantically. Such semantic representation has been then used for supporting the

Figure 10. The Poseacle Converter

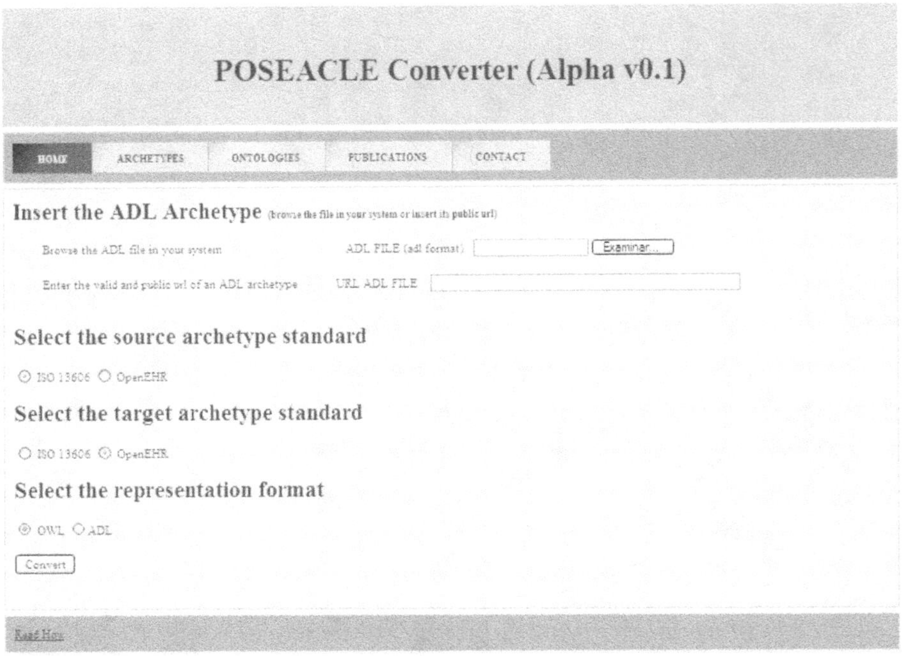

development of methods for semantic archetype interoperability. There, we mentioned that EHR systems are expected to exchange archetyped data. Consequently, ensuring the existence of archetyped EHR extracts is also important for achieving practical semantic interoperability. However, despite the increasing relevance of standards such as OpenEHR and ISO EN 13606, the availability of such tools is limited.

In this section we describe an approach for the automatic generation of applications based on ADL archetypes. The resulting applications, which will be called ArchForms applications, would allow professionals to input clinical data and generating EHR extracts in XML format to exchange data with other systems and to facilitate the insertion of data in the already existing databases. The generic approach here described has successfully been applied to ISO 13606 so far. We are not aware of any system that provides a similar functionality, although related efforts can be found in the OpenEHR community as the Ocean archetype editor (Ocean-editor, n. d.; the work described in Schuler et al., [2006]; or the LiU archetype editor, LiU, [n. d.]).

THE ARCHFORMS GENERATOR

The Archforms generator automatically generates the Archforms applications. This generator has been developed and validated following a MDE software process (Stahl, 2006). The architecture of such applications is based on the model-view-controller pattern (see Figure 11) that isolates the business logic from the input and presentation layers. It consists mainly of the following components:

- **Controllers:** They implement the business logics of the application. There is a main controller and secondary ones.

Figure 11. Architecture of the Archforms applications

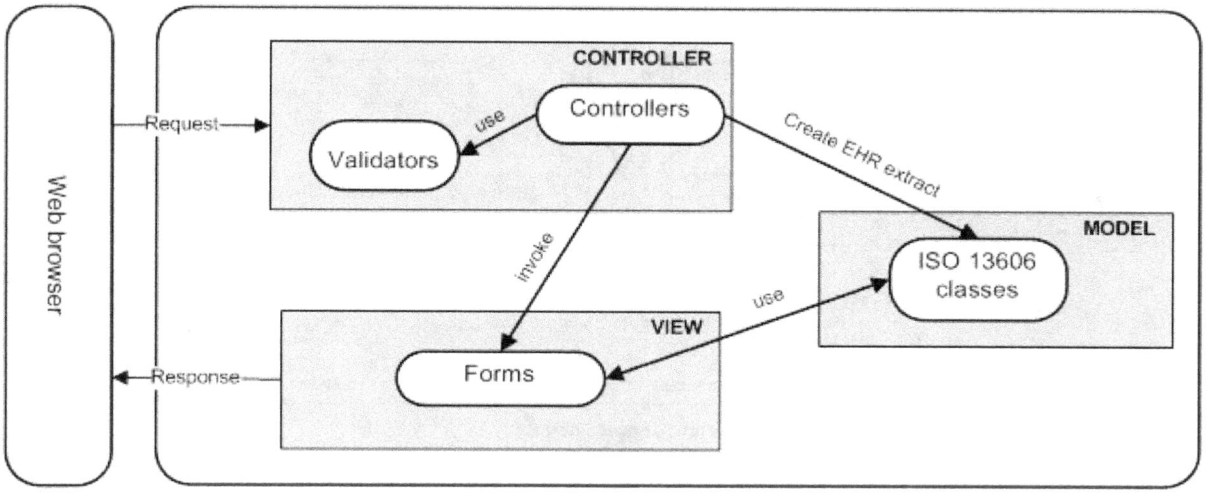

The main controller represents the root concept of the archetype and secondary controllers are created for each ENTRY restricted by the archetype. Among others, they all are responsible of implementing the validation of the constraints defined for the data structures and types in the archetype, and the generation of EHR extracts.

- **Views:** They are the interfaces that will be exploited by the users and are built from the view representation associated to the Reference Model data structures and types.
- **Model:** It contains the ISO 13606 Java classes used for the EHR extract generation.

In order to generate the web application, the controllers and views have to be dynamically created for the input archetype. Figure 12 depicts the architecture of the generative solution. This architecture provides a transformation process which has two steps, one step is independent of the technology and another one is technology-dependent. Thereby, the user interfaces are represented in a platform-independent way by means of the W3C standard XForms (XForms, n. d.) that also allows including validation restrictions of data to be collected by the views. The automatic generation of those user interface models rely on the existence of a mapping between the data structures and data types of the reference model of the EHR standard and the XForms components. In our architecture, this mapping is not defined from the components of the ADL archetype, but from the components of the semantic representation of the archetype. This decision is due to its more comprehensible representation provided by the semantic models and ontologies presented in previous sections have been used. The technology independent generation process is implemented in four main modules:

1. Archetype2XForms, which generates the XForms representation of the archetype.
2. Forms2Code, which generates the controllers and the validation code of the application.
3. XForms2View, which derives the interfaces from the XForm views.

Figure 12. The generative architecture

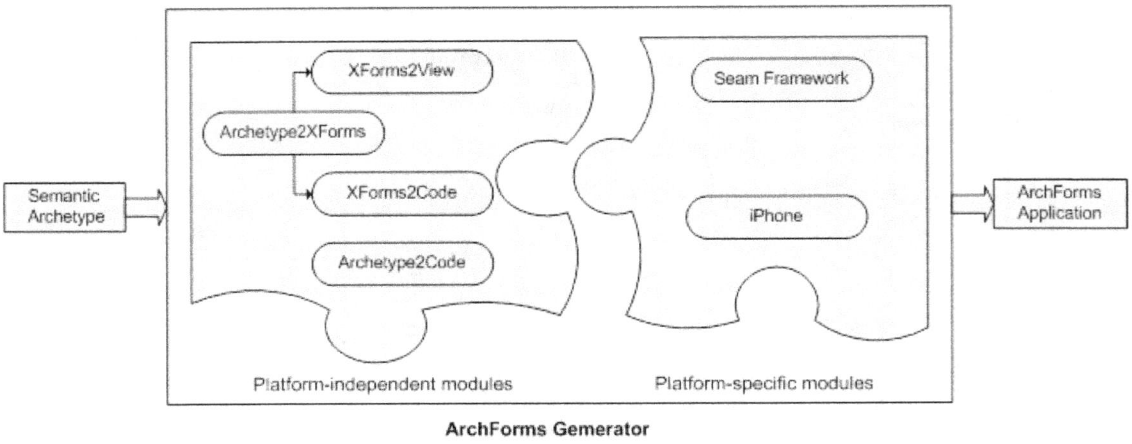

4. Archetype2Code, which is in charge of obtaining the remainder supporting code.

These generative modules define *hooks* that are to be completed by platform-specific modules. At the moment, Archforms applications can be implemented in two platforms based on Java technology: the Seam framework (Seam, n. d.) and iPhone.

ARCHFORMS APPLICATIONS

The applications generated by ArchForms generator for the blood pressure archetype used as running example in this chapter are described next. First, the Seam web application is shown in Figure 13. There, the systolic, diastolic and mean pressures are represented as Physical Quantities. The attributes *magnitude* and *units* define this data type. The value of *magnitude* must be within an interval (e.g., [0,1000]) and the *units* must be mmHg. Thus, the application will check that the introduced values satisfy the constraints. The position is represented as a Coded Text data type. It is defined by the attributes *coding*, which represents the coding schema, and *position*, which defines the possible values. In the example, the coding system is SNOMED-CT and the position must be a value of the list {Sitting, Standing, Lying, Reclining}. The left side of the window includes the application navigation tree, which provides access to the different forms that are defined in the application. In the example, there is an only node, the one that corresponds to the Blood Pressure ENTRY.

Two screenshots of the iPhone application for the same archetype are shown in Figure 14. The left part shows the graphical representation of the systolic measure and the right one shows in which position it has been measured by selecting the SNOMED-CT term.

Note that the two types of applications share the semantic model and the functionality but they differ in how the user interacts with the particular device. Both applications allow the generation of XML extracts from the input data. An example of such XML extract is shown in Figure 15. That extract shows the values for the systolic, diastolic and mean pressures and the position.

Figure 13. Blood pressure ISO 13606 graphical representation

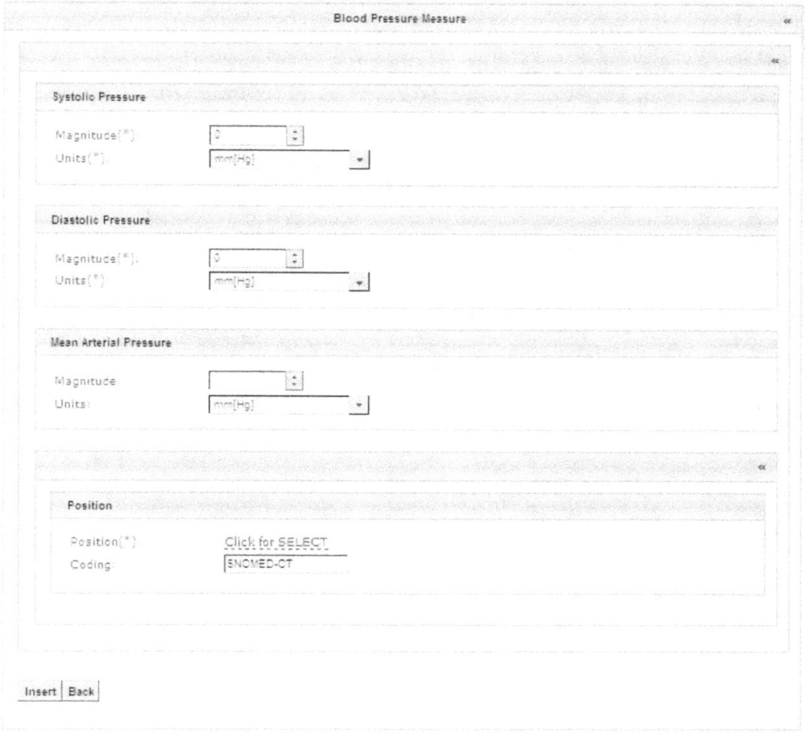

Figure 14. Blood pressure ISO 13606 iPhone application

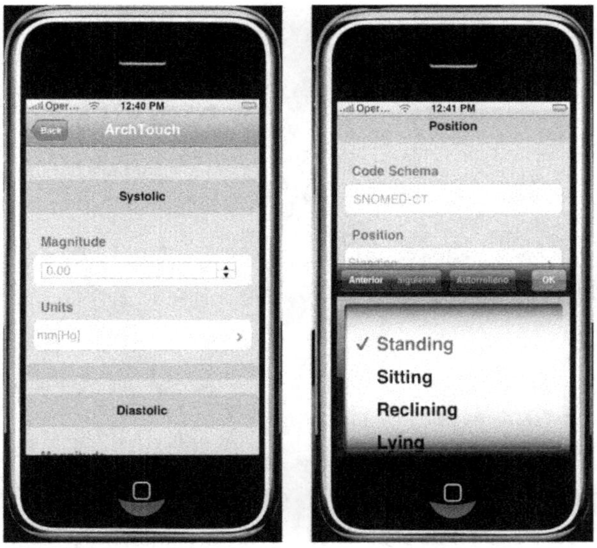

Figure 15. Blood pressure ISO 13606 extract

```
<?xml version="1.0" encoding="UTF-8"?>
  <EXTRACTS xmlns:xsi="http://www.w3.org/2001/XMLSchema-instance" xmlns="CEN/13606/ISO-RM"
  xsi:schemaLocation="CEN/13606/ISO-RM
  http://miuras.inf.um.es/~researchehr/CEN-Schemas\ExtractEHR.xsd">
    <archetype_ID>CEN-EN13606-ENTRY.Blood_pressure.v1</archetype_ID>
    <extract>
    <id_pat>0012</id_pat>
    <items xsi:type="ENTRY" archetypeId="at0000">
      <parts xsi:type="CLUSTER" archetypeId="at0001">
        <parts xsi:type="CLUSTER" archetypeId="at0006">
          <parts xsi:type="CLUSTER" archetypeId="at0003">
            <parts xsi:type="ELEMENT" archetypeId="at0004">
               <value xsi:type="PQ">
                <archetypeId>at0047</archetypeId>
                 <value>120.0</value>
                 <units xsi:type="CS">
                   <archetypeId>at0063</archetypeId>
                   <codingSchemeName>UCUM</codingSchemeName>
                   <codeValue>mm[Hg]</codeValue>
                 </units>
               </value>
            </parts>
            <parts xsi:type="ELEMENT" archetypeId="at0005">
               <value xsi:type="PQ">
                <archetypeId>at0048</archetypeId>
                 <value>80.0</value>
                 <units xsi:type="CS">
                   <archetypeId>at0064</archetypeId>
                   <codingSchemeName>UCUM</codingSchemeName>
                   <codeValue>mm[Hg]</codeValue>
                 </units>
               </value>
            </parts>
            <parts xsi:type="ELEMENT" archetypeId="at0013">
               <value xsi:type="PQ">
                <archetypeId>at0049</archetypeId>
                 <value>75.0</value>
                 <units xsi:type="CS">
                   <archetypeId>at0065</archetypeId>
                   <codingSchemeName>UCUM</codingSchemeName>
                   <codeValue>mm[Hg]</codeValue>
                 </units>
               </value>
            </parts>
          </parts>
          <parts xsi:type="ELEMENT" archetypeId="at0017">
            <value xsi:type="CODED_TEXT">
              <archetypeId>at0036</archetypeId>
             <codedValue  xsi:type="CD">
                <codingSchemeName>SNOMED-CT</codingSchemeName>
               <codeValue>33586001</codeValue>
             </codedValue>
            </value>
          </parts>
        </parts>
      </parts>
    </items>
  </extracts>
</EXTRACT>
```

FUTURE RESEARCH DIRECTIONS

The development and application of the semantic representation and transformation models have contribute to ease the development and maintenance of the solutions for interoperability based on EHR standards, and opens a series of new research lines that need to be researched in the future. An important issue is to guarantee the validity of archetypes. Most systems do not check the correctness of specializations in archetypes properly, which could be efficiently supported by Semantic Web technologies such as OWL and reasoners. The semantic representation of archetypes would also simplify the development of semantics rich archetype editors. The semantic transformation models for archetypes can be used as a reference for supporting the interoperability at data level, that is, the exchange of instances of archetyped data. The semantic querying of clinical knowledge and archetypes should also be researched. We are currently working on making the query design easier for the users by abstracting the concepts of the reference model and using the terminological information and the labels, which are simpler for the users.

So far, good solutions for the proper combination of archetypes and terminologies have not been provided. SNOMED-CT is the most important terminology, and it has become the official terminology in a few countries. This makes the research of its integration with archetypes a very important challenge that would certainly increase the impact of dual EHR approaches and OWL seem to be promising as technological space for such integration. Finally, researching the interoperability with non-dual EHR standards is also a major challenge.

CONCLUSION

The semantic interoperability of EHR systems is a major challenge in healthcare since it would contribute to increase the quality of health care and patient safety. In this chapter, the achievement of such interoperability is based on the usage of different types of standards, that is, EHR standards such as ISO EN 13606 and OpenEHR, standards for the representation of archetypes and knowledge such as ADL and OWL respectively, and standards for the representation of interfaces such as XForms. The use of standards is fundamental since they provide norms that are shared by a community, and this makes easier to achieve the desired goal.

We have described an approach for the semantic interoperability of dual model EHR standards at archetype level, which can be extended to cover the data level. Our solution does not only provides the possibility of communicating semantically precise knowledge items between EHR systems, but also opens the possibility of applying advanced Semantic Web techniques to standardized clinical knowledge. Our technological architecture makes proper use of two basic elements for achieving the semantic interoperability in healthcare, that is, archetypes and ontologies, whereas terminologies are not exploited in this architecture yet.

REFERENCES

AQL. (n. d.). Retrieved November 2013, from http://www.openehr.org/wiki/display/spec/Archetype+Query+Language+Description

Beale, T. (2001). *Archetypes constraint-based domain models for futureproof information systems*. Retrieved November 2013, from: http://www.oceaninformatics.biz/publications/archetypes_new.pdf

Blobel, B. (2006). Advanced and secure architectural EHR approaches. *International Journal of Medical Informatics*, *75*(3-4), 185–190. doi:10.1016/j.ijmedinf.2005.07.017 PMID:16112891

Brewster, C., & O'Hara, K. (2007). Knowledge representation with ontologies: Present challenges-future possibilities. *Journal of Human-Computer Studies*, *65*(7), 563–688. doi:10.1016/j.ijhcs.2007.04.003

CEN/TC 251 (TC251). (n. d.). Retrieved November 2013, from http://www.centc251.org

Dogac, A., Bicer, V., & Okcan, A. (2006), Collaborative business process support in IHE XDS through ebXML business processes, In *Proceedings of the 22nd International Conference on Data Engineering ICDE '06,* p. 91.

European Community. (2009). *Semantic interoperability for better health and safer healthcare. deployment and research roadmap for Europe*. EC Roadmap.

Health Level Seven (HL7). (n. d.). Retrieved November 2013, from: http://www.hl7.org

ISO/EN 13606 (ISO13606). (n. d.). Retrieved November 2013, from http://www.iso.org/iso/home.htm

LiU EHR GUI. (n. d.). Retrieved November 2013, from https://github.com/LiU-IMT/EEE

MEDCIN. (n. d.). Retrieved November 2013, from http://www.medicomp.com/

MOFScript. (n. d.). Retrieved November 2013, from http://www.eclipse.org/gmt/mofscript/

Object Management Group (OMG). (n. d.). Retrieved November 2013, from http://www.omg.org/

Ocean OpenEHR Archetype Editor. (n. d.). Retrieved November 2013, from http://www.oceaninformatics.com/Solutions/ocean-products/Clinical-Modelling/ocean-archetype-editor.html

OMG. (2006) *Meta object facility (MOF) 2.0 core specification* (OMG Document Formal). Retrieved from: http://wwwomgorg/cgi-bin/doc?formal/2006-01-01. 2006

OpenEHR (OpenEHR). (n. d.). Retrieved November 2013, from http://www.openehr.org

OpenEHR repository. (n. d.). Retrieved November 2013, from https://github.com/openEHR

OWL Web Ontology Language Reference (OWL). (2004). Retrieved November 2013, from http://www.w3.org/tr/owl-ref/

Paterson, G. I. (2004). Semantic interoperability for decision support using case formalism and controlled vocabulary. In *Proceedings of the e-Health 2004 Conference*.

Poseacle repository. (n. d.). Retrieved November 2013, from http://miuras.inf.um.es/~researchehr/websvn/

Sánchez-Cuadrado, J., García-Molina, J., & Menárguez-Tortosa, M. (2006). RubyTL: A practical, extensible transformation language. *Proceedings of ECMDA-FA*, *2006*, 158–172.

Schuler, T., Garde, S., Heard, S., & Beale, T. (2006). Towards automatically generating graphical user interfaces from openEHR archetypes. In MIE2006, 221-226.

Seam. (n. d.). Retrieved November 2013, from http://www.seamframework.org/

SNOMED-CT. (n. d.). Retrieved November 2013, from http://www.snomed.org

SPARQL. (n. d.). Retrieved November 2013, from http://www.w3.org/TR/rdf-sparql-query/.

Stahl, T. M. V. (2006). Model-driven software development. Hoboken, NJ: John Wiley and Sons.

UMLS. (n. d.). Retrieved November 2013, from http://www.nlm.nih.gov/research/umls/

Van Heijst, G., Schreiber, A. T., & Wielinga, B. J. (1997). Using explicit ontologies in KBS development. *International Journal of Human-Computer Studies*, *46*(2), 183–292. doi:10.1006/ijhc.1996.0090

XForms. (n. d.). Retrieved November 2013, from http://www.w3.org/TR/xforms11/

ADDITIONAL READING

Berners-Lee, T., Hendler, J., & Lassila, O. (2001). The Semantic Web. *Scientific American*, *284*(5), 34–43. doi:10.1038/scientificamerican0501-34 PMID:11396337

Brewster, C., O'Hara, K., Fuller, S., Wilks, Y., Franconi, E., & Musen, M. A. et al. (2004). Knowledge Representation with Ontologies: The Present and Future. *IEEE Intelligent Systems*, *19*(1), 72–81. doi:10.1109/MIS.2004.1265889

Chen, R., Klein, G., Sundvall, E., Karlsson, D., & Ahlfeldt, H. (2009). Archetype-based conversion of EHR content models: pilot experience with a regional EHR system. *BMC Medical Informatics and Decision Making*, *9*(33). PMID:19570196

Commission Recommendation of 2 July 2008 on cross-border interoperability of electronic health record systems (notified under document number C(2008) 3282) 2008.

Della Valle, E., Cerizza, D., Celino, I., Estublier, J., Vega, G., & Kerrigan, M. et al. (2007). SEEMP: A Semantic Interoperability Infrastructure for e-Government Services in the Employment Sector. *Lecture Notes in Computer Science*, *4519*, 220–234. doi:10.1007/978-3-540-72667-8_17

Eichelberg, M., Aden, T., Riesmeier, J., Dogac, A., & Laleci, G. B. (2006). Electronic Health Record Standards- A brief overview. 4th International Conference on Information and Communications Technology, Cairo, Egypt, December 2006

epSOS European eHealth project. [cited 2013 November], Available from: http://www.epsos.eu/

Fernández-Breis, J. T., & Martínez-Béjar, R. (2002). A Cooperative Framework for Integrating Ontologies. *International Journal of Human-Computer Studies*, *56*(6), 662–717. doi:10.1006/ijhc.2002.1010

Fernandez-Breis, J. T., Menarguez-Tortosa, M., Martinez-Costa, C., Fernandez-Breis, E., Herrero-Sempere, J., Moner, D., et al. (2008). A semantic web-based system for managing clinical archetypes. 2008, Vancouver, BC, 1482-5.

Fernández-Breis, J. T., Vivancos-Vicente, P. J., Menarguez-Tortosa, M., Moner, D., Maldonado, J. A., Valencia-García, R., et al. (2006) Towards the semantic interoperability of EHR information systems. Pacific Rim Knowledge Acquisition Workshop 2006, Guilin, China.

Garde, S., Knaup, P., Hovenga, E. J. S., & Heard, S. (2007). Towards semantic interoperability for electronic health records. *Methods of Information in Medicine*, *46*(2), 332–343. PMID:17492120

GEHR. [cited 2013 November], Available from: http://www.chime.ucl.ac.uk/work-areas/ehrs/GEHR/index.htm

Gruber, T. R. (1993). A Translation Approach to Portable Ontology Specifications. *Knowledge Acquisition*, *5*(2), 199–220. doi:10.1006/knac.1993.1008

ISO/FDIS 21090. Harmonized data types for information interchange. [cited 2010 February], Available from: http://www.iso.org/iso/catalogue_detail.htm?csnumber=35646

Joseph, F. C., Angelo Rossi, M., & Stanley, M. H. (2003). Standards for detailed clinical models as the basis for medical data exchange and decision support. *International Journal of Medical Informatics*, *69*(2), 157–174. PMID:12810120

Kalra, D., & Archana, T. (2008). The EHR and Clinical Archetypes: time for clinical engagement! eHealth Planning and Management Symposium, Copenhagen, Denmark

Martínez-Costa, C., Menárguez-Tortosa, M., Fernández-Breis, J. T., & Maldonado, J. A. (2009). A model-driven approach for representing clinical archetypes for Semantic Web environments. *Journal of Biomedical Informatics*, *42*(1), 150–164. doi:10.1016/j.jbi.2008.05.005 PMID:18590985

Martínez-Costa, C., Menárguez-Tortosa, M., Maldonado, J. A., & Fernández-Breis, J. T. (2009). *Semantic Web technologies for managing EHR-related clinical knowledge*. Semantic Web.

Martínez-Costa, C., Miñarro-Giménez, J. A., Menárguez-Tortosa, M., Valencia-García, R., & Fernández-Breis, J. T. (2010). *Flexible Semantic Querying of Clinical Archetypes. KES 2010*. Special Session on Application of Knowledge Models in Healthcare.

Moner, D., Maldonado, J. A., Bosca, D., Fernández-Breis, J. T., Angulo, C., Crespo, P., et al. (2006) Archetype-Based Semantic Integration and Standardization of Clinical Data. 28th Anual International Conference IEEE Engineering in Medicine and Biology, New York, EEUU.

Nardon, F. B., & Moura, L. A. (2004). Knowledge sharing and information integration in healthcare using ontologies and deductive databases. *Medinfo*, *11*(Pt 1), 62–66. PMID:15360775

Partridge, C. (2002) The Role of Ontology in Semantic Integration

Rose, J.S., Fisch, B.J., Hogan, W.R., Levy, B., Marshal, P., Thomas, D.R., Kirkley, D. (2001) Common medical terminology comes of age, Part One: Standard language improves healthcare quality. Journal of Healthcare Information Management, Fall, 15(3), 307-18.

Schulz, S., & Hahn, U. (2005). Part-whole representation and reasoning in formal biomedical ontologies. *Artificial Intelligence in Medicine*, *34*(3), 179–200. doi:10.1016/j.artmed.2004.11.005 PMID:15993045

Semantic Health Project. [cited 2013 November], Available from: http://www.semantichealth.org/

Smith, B. (2006). From concepts to clinical reality: an essay on the benchmarking of biomedical terminologies. *Journal of Biomedical Informatics*, *39*(3), 288–298. doi:10.1016/j.jbi.2005.09.005 PMID:16293444

Smith, B., & Ceusters, W. (2005) An ontology-based methodology for the migration of biomedical terminologies to electronic health records. AMIA Annual Symposium Proceedings, 704-708.

KEY TERMS AND DEFINITIONS

Archetype: Formal re-usable model of a domain concept.

Electronic Healthcare Record: Collection of electronic health information about individual patients, stored in digital format.

Model-Driven Engineering: Software development methodology focused on creating domain models.

Ontology: Formal representation of the knowledge by a set of concepts within a domain and the relationships between those concepts.

Semantic Interoperability: Ability of systems to share and exchange information with unambiguous meaning.

Semantic Web: Technological evolution of the Web in which the meaning of content is provided for being used by machines.

Chapter 5
On the Integration of Clinical Archetypes with Ontologies and Rules

Leonardo Lezcano
University of Alcalá, Spain

ABSTRACT

This chapter presents an approach to translate definitions expressed in openEHR Archetype Definition Language (ADL) to a formal representation using ontology languages. The approach is implemented in the ArchOnt framework, which is also described. The integration of those formal representations with clinical rules is then studied, providing an approach to reuse reasoning on concrete instances of clinical data. Sharing the knowledge expressed in the form of rules is coherent with the philosophy of open sharing underlying clinical archetypes, and it also extends reuse to propositions of declarative knowledge as those encoded for example in clinical guidelines. Thus, this chapter describes the techniques to map archetypes to formal ontologies and how rules can be attached to the resulting representation. In addition, the translation allows specifying logical bindings to equivalent clinical concepts from other knowledge sources. Such bindings encourage reuse as well as ontology reasoning and navigability across different ontologies. Another significant contribution of the chapter is the application of the presented approach as part of two research projects in collaboration with teaching hospitals in Madrid. Examples taken from those cases, such as the development of alerting systems aimed at improving patient safety, are explained. Besides the direct applications described, the automatic translation of archetypes to an ontology language fosters a wide range of semantic and reasoning activities to be designed and implemented on top of a common representation instead of taking an ad-hoc approach.

DOI: 10.4018/978-1-4666-3000-0.ch005

1. INTRODUCTION

Clinical practice can be represented as an iterative care delivery process that starts with *observations* of the status of the patient. Such *observations* lead to informed *opinions* on the part of a health care professional, including assessment of the current situation, goals for a future situation and plans for achieving the goals. Such plans then turn into detailed *instructions* for clinical practice that eventually trigger the appropriate *actions*. At this stage, we may need to repeat the whole iteration until the problem is solved. These four kinds of information are breakpoints where communication between independent healthcare systems is frequently lost because of data ambiguity and incompatibility.

In the last years, the paradigm of archetypes (Garde, Knaup, Hovenga, & Heard, 2007) has brought a new way to define the models of electronic health records and to normalize the information transfer between such heterogeneous healthcare systems, making them more interoperable. Archetypes are formal clinical specifications, expressed in terms of constraints on a generic reference model. They can be combined together through templates, and used at runtime to extract data, to enable querying, and to support legacy data transformation. Thus, archetypes serve as a shared language for common and specialised clinical concepts. In other words, the reference model encloses the stable features like the set of classes that make up the blocks constituting an electronic health record and the basic syntax of statements, while archetypes allow for sharing a wide variety of combinations of those classes corresponding to record fragments created for specific clinical situations. For example, *Blood Pressure*, *Medication Order* and *Transfusion* are clinical statements that have already been specified as archetypes, so they can be used or refined as reference data structures for the interchange of clinical data.

However, improving interoperability requires different systems to have the ability to exchange every possible information related to healthcare, including propositions of *declarative knowledge* as those encoded for example in clinical guidelines. The archetypes paradigm and the underlying two-level model (which are detailed in the Background Section) allow reaching this understanding at syntactic, structural and semantic levels (Garde et al., 2007). Nevertheless, when it comes to clinical rules, archetypes and the languages used to define them show themselves insufficient, at least to guarantee a seamless exchange of the underlying semantics.

The consideration of semantic interoperability introduces the need for computational semantics. For example, a health care information system that receives some observation entry like *Body Temperature* (no matter from where but conforming to some archetype specification) should be able to deliver it to the appropriate professional, who would eventually proceed to deal with the assessment of the observation. This is clearly a significant advance for the interoperability of health systems, but it could be further enhanced with semantics attached to the archetypes. If the archetype is linked to knowledge representations, then the system would be able to act upon the information directly (e.g. by triggering an alert or notification), or to suggest the clinician some courses or action or relationships with other existing information. This additional processing on the data requires shared representations as those that can be found in formal *ontologies* (Gruber, 1993). A further step would be that of being able to infer knowledge on how to assess, evaluate and act upon the information, using rules or other automated reasoning systems.

As clinical archetypes currently support neither inference nor rules, a proposed solution is to translate archetype definitions to an ontology language as OWL that supports integration with rules, for example, SWRL rules (both languages are described in the Background Section). The integration with OWL and SWRL gives the archetype paradigm the capacity to reach many systems and development tools that are already designed for the Semantic Web technologies (Golbreich & Imai, 2004). Besides, this research is oriented to evaluate the description logic capabilities offered by OWL when expressing the structural and semantic constraints contained in clinical archetypes.

Going a step beyond, this chapter recommends a flexible approach for reusing declarative knowledge in the form of rules. That form of knowledge is commonly found in clinical guidelines (some examples are provided in section 2.3.2). Then, the representation of the decision points that drive the execution of clinical guidelines can be approached as a complement to existing archetype models. Moreover, attaching rules and reasoning on archetypes can offer consistency checks that help detecting data representation errors and validating archetypes. From a wider perspective it represents a step towards level 3 of Semantic Interoperability, introduced in the last SemanticHEALTH report (Stroetmann et al., 2009) and described in section 2.1. For example, a reasoner can detect inconsistent restrictions included in some archetype according to the RM or a parent archetype that is being specialised.

One of the greatest advantages of the philosophy of two–level modelling with archetypes resides is allowing the definition and sharing of archetype expressions as a *decentralized process*, that is, a process where large repositories of archetypes are updated and maintained by a variety of cooperating groups of experts or institutions, working on the same or different domains. Following the same philosophy, this research will develop an approach to allow for the collaborative definition of the SWRL rules associated to archetypes.

For example, having the *Blood Pressure* archetype translated to OWL allows any group of experts to define and publish some SWRL rules that detect and evaluate measures' anomalies from a *Hypertension* perspective. At the same time, a different group completely unconnected from the first one can do the same but from a *Hypotension* perspective. As well as an archetype repository, the clinical rule repository will hold the bindings between the SWRL definitions and the OWL version of the archetypes they refer to. It should be noted that SWRL rules can be inserted in the same OWL file as the archetype, as well as in a different one via ontology import. Such Clinical Rule Repository will provide typical repository functionalities, like management, searching, browsing, etc.

In this manner, the goals of present research are oriented to fulfil the semantic interoperability requirements that were pointed out in the European Commission report titled "Semantic Interoperability for Better Health and Safer Healthcare" (Stroetmann et al., 2009). The report defines semantic interoperability as "the ability, facilitated by ICT applications and systems, to exchange, understand and act on citizens/patients and other health-related information and knowledge among linguistically and culturally disparate health professionals, patients and other actors and organizations within and across health system jurisdictions in a collaborative manner".

1.1 Chapter Structure

Section 2 provides a summary of SIOp when applied to the healthcare environment. Goals, trends and requirements for a full SIOp are described. The section also provides an overview of used languages and models, introducing ADL, OWL, SWRL, openEHR models in addition to the SNOMED-CT clinical terminology. Then Section 3 gives a review of related work, contrasting existing approaches to archetype translation with the one presented in the present research. Some approaches to clinical guidelines execution and bindings between archetypes and clinical terminologies are also analysed.

The main contributions of the work described in this chapter are covered in the next four sections. Section 4 details the principles of the ADL to OWL translation approach. It should be noted that the new features of OWL 2.0 are considered here in order to properly translate some archetype constraints that were abstrusely translated with previous OWL versions. These principles are put into practice in Section 4.7, where the ADL2OWL translator implementation is described. Section 5 subsequently reports on a method for attaching reusable clinical rules to the OWL representation of archetypes, providing case studies that are useful for implementing patient safety mechanisms. Another field of application of expressing archetypes through OWL is that of terminology integration and bindings to existing clinical ontologies. Such subject is covered in Section 6.

Section 7 addresses the evaluation of the ADL2OWL translator as well as the proposed rule system. Finally, Section 8 concludes the chapter with an outline of the research performed in the preceding sections. Suggestions for future work to take the research forward are also provided in the last section.

2. BACKGROUND

Since the beginning of the work on health informatics, one of the most important factors has been the quality of the data. There have been several efforts and studies directed to encourage clinical professionals to use computer systems to distribute and collect patient data, for example, Collen, Van Brunt and Davis (1976), Rogne (1984) and Kuhn et al. (1982). Nevertheless, most of the quality of the data from these researches has been below the expected standard of completeness and consistency, needing additional efforts to improve health systems.

Then an important advance in the field of health informatics was carried out by the health services in the UK. In 2000 the Department of Health UK published the "Information for Health" document to analyze the issues of developing a strategy for Information Management and Technology at the local level of the National Health Service (NHS) (Preston, 2000). This led to further development of electronic health records (EHRs), which has then created a growing need to integrate the various EHRs.

The fact that health care is near a decade behind many other high-risk industries in its attention to ensuring basic safety is partly due to the lack of a single designated government agency devoted to improving and monitoring safety throughout the health care delivery system. In addition, it is due to the existence of several approaches to the same problem, none of which has been yet accepted as a worldwide standard. According to Rector (1999), the problems of standardising the medical language and terminology have been a major concern in health informatics efforts for over a decade. Another reason for this backwardness is that health care data has a number of distinctive characteristics that differentiate it from other industries. The research analysis by Pedersen and Jensen (1998) includes a comparison showing that conventional data warehouses are more complex in general than EHR, see Table 1.

In addition to the quality of the data, it is also challenging to get doctors to use knowledge-based systems as an aid to the process of data collection and usage. The main reason for the lack of a widespread use of knowledge systems for decision making and data collection, especially in hospitals, is the severe time pressure under which clinicians work. The success of a system is only possible if many people agree to use it for the purposes for which they are conceived. Besides, financial pressures, particularly in secondary care, often lead to cut government budgets on hardware and software. Subsequently, this leads to breakdowns in consistently seeking for the computerization of the health care process (Rector, 1989). Some of the limitations have gradually declined over the last 20 years and there is increasing computerization of the systems of health care. Nevertheless, the need to improve the quality and accuracy of "data" remains alive.

Table 1. Conventional versus Clinical Data warehouses. Taken from Pedersen and Jensen (1998).

	Clinical	Conventional
Data Model	Simple	Complex
Temporal Support	Medium	Advanced
Classifications	Simple	Advanced
Continuously Valued Data	No	Yes
Dimensionally Reduced Data	No	Yes
Very Complex Data	No	Yes
Advanced Business Rules	Maybe	Yes(Protocols)
Data Mining	Maybe	Yes(Medical Research)

The following sections in this section describe the role that clinical data models, ontologies and terminologies play in reaching such quality and accuracy in the healthcare environment. It is also explained why semantic interoperability has become a key goal to achieve an adequate functionality of healthcare systems.

2.1 Interoperability in Health Systems

The term "semantic interoperability" (SIOp) has been used for more than a decade in computer science as the ability to exchange services and data between components of large-scale, distributed systems in way that ensures the requesters and providers to have a common understanding of the meanings of the requested services and data (Heiler, 1995). With regard to the medical domain, SIOp is mainly associated to the speed and consistency of accessing meaningful health related data. The term has rapidly gained importance since researches like Kalra, Blobel, and Regensburg (2007) and Aspden (2004) pointed out that SIOp is essential if we aim to enable electronic health record information to be shared seamlessly and meaningfully, and computational services are to be able to interpret safely clinical data that has been collected from different sources.

Then a milestone was reached when the "Semantic interoperability for better health and safer healthcare" report was published by the SemanticHEALTH project (Stroetmann et al., 2009). It is a comprehensive report including the goals, trends and technical challenges to achieve SIOp between heterogeneous healthcare systems. A definition of the term according to this specific domain is provided: "the ability, facilitated by ICT applications and systems, to exchange, understand and act on citizens/patients and other health-related information and knowledge among linguistically and culturally disparate health professionals, patients and other actors and organizations within and across health system jurisdictions in a collaborative manner".

SIOp not only offers means for new methods and services in the health domain but also contributes to maximise all the benefits from the relation between medicine/healthcare and information technology, given the constraints in resources. These efficiency gains have been emphasized by studies such as Walker et al. (2005) that estimates that US$77.8 billion per year could be saved by implementing fully standardized electronic health care information exchange and interoperability (HIEI) between providers and independent laboratories, radiology centres, pharmacies, payers, public health departments and other providers in the US. Another study from the RAND Corporation (Girosi, Meili, & Scoville, 2005) considered that standardised information exchange systems could result in net savings of as much as 5% of current US healthcare expenditure.

As interoperability is not a binary variable but rather a scale reaching from zero to full IOp, it should be noted that the benefits can be achieved to a greater or lesser extent depending on the degree of level of interoperability present. The definition of such levels has evolved from a general perspective oriented to any kind of information system (Sheth, 1999) to a more specific definition in accordance to the requirements of a particular domain. In this manner, Garde et al. (2007) provided three levels adapted to the healthcare environment.

However, reaching high levels of interoperability is a resource intensive task while nowadays it is difficult to associate the benefits of interoperability with those who pay for it. Therefore, one of the objectives of this research is to provide a convincing demonstration of the benefit of migration from ad-hoc to interoperable systems.

For the purpose of increasing the level of IOp and attain full SIOp, certain technological trends and challenges have been identified by the SemanticHEALTH report. They revolve around some key information and knowledge artefacts such as *clinical archetypes*, *ontologies*, *terminologies* and *rules*[1]. In general, these artefacts must be combined, integrated and enhanced in order to ensure precision of meaning, consistency, understandability and reproducibility of clinical data and information. Narrowing down to more precise recommendations, the following list contains the ones which are directly encouraged by this chapter:

- Adopt a standardised approach for representing and sharing of clinical data structure specifications: agree to use archetypes.
- Develop and integrate ontologies into decision support and knowledge management software.
- Collaborate on key use cases for shared care and patient safety, and on defining and tidying the corresponding SNOMED CT subsets.
- Seed clinical forums to develop care pathways and archetypes to meet the needs of safe and evidence based care in different medical domains and disciplines.
- Enable guidelines, care pathways, alerting/monitoring and decision support

components to function effectively and safely across heterogeneous systems.

- Archetype indexing, ontology binding to archetypes, and archetype/template repository services.
- Development of methodologies and tools for binding of archetypes and HL7 v3 messages to terminologies and ontologies.
- The use of SNOMED CT with archetypes and HL7 v3.
- Research on ontology driven architectures for clinical medicine.

2.2 The Two-Level Paradigm and the OpenEHR Approach

For decades, patient data was stored in the form of free text narratives in clinical notes, or in prescription notes. As this kind of documents are abundant in the healthcare domain and they need to be mapped to specific terminologies, there are projects such as the Medical Subject Headings (MeSH) that work with clinical narratives to extract relevant information for storage in EHRs or for coding to standard terminologies (Lowe & Barnett, 1994). However, poor and incomplete quality data that may lead to negligence and medical errors has brought about awareness to improve the methods employed to record data. Besides, the field is difficult due to lack of context. It is difficult to trust the results without knowing the context in which a particular clinical statement was carried out. In recognition of the importance of context, efforts are being made to increase the utilization of structured data entry, in the form of electronic health records (EHRs), which can control the quality and context of data. EHRs also provide sufficient traceability and reduction of omissions and errors.

Thus, EHRs have been developed mainly to address the limitations of most existing systems to record the fine grained elements in a structured way, which are required for health care and clinical decision making (Rector, Nowlan, Kay, Goble, & Howkins, 1993). Coiera (1997) asserts that if the data contained in EHRs are to be analysed they need to be accessible in some regular way.

It should be also noticed that healthcare systems development have classically followed similar steps to those of other IT domains. That is, requirements are gathered via ad-hoc discussions with users (typically based on the well-known "use case" methodology), designs and models built from the requirements, implementation proceeds from the design, followed by testing and deployment and ultimately the maintenance part of the lifecycle. This procedure is usually characterised by ongoing high costs of implementation change and a widening gap between system capabilities and the requirements at any moment. The approach also suffers from the fact that ad-hoc conversations with systems users frequently fail to reveal underlying content and workflow. Besides, the collaboration is rarely effective between the main two groups of professionals interacting in this domain, i.e. information science experts and health professionals. Without such collaboration it is not possible to achieve any efforts at developing safer health information systems that interoperate seamlessly at different levels of granularity. On one hand, clinical experts may not be well-versed in the field of information technology, thus being unaware of the technical limitations of certain solutions proposed by them. On the other hand, information science experts do not have the clinical background and expertise to independently develop systems that meet the requirements of the health professionals, and the simplicity and understandability ones. Further problems with the classical modelling approach are pointed out by Beale (2002).

A promising solution to these inconveniences is to model the clinical domain using the so called two-level modelling approach (J. Grimson et al., 1998; Beale, 2002; Garde et al., 2007). The openEHR Foundation[2] is an international organization comprising a non-for-profit company and an online community supporting the development of specifications and tools for EHR interoperability according to the archetype methodology and the two-level approach. Another initiative supporting archetypes is the European Committee for Standardization (CEN)[3], Technical Committee 251 (CEN/TC 251)[4], that has produced CEN 13606, an electronic health record (EHR) extract standard based on archetypes. Currently the standard is also approved by ISO[5] so it is known as CEN/ISO 13606. This chapter is based on openEHR instead of CEN/ISO 13606 since the first can be considered a superset of the latter (Schloeffel, Beale, Hayworth, Heard, & Leslie, 2006) thus providing richer built-in semantics.

According to the openEHR approach, the two-level model contains a generic RM that defines a logical information architecture for the interoperability of EHR systems, constituting a base representation framework. The RM represents the general features of the components of the EHR, how they are organized and the context information needed to satisfy both the ethical and legal requirements of the record. It includes a flexible syntax and some generic types of clinical information as *observations*, *evaluations*, *instructions* and *actions*. Then, instances or specialisations of that RM are devised in the form of constraints expressed through more concrete "archetypes", which serve as a shared language for common and specialised clinical concepts. In other words, the RM encloses the stable features like the set of classes that make up the blocks constituting an EHR and the basic syntax of statements, while archetypes allow for sharing a wide variety of combinations of those classes corresponding to EHR fragments created for specific clinical situations. For example, "blood pressure", "medication order" and "transfusion" are clinical statements that have already been specified as archetypes, so they can be used or refined as reference data structures for the interchange of clinical data.

Predecessors of the current openEHR archetype approach were first proposed and developed across Europe in 1996-1998, through the *Synapses Project* (W. Grimson et al., 1998) and in Australia in 1997-1999 within the *Good Electronic Health Record Project* (Beale, 1999; Heard, 2000). Both approaches stated that generic information models to represent EHR data gave considerable freedom to clinicians and implementers. They could define hierarchical representations of specific clinical record entries in potentially different ways. These archetypes ancestors sought to standardise the way in which concepts should be represented in the clinical health record within generic EHR models, to fulfil clinical requirements and guarantee interoperability.

As said before, the OpenEHR Model is separated in two layers, a variable one described by AM and a stable one described by the RM. Both of these models are different in the levels of abstraction from the models of reality such as classifications and ontologies which are describing the real phenomena. However, in spite of the fact that they have different types of authors, representations and purposes, they are complementary knowledge artefacts that can and should be integrated, in order to allow for SIOp and improve patient safety.

One of the greatest advantages of the philosophy of two–level modelling with archetypes resides in that it allows the definition and sharing of archetype expressions as a *decentralized process*, that is, a process where large repositories of archetypes are updated and maintained by a variety of cooperating groups of experts or institutions, working on the same or different domains. An example of such repositories is the one provided by openEHR[6].

Nevertheless, as this approach is becoming widely accepted, it is certain that the number of available archetypes will become very large and hard to manage. Besides, such decentralized development of archetype definitions is exposed to content overlapping and limitations in the normalization scope. The translation approach proposed in this chapter encourages the development of better integration and management environments for archetypes by supporting semantic metadata and classification.

2.2.1 The OpenEHR Reference Model, Archetypes and Templates

The formal definition provided by openEHR (Beale & Heard, 2007) is that an archetype is a computable expression of a domain content model in the form of structured constraint statements, based on a reference (information) model. OpenEHR archetypes are based on the openEHR RM. Archetypes are all expressed in the same formalism. In general, they are defined for wide reuse; however, they can be specialised to include local particularities. They can accommodate any number of natural languages and terminologies.

As an example of the two-level modelling approach consider the *Systolic Blood Pressure (SBP)* included in the *Blood Pressure* archetype. The SBP is a clinical concept defined at the archetype level and representing the peak systemic arterial blood pressure of a patient in a given moment. However, its definition is a specialisation of the DV_QUANTITY class that belongs to the RM level. In general, DV_QUANTITY instances can store any magnitude and its unit, among other attributes, but in the *SBP* specialisation, the magnitude is constrained to the values less than 1000 and not less than cero, measured in millimetres of mercury (*mmHg*) as the mandatory unit. The *Blood Pressure* archetype is in turn a specialisation of a wider RM class OBSERVATION.

An archetype gives specifications of predefined constraints on the data recorded and also of the data structure including multiplicity, optionality and relevant bindings to terminology systems and natural language. An archetype definition can specialise or contain other archetypes, and can reuse or import blocks of elements occurring previously in the same archetype or in another archetype. Archetype specialisation allows including local peculiarities. For example, the *Examination of the fetus* archetype and the *Examination of the uterus* archetype are both specialisations of the *Examination* archetype, according to the openEHR Clinical Knowledge Manager[7]. Beale and Heard (2008a) summarizes the openEHR Health Computing Platform where archetypes are combined together through templates, and used at runtime to extract data, to enable querying, and to support legacy data transformation.

With regard to clinicians' perspective, OBSERVATIONs and ACTIONs are used to record information about the past while EVALUATIONs are about the present and INSTRUCTIONs describe events to be carried out in the future. As described by Beale, Heard, Kalra, and Lloyd (2008), OBSERVA-

TIONs are distinguished from ACTIONs in that ACTIONs record interventions whereas OBSERVATIONs record only information relating to the situation of the patient, not what is done to him/her. An EVALUATION may say that "*oral cortico-steroids are indicated at a peak flow of 200 l/m*". A corresponding INSTRUCTION would be issued to indicate the actual drug, route, dose, frequency, and so on.

The separation of clinical information in categories or types is essential for achieving semantic interoperability. Take as example that the "high blood pressure" statement can be related to a finding (OBSERVATION), but can also be a diagnosis of *hypertension* disease included in an EVALUATION entry. There is an important semantic difference that can be represented in this case by using different RM classes.

2.2.2 The Archetype Definition Language and the AOM

The openEHR Archetype Definition Language, or ADL, is a formal language for expressing archetypes that can be categorized as a knowledge description language. It provides a formal, abstract syntax for describing constraints on any domain entity whose data is described by an information model. The syntax is congruent with Frame Logic queries (Kifer, Lausen, & Wu, 1995). It is primarily useful when very generic information models are used for representing all data in a system, for example, where the logical concepts Patient, Doctor and Hospital might all be represented using the class Party, Address, and related generic classes. Archetypes are then used to constrain the valid structures of instances of these generic classes to represent the desired domain concepts. In this way, future-proof information systems can be built and relatively simple information models and database schemas can be defined while archetypes supply the specific modelling, completely outside the software.

An ADL file starts with a header section followed by a definition section and an ontology section (Beale & Heard, 2008b). ADL is divided into two main syntaxes: the data definition syntax or *dADL*, and the constraints definition syntax or *cADL*. The header and ontology sections of the archetype are written in *dADL* and the main definition section of an ADL archetype is written in *cADL*, containing constraints on the data. The header section uniquely identifies the archetype and the clinical concept involved, and includes metadata about the archetype (e.g. its purpose and use). The definition section contains constraints in a tree-like structure created from the reference information model. Finally, codes representing the meanings of nodes and constraints on text or terms as well as bindings to terminologies such as SNOMED-CT (see section 2.4), are stated in the ontology section of the archetype. However, these are optional and they are not available in most of the archetypes openly published on the Web nowadays. Archetypes should fulfil a set of design principles[8], like for example that an archetype can be a specialisation of another archetype and they must be neutral with respect to terminologies.

Archetypes are themselves instances of the openEHR Archetype Object Model (AOM) that specifies the formalism for their definition. The AOM is a model of the semantics of archetypes that defines an equivalent object model in terms of a UML[9] model. Within such model, the archetype definition is an instance of the C_COMPLEX_OBJECT class, which is the root of the constraint structure of an archetype. The last section of an archetype, the ontology, is represented by its own class, and is what allows the archetypes to be natural language-and terminology-neutral.

Therefore, the AOM is a generic model, meaning that it can be used to express archetypes for any reference model in a standard way. The ADL and the AOM are supported by an ADL parser that can read ADL archetype texts, and whose parse tree results in memory object representation. A parser implementation to handle ADL archetypes is provided by the openEHR Java Implementation Project (R. Chen & Klein, 2007). The ADL to OWL translation implementation described in Section 4, which is Java based, is been integrated as a module of that openEHR project[10,11].

2.3 Semantic Web Ontologies and Rules

There is an evolving extension of the World Wide Web known as the *Semantic Web*[12] (Berners-Lee, Hendler, & Lassila, 2001) which provides a common framework that allows data to be shared and reused across application, enterprise, and community boundaries. It is a collaborative effort led by the W3C with participation from a large number of researchers and industrial partners. "The Semantic Web is an extension of the current Web in which information is given a well defined meaning, better enabling computers and people to work in cooperation" (Guha, McCool, & Miller, 2003).

The Semantic Web is envisioned as the next generation of the WWW, according to Christiaens (2006), it is a Web in which all content has machine-processable meaning. This Semantic Web provides all the functionality needed to build the Pragmatic Web on top of it. Communities will no longer search, but rather find and use information in this Pragmatic Web. The explicit meaning, understandable by both human and machine agents, attached to content is necessary for proper information retrieval and usage.

Ontologies are considered one of the pillars of the Semantic Web. The technical term was introduced in computer science by Gruber (1993). In the context of computer and information sciences, an ontology defines a set of representational primitives with which to model a domain of knowledge or discourse. The representational primitives are typically classes, attributes and relationships. The definitions of the representational primitives include information about their meaning and constraints on their logically consistent application (Gruber, 2009)..

Ontologies are used in artificial intelligence, the Semantic Web, software engineering, library science and information architecture as a form of knowledge representation about the world or some part of it. It is been several years since ontologies began to be used for representing biomedical knowledge. For example, researches such as Schulz and Hahn (2005) and Smith (2006) formalized medical concepts by means of ontologies. One of the most important advances in bioinformatics was the development of the Gene Ontology (Ashburner et al., 2000), which popularized the development of bio-ontologies. Currently there are large projects and consortiums like the OBO Foundry[13] ensuring the coordinated development of these ontologies and also the United States have established research centres in biomedical ontologies such as the National Center for Biomedical Ontology[14]. There are other previous works that make use of ontologies for tasks related to electronic medical records management (Rose et al., 2001; Nardon & Moura, 2004; Smith & Ceusters, 2005).

Ontologies are usually accompanied by some document in a formal ontology language. With regard to the semantic web, there have been several approaches (Pulido et al., 2006). Among those, the Ontology Web Language (OWL)[15] is a W3C recommendation for an ontology description language that has gained widespread adoption and for which a considerable number of tools have been developed. It has more facilities for expressing meaning and semantics than XML, RDF, and RDF-S, and thus OWL goes beyond these languages in its ability to represent machine interpretable content on the Web.

2.3.1 The Protégé-OWL API

Protégé[16] is a flexible, configurable platform for the development of arbitrary model-driven applications and components. It has an open architecture that allows programmers to integrate plug-ins, which can appear as separate tabs, specific user interface components (widgets), or perform any other task on the current model. The Protégé-OWL editor provides many editing and browsing facilities for OWL models, and therefore can serve as an attractive starting point for rapid application development. Developers can initially wrap their components into a Protégé tab widget and later extract them to distribute them as part of a stand-alone application.

The Protégé-OWL API[17] is an open-source Java library for OWL and RDF(S). The API provides classes and methods to load and save OWL files, to query and manipulate OWL data models, and to perform reasoning based on Description Logic engines. Furthermore, the API is optimized for the implementation of graphical user interfaces.

The translator implementation that is described in Section 4.7 was originally based on the Protégé 3.4 open source platform that provides both an ontology editor and the Protégé-OWL API (v 3.4) allowing for the creation, visualization and manipulation of ontologies in the OWL 1.0 format. As the new Protégé 4 has reimplemented its interface on top of the OWLAPI[18], which is already designed to support OWL 2[19], the ADL to OWL translator is also being adapted to the new API in order to get the benefits from the OWL 2 new features like Qualified Cardinality Restrictions (QCRs), see section 4.3.

2.3.2 SWRL Rules

Besides the biomedical interest in OWL, many health care processes such as computer aided decision making or disease diagnosis and treatment, are often best modelled using a declarative approach and rules, leading to a very active interest in rule-based systems (O'Connor et al., 2005). However, interoperability among the multitude of current rule-based systems is limited. The Semantic Web Rule Language (SWRL)[20] has emerged as a first step solution to increase rule-based systems interoperability from the Semantic Web perspective. It is based on a combination of OWL with the Rule Markup Language[21]. The combination of OWL and SWRL provides inference capabilities beyond the classification capabilities built-in the description logics implemented by OWL (Baader, Calvanese, McGuinness, Nardi, & Patel-Schneider, 2003). In the clinical environment, different kinds of rules can be expressed with this logic. For example, *standard-rules* allow for chaining ontologies properties as well as *mapping-rules* between ontologies contribute to data integration and navigability, as pointed out by Golbreich and Imai (2004). Currently SWRL provides a set of built-ins to deal with comparisons, math operations, strings and date/time among others. This modular approach to built-ins will allow further extensions in future releases and provides the flexibility for various implementations to select the modules to be supported with each version of the language. For instance, a SWRL extension to overcome complex scenarios that include mathematical relationships and formulas that exceed current SWRL capabilities is proposed by Sánchez-Macián, Pastor, Vergara, and López (2007).

2.3.3 SWRL Rules and Clinical Guidelines

Clinical guidelines, also called medical guidelines, contain "systematically developed statements to assist practitioner and patient decisions about appropriate health care for specific clinical circumstances" (Field & Lohr, 1990). Examples of decision points and declarative knowledge contained in clinical guidelines that can be entirely or partially represented and shared by merging archetypes and rules are the following:

- **Antibiotic prescribing:** A complete example on respiratory tract infections is described by Lezcano, Sicilia, and Rodríguez-Solano (2011).
- **Risk assessment of pressure ulcers:** A key element in the Prevention and Treatment of the Pressure Ulcers guideline from NICE[22,23]. Figure 37 depicts some of the most important SWRL rules that were used in the CISEP project (see section 7.2) to evaluate pressure ulcers.
- **Alerts and risk of CVD:** Included in the key messages of the Seventh Report of the Joint National Committee on Prevention, Detection, Evaluation, and Treatment of High Blood Pressure[24,25].
- **Transverse Sinus Ligation:** The research by Lezcano, Sicilia and Serrano-Balazote (2008) was specifically oriented to aid intraoperative monitoring on *Transverse Sinus Ligation* by combining SWRL rules, like the one in Figure 23, with the OWL version of the *Intravascular Pressure* archetype.
- **Stages of COPD:** Defined in the Pocket Guide to COPD Diagnosis, Management, and Prevention[26,27]. SWRL rules to infer the stage of COPD according to such guideline are shown in Figure 38.

2.4 Clinical Terminologies

The consistent use of *clinical terminologies* and the development of good practice in archetype design and terminology binding to them play an important role in building structured EHRs and reaching semantic interoperability, as alleged by the European Commission (Stroetmann et al., 2009). The primary objective of clinical terminologies for interoperability is to enable the faithful exchange of meaning between machines and between machines and people. Therefore, a lot of research has to be done in order to integrate clinical terminologies with data models, ontologies, archetypes and the rest of knowledge artefacts involved in level 3 of SIOp. Some efforts have been already made to align the use of content in structured data models to one or more chosen terminologies (Markwell, Sato, & Cheetham, 2007; Smith & Ceusters, 2005).

In most cases the data and terminology models are developed independently by separate professional groups. While data modelling techniques are developed by IT professionals, terminologies are primarily dominated by clinicians and other clinical experts. Therefore, integration will be best achieved for terminologies by starting with areas where there is a high consensus on the need and the content. Translational medicine and *adverse drug reactions* are examples of such areas.

2.4.1 Relevant Clinical Terminologies and Ontologies

2.4.1.1 SNOMED-CT

SNOMED-CT[28] is a comprehensive clinical terminology, originally created by the College of American Pathologists (CAP) and, as of April 2007, owned, maintained, and distributed by the International Health Terminology Standards Development Organization (IHTSDO), a non-for-profit association in Denmark. It provides the core general terminology for the EHR and contains more than 311,000 active concepts with unique meanings and formal logic-based definitions organized into hierarchies (Schulz, Suntisrivaraporn, Baader, & Boeker, 2009).

SNOMED-CT was selected for this research study because of the following reasons:

- As it is widely used in Europe and all over the world, this chapter could be significant for several researches in the EHR community. Spain has become the eleventh country to join the IHTSDO[29].
- SNOMED-CT has a large coverage of the clinical concepts required for the case studies that were carried out here.
- It is simple to use and query, in spite of its large size.
- At least part of the terminology has been classified by DL reasoners, making it more reliable when compared to completely unclassified terminologies. The reliability is based on the assumption that logical errors would have been resolved during classification. The semantic completeness of SNOMED-CT has been audited by Jiang and Chute (2009).

2.4.1.2 OpenGALEN

OpenGALEN[30] is a not-for-profit organisation providing another medical terminology. The GALEN programme of research into medical terminology began in 1991. In 1999 OpenGALEN was formed to provide an open source route both for disseminating the results of that programme and as a framework for its future development (Rector, J. E. Rogers, Zanstra, & Van Der Haring, 2003).

2.4.1.3 UMLS

The Unified Medical Language System (UMLS) is a compendium of three knowledge sources in the biomedical sciences, which are distributed with several tools that facilitate their use (Bodenreider, 2004; Lindberg, Humphreys, & McCray, 1993).

2.4.1.4 ICD

The International Classification of Diseases (ICD)[31] is a standard diagnostic classification for all general epidemiological, many health management purposes and clinical use. These include the analysis of the general health situation of population groups and monitoring of the incidence and prevalence of diseases and other health problems in relation to other variables such as the characteristics and circumstances of the individuals affected, reimbursement, resource allocation, quality and guidelines.

In addition, there are other clinical terminologies and sources of knowledge that address specific areas of medicine. For example, the Logical Observation Identifier Names and Codes database (LOINC) is a naming structure for laboratory test (Forrey et al., 1996); RxNorm[32] is a standardized nomenclature for clinical drugs and drug delivery devices, produced by the National Library of Medicine (NLM); the Digital Imaging and Communication in Medicine (DICOM)[333] is a standard for medical imaging; and the Foundational Model of Anatomy (FMA)[34] is a reference ontology for the human anatomy. The BioPortal[35] allows to access and share ontologies that are actively used in biomedical communities, and RadLex[36] is a lexicon for uniform indexing and retrieval of radiology information resources.

2.4.2 Integrating Archetypes and Clinical Terminologies

The term binding section in archetypes enable elements to be mapped to one or more terminology concepts, allowing to comply with terminology standards. This provides a means for a controlled method of data entry to enable reuse and lead to semantic interoperability. At present, such semantic mapping task is carried out manually to bind with external terminology systems such as ICD, SNOMED-CT and GALEN. Three main parts are required to create a term mapping statement in ADL. These are: (a) the internal fragment identifier, (b) the name of the terminology model such as LOINC, ICD or SNOMED, and (c) the terminology concept code.

Some of the terminology systems conceived by openEHR to be used with archetypes include: (a) SNOMED-CT, so that reliable inference and decision support based on EHR data can be made possible, (b) LOINC, so that traceability and sharing of laboratory data can be achieved, and (c) ICD and ICPC classifications, so that reliable reimbursement, management, and public health studies can be made possible (Beale, Heard, Kalra, Lloyd, & Schloeffel, 2006).

This chapter combines archetypes with the OWL version of several SNOMED subsets including allergies, drugs and respiratory tract infections, among others. As recommended by Wroe (2006), the SNOMED concepts are considered as OWL classes that conform a subsumption hierarchy while nontaxonomic relations are represented by means of quantifier restrictions. A specific subset of SNOMED including allergies, drugs and respiratory tract infections is used. Clinical concepts that represent allergies are considered as OWL classes, as well as substances and drugs concepts. Then, the codes of those concepts will be considered as individuals or instances of the classes and used within SWRL rules.

3. RELATED WORK

Many efforts have been made in the last decade to achieve interoperability of heterogeneous healthcare systems by means of terminologies, EHR models, clinical archetypes, templates, etc. Then ontologies and rules have also become an instrument to achieve such interoperability as the Semantic Web has progressively been adopted. More recently, the experience gained from those works have shown that dealing with SIOp requires the combination and seamless integration of several knowledge artefacts as none of them is able to completely fulfil the SIOp requirements when used in isolation. Thus, integration methods have started to appear in different areas of the clinical and biomedical domains. Some of them specifically designed to address a concrete necessity within current conditions, while other approaches have a wider scope and/or a future oriented application.

This section presents a range of research projects already completed or still being carried out to achieve semantic interoperability in EHR systems. Accordingly, references for three main combinations will be analysed. Firstly, those related to translating clinical archetypes to ontologies are presented. Then, some recently developed approaches to aid clinical guideline execution by combining ontologies and rules are described. Finally, the section concludes with the analysis of some projects addressing the integration of clinical terminologies and ontologies, as well as archetypes and terminologies bindings by means of ontologies. The discussion of each of the related works is completed with a comparative analysis with respect to this chapter' approach.

3.1 Translating Clinical Archetypes to Ontologies

Translating ADL definitions to OWL can be done in two different ways. In the "*translating archetypes as classes*" method, ADL definitions can be considered as ontology classes that specialise the OWL representation of the RM. Therefore, the data about patients and clinical facts is represented as instances of those classes. Taking as example the *Heart_Rate-Pulse*[37] archetype, we can translate its components into a group of RM specialised classes (e.g. specialising the OBSERVATION class, the ITEM_TREE class, etc.

A different approach or "*translating archetypes as instances*" takes archetypes as instances of an OWL representation of the AOM, leaving no room for patient data instances. When considering archetypes themselves as instance data, ELEMENTs, ITEM_TREEs, CLUSTERs, etc. are translated into instances of classes in the Constraint_model package. For example the OBSERVATION statement included in the *Heart_Rate-Pulse* archetype can be translated into an instance of the OWL representation of the C_OBJECT class (*complex object*) defined in the AOM. The POSEACLE approach by Martínez-Costa, Menárguez-Tortosa, Fernández-Breis, and Maldonado (2009) has selected the second method, in which archetypes are translated into instances of some classes representing an archetype model. The main objectives of that project include facilitating semantic search at the archetype specification level, as well as other semantic tasks that improve EHR management.

In contrast with the POSEACLE approach, inference execution over recorded clinical data is the main final goal of the ADL to OWL translation method described in this chapter. Therefore, the former perspective (i.e. "*translating archetypes as classes*") is designed and explained in the following sections, thus storing patient data as instances of RM specialised classes. The translation starting point is then an OWL representation of the RM instead of the AOM representation used in the POSEACLE approach.

Clinical archetypes were also translated to OWL, within the scope of the ARTEMIS project (Dogac et al., 2006), for the purpose of achieving the interoperability of Web Service messages exchanged in the health care domain. Interoperability issues like creating semantic mappings between classes in different reference models (e.g. the EHRcom and the HL7 CDA) were addressed in the project. Thus, the OWL representation of archetypes was used to semantically annotate the Web Service messages and then provide the mapping between the OWL representations of archetypes through an OWL ontology mapping tool (OWLmt).

The translation principles explained in this chapter are consistent with the ones applied in the ARTEMIS project (Kilic, Bicer, & Dogac, 2005; Bicer, Kilic, Dogac, & Laleci, 2005). Going further, this chapter proposes workarounds to the translation issues that remain unsolved in those publications and, in addition, provides new translation mechanisms that take advantage of the improved potential of OWL 2. For example, regarding the translation of the data constraints contained in archetypes, a complete description containing the limitations of OWL 1 datatyping can be found in a study by J. Z. Pan and Horrocks (2005). They proposed an extension to OWL DL, called OWLEu, which integrates a large family of decidable Description Logics with unary datatype groups, so as to support user defined datatypes. However, the emerging OWL 2 adopted a different approach that is used in section 4.2 to capture the quantitative constraints of archetypes. Another significant difference with the ARTEMIS approach to archetypes translation is that the methods in Section 4 explain not only how to represent the ADL constraints and semantics in OWL but also how to accomplish such task without human intervention. Thus, they were conceived as completely automatic processes that support the implementation of the automatic ADL to OWL translator described in Section 4.7.

3.2 Clinical Guidelines Integration

Given the each day more important interoperability feature between healthcare systems and the increasing use of Semantic Web technologies within services integration, there have been a few approaches addressing the incorporation of clinical guidelines in healthcare systems to support the decision making process by means of these technologies. For example, the approach by Argüello and Des (2008) explains how to facilitate the use of a clinical guideline for the diagnosis and clinical management of Diabetic Retinopathy by means of web services. The approach outlines the use of the OWL's XML syntax to obtain web services that provide reasoning and easily deal with fact and rules, which are defined in SWRL. Authors argue that having inference mechanisms and descriptive knowledge combined under the same syntactic structure provides means for the interoperability of rule systems.

The more recent work by C. Chen, K. Chen, Hsu, and Li (2010) has also been carried out to integrate clinical guidelines by means of ontologies and rules. The research describes an application based on Protégé and Java technologies aimed at translating the visual representation of clinical guidelines rules to a representation in XML, which in turn is transformed to Jess rules for execution. Although their results show high levels of effectiveness when tested against historical data, the rules derived from the guidelines and the used data instances are not expressed in a language that is independent from their particular implementation.

In parallel to these Semantic Web based approaches, traditional designs have been also appearing. The system presented by Rossille, Laurent, and Burgun (2005) is meant to be a data warehouse in oncology, storing valuable information for treating, for instance, patients with rare tumours, or not reacting normally to a treatment. It is a multi-modal decision-support system as it is based on both rule-based reasoning (with GLIF3[38] guidelines) and case-based reasoning (with individual cases).

As can be seen, the approaches introduced in this section had to select a mechanism to represent guidelines steps and structures as well as a knowledge representation mechanism to represent patients' data. GLIF is sometimes used to model clinical guidelines while mappings to clinical terminologies like UMLS and ICD is used in other cases to reduce discrepancies with regard to clinical concepts meanings. However, even when some importance has been given to knowledge normalization, standards are not equilibrated in none of above mentioned works. As a result, either patients' data or clinical guidelines are always implemented through a specific or ad-hoc approach the makes the overall implementation dependant from a particular context, underlying systems and locally agreed semantics. This entails sharing and reusing difficulties that preclude reaching level 3 of SIOp (Stroetmann et al., 2009). In contrast, the research described in this chapter is addressed to avoid these inconveniences by completely relying on the integration of widely accepted models and standards.

3.3 Binding Terminologies to Clinical Archetypes

Previous work on terminology mappings includes two separate tracks. On one hand is the problem of finding suitable terminology codes to map to the archetype terms, while on the other hand is the problem of testing the logical correctness of these mapped codes. A relevant research addressing the first issue is the Model Standardisation using Terminology (MoST) (Qamar, 2008), which is largely involved with finding the semantically correct SNOMED codes to bind to the archetype fragments.

Significant works in the other line of research include a general methodology for defining a code binding interface in OWL (Rector, Qamar, & Marley, 2009). Such Code Binding Interface constrains and specifies how coding systems are to be used in EHR data structures. The approach presents the development of an ontology that acts as a meta-model of meaning, defining the codes that can be logically included in place of the archetype fragments, to retain the semantic and logical correctness of the original data model. The intention is to classify the ontology to indicate any inconsistencies in the integrated model. It should be noted that this task is essentially syntactic as it is concerned with the reliable processing of data structures and not with whether the information conveyed is accurate and correct. The authors argue that many controversies around coding systems and EHR standards arise from the lack of a clear distinction between validity and accuracy. The approach needs to be further evaluated in order to become widely accepted as a key step towards semantic interoperability.

In that second direction, Section 6 illustrates several applications and advantages that arises from a similar binding when applied to the case of openEHR, OWL and SNOMED. Such benefits are supported by the ADL to OWL translation approach that is explained in this chapter before arriving to Section 6. Also some issues related to the connections between Information, Terminology and Inference Models have been studied by Rector, Johnson, S. Tu, Wroe, and J. Rogers (2001).

Taking the OWL version of archetypes as metadata allows for ontologies to be used to index these clinical statements and provide better tools of retrieval. There have already been several research efforts that address the indexing of information by means of ontologies (Tzitzikas, 2002), and according to Kalra (2008), archetypes indexing and archetypes repository services fall into the areas needing research inside the semantic interoperability domain. With the increase in the amount of definitions, archetypes management will become a key matter of concern.

4. OVERALL APPROACH TO THE TRANSLATION

This section describes the approach resulting from this research to translate the representation of clinical archetypes in ADL to an ontology language like OWL. Section 4.1 exposes general aspects of the automatic translation from ADL to OWL. Then section 4.2 details the mappings of quantitative constraints to the ontological version of the archetype. Section 4.3 gives a recommendation on how to translate the occurrences constraints. Then, section 4.4 describes the importance of annotation properties as a means for a reusing technique and section 4.5 shows a method for constraining an archetype term to a small and finite set of values. Finally, section 4.6 provides a list of the basic translations and mapping rules applied in the translation of leaf data and ADL constraints keywords.

4.1 Overview of the ADL to OWL Translation

ADL files express clinical archetype definitions by means of constraint definitions (*cADL*) and data definitions (*dADL*) as explained in section 2.2.2. Therefore, translating ADL files to OWL implies rendering each and every *cADL* and *dADL* definitions using the OWL syntax. Main difficulties underlying this process come from the fact that there are different ways to represent the same information in OWL. This research requires a proper mechanism to be selected in order to support further tasks like adding SWRL rules and launching inference, setting bindings to terminologies, validating archetypes, etc. Thus, it should be noted that describing constraints as human-readable comments should be avoided as far as possible given that they cannot be used by semantic reasoners. For example, numerical range constraints, which are very common in archetype definitions, should not be translated as annotation properties but as user-defined datatypes (see section 4.2).

The two-level modelling paradigm and the knowledge representation mechanism followed by archetypes are analogous to some Object-Oriented Programming (OOP) patterns. As well as a *Student* class is frequently defined in an OOP context as a specialisation of a more general *Person* class, archetypes define clinical concepts by specialising more general ENTRY types and other classes from the RM. Therefore, the applied ADL to OWL translation implements such *inheritance* relation between the AM and the RM by means of the fundamental taxonomic constructor *rdfs:subClassOf*. It relates a more specific class to a more general class. If an OWL class A is a subclass of B, then every instance of A is also an instance of B. The *rdfs:subClassOf* relation is transitive and reflexive (i.e. every class is its own subclass, for example every person is a person). As with OOP inheritance, the OWL version of an archetype inherits all attributes and properties from its parent RM class and is able to overwrite them by adding new restrictions. For example, narrowing the allowed *Blood Pressure* numerical values to the range of integers between 0 and 250 follows similar purposes to those of the bundling data mechanism provided by OOP *encapsulation*.

Given the archetypes capability of being defined as specialisations of more general archetypes, the translation mechanism encourages the compatibility of SWRL across hierarchies. Thus, an SWRL rule originally designed according to the OWL version of a parent archetype will be suitable for all its descendants. This "*Inheritable compatibility*" as well as other benefits of the OWL + SWRL integration proposed in this chapter are all listed in section 5.1. The principles of this "*translating archetype as classes*" approach will be detailed throughout the current section. Existing alternative approaches are commented in the Related Work Section.

During translation we deal with two different information hierarchies. One of them is defined by the archetype level in an ADL file as shown in section 2.2.2. This one is composed of RM containers and classes from the constraint model package. This containers-tree has a variable structure because it depends on the objectives of specific clinical situations. The other one is the hierarchal tree conforming the RM, which has the same structure across different archetypes. The approach proposed in this chapter considers that each level of the archetype tree defines a subclass of an entity belonging to the RM tree. So, to map the archetype tree to OWL we need to specialise the corresponding RM classes while preserving the archetype tree interconnections between new classes.

It should be noted that both trees are mixed in a way that remains compatible with the RM original structure. The point of departure is the mapping developed by Román, Roa, Reina-Tosina, and Madinabeitia (2006). Archetype definitions start with an ENTRY subtype like EVALUATION, INSTRUCTION, ACTION or OBSERVATION. Essentially, an archetype constrains the instances of such categories, so a main translation principle is having those ENTRY categories as classes and each archetype definition becoming a subclass depending on the subtype.

This section takes as example the translation process of the *Heart rate and rhythm* archetype. It is an OBSERVATION to record the measured characteristics related to the rate and rhythm of the heart, including a simple statement of presence of heart rate. These are not recorded by direct observation of the heart itself but inferred from alternative sources including the direct auscultation of the heart or an electrocardiograph reflecting the electrical activity of the heart.

In general, the OBSERVATION type is used to record the observation of any phenomenon or state of interest related to the patient. It only records information relating to the situation of the patient, not what was actually done while treating him/her. Among other things, observations also include pathology analysis results as well as the family history and social circumstances of the patient as told to the clinician. *Heart rate and rhythm* (or its specialisation, *Pulse*) are commonly recorded as one component of *Vital signs*, which includes: *Blood Pressure*, *Respirations*, *Temperature* and *Oximetry*. There are additional specific OBSERVATION archetypes for each of these concepts.

In addition to the attributes inherited from ENTRY and CARE ENTRY, the OBSERVATION type has only two attributes, data:HISTORY and state:HISTORY. The translation process and principles illustrated through an OBSERVATION can be then applied to any sort of archetypes.

The code fragments provided in Figure 1, Figure 2 and Figure 3 illustrate the mapping from the archetype root definition to the *Heart rate and rhythm* OWL class. The *rdfs:subClassOf* property is being used to inherit all the OBSERVATION features. The name of the new OWL class is retrieved from the ADL ontology section using the ADL node identifier, in the case of the example, [at0000]. This code is attached to the class by an *annotation property* named *NodeID*. Annotation properties are pieces of metadata that can place annotations on classes. Other groups of properties can only relate data values, individuals and ontologies[39].

As well as translating each ADL node to an OWL class we need to preserve the connections established by ADL relations like data. By translating these ADL relations to OWL individual-valued properties and restricting them by means of an *owl:allValuesFrom* property, we guarantee that defined classes exactly map the configuration of the structure in the archetype specification. Also known as *universal* restriction, the *owl:allValuesFrom* is a built-in OWL property that constrains the relationships along a given property to individuals that are members of a specific class (Horridge, 2009).

Figure 4 illustrates how the OWL root class have a restriction on its *data* property that forces class instances to be related only to *History* instances, which is the next downwards archetype definition. At the same time, each OWL class is created as a specialisation of its RM category. Because archetypes have a tree like structure the above steps are repeated for each level until the whole hierarchy is mapped.

Considering the ADL tree as a graph, the traverse method applied by the translation process resembles the *Depth First Search* pattern or *DFS*. It extends the current path as

Figure 1. Heart rate and rhythm archetype (ADL root)

```
definition
  OBSERVATION[at0000] matches {        -- Heart rate and rhythm
    data matches {
      HISTORY[at0002] matches {        -- history
```

Figure 2. Heart rate and rhythm archetype (OWL XML/RDF syntax)

```
<owl:Class rdf:ID="Heart_rate_and_rhythm">
  <NodeID rdf:datatype="http://www.w3.org/2001/XMLSchema#string"
  >at0000</NodeID>
  <rdfs:subClassOf>
    <owl:Restriction>
      <owl:allValuesFrom rdf:resource="#HISTORY"/>
      <owl:onProperty rdf:resource="http://.../EHR/EHR_RM.owl#data"/>
    </owl:Restriction>
  </rdfs:subClassOf>
  <rdfs:subClassOf rdf:resource="http://.../EHR/EHR_RM.owl#OBSERVATION"/>
</owl:Class>
```

Figure 3. Heart rate and rhythm archetype (OWL Manchester syntax)

```
CLASS Airway_assessment_anaesthesiology
  ANNOTATIONS: NodeID "at0000"
  SUBCLASSOF: OBSERVATION THAT data ONLY HISTORY
```

Figure 4. Restriction of inherited properties to guarantee OWL and ADL structure compatibility

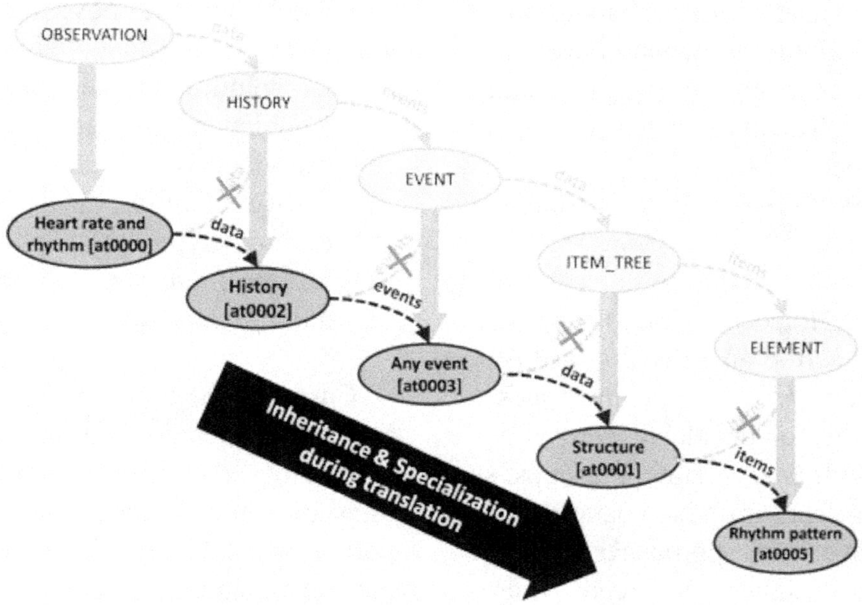

far as possible before backtracking to the last choice point and trying the next alternative path. A deeper explanation can be found in Cormen, Leiserson, Rivest, and Stein (1990).

In this particular example, the yellow ovals represent the RM classes being restricted by the *Heart rate and rhythm* archetype. The blue ovals represent the OWL subclasses implementing those restrictions. The Xed out yellow dotted lines and the blue dotted lines represent the addition of new *owl:allValuesFrom* restrictions that override the inherited ones and confine the bindings to the subclasses defined for this archetype. Thus, the archetype tree-like structure is being simulated on top of the RM.

At the ADL's bottommost level we find several types of data-valued constraints (e.g. C_DATE, C_BOOLEAN, etc.) that are translated to their counterparts in the RM ontology whose names start with DV (e.g. DV_BOOLEAN, DV_DATE). The following sections explain the particular cases where translation is more complicated.

A mapping reference including the formal rules for these translation techniques is listed in section 4.6.

4.2 User-Defined Datatypes to Represent Restrictions on Quantified Values

Archetypes allow a wide variety of constraints to be applied on the primitive types located at the ADL's bottommost level. For example, in the case of indicators like rates, temperatures, indexes and pressures, constraints are commonly needed to represent limits in measurement. The OWL 1.0 language presents serious disadvantages to cover this kind of restriction. It allows controlling the cardinality of relations using the *owl:cardinality* built-in[40] and also it may guarantee the link with a certain value using the *owl:hasValue* built-in[41]. By combining both restrictions we can constrain a primitive type to a small and discrete set. However, it is not enough to deal with a continuous range defined by a minimum and a maximum value. A complete description containing the limitations of OWL 1.0 datatyping can be found in Pan and Horrocks (2005).

To overcome this issue, there are a number of approaches:

- Pan and Horrocks (2005) and Pan (2004) describe an extension to OWL DL, called *OWLEu*, that integrates a large family of decidable *Description Logics* with unary datatype groups, so as to support user defined datatypes.
- There have been approaches from the language designers that tend towards reusing the mechanism for user defined datatypes in the XML Schema specifications[42]. Since the XML Schema blocks are not in RDF format, there is no consensus on what URI should be used to identify the defined datatypes. Therefore they cannot easily be integrated in the ontology. Options to this problem have been drafted by Carroll and Pan (2006).
- Another approach is provided by Knublauch (2005), explaining a Protégé-OWL implementation of user defined datatypes. It involves the use of a small extension ontology *xsp.owl* that defines RDF properties to represent XML schema facets. Once imported in our ontology file, user-defined datatypes can be embedded into the same file in contrast with the two files required by the above proposal.
- OWL 2 has adopted a very similar solution to the one proposed by Knublauch, in order to deal with user-defined datatypes. The normative constraining facets[43] for the datatype are *xsd:minInclusive*, *xsd:maxInclusive*, *xsd:minExclusive*, and *xsd:maxExclusive*.

Currently the translation implementation applies the penultimate solution given its simplicity and consistency for the automatic translation process and because it is fully supported by the Protégé-OWL API. However, the implementation is being migrated in order to apply the last solution.

An example from the *Pulse* archetype can be appreciated in Figure 5. The *Pulse* contains the ELEMENT[at0.11] that outlines the *Missed beats per minute* as an integer greater than or equal to 0. Its corresponding OWL code according to Knublauch recommendation is given in Figure 6 and 7.

4.3 Representing *Occurrences* Restrictions in OWL

The ADL syntax includes the occurrences{...} statement that is used only with cADL object nodes (not attribute nodes) to restrict the times that a particular piece of information is recorded as part of a more general container. For example, occurrences ∈ {1..1} indicates

Figure 5. A DV_COUNT constraint from the Pulse archetype (ADL)

```
ELEMENT[at0.11] occurrences matches {0..1} matches {    -- Missed beats per minute
  value matches {
    DV_COUNT matches {
      magnitude matches {|>=0|}
    }
  }
}
```

Figure 6. A DV_COUNT constraint from the Pulse archetype (OWL XML/RDF syntax)

```
<rdf:datatype="http://www.w3.org/2001/XMLSchema#int"
  <xsp:minInclusive rdf:datatype="http://www.w3.org/2001/XMLSchema#int"
  >0</xsp:minInclusive>
  <xsp:base rdf:resource="http://www.w3.org/2001/XMLSchema#int"/>
</rdfs:Datatype>
```

Figure 7. A DV_COUNT constraint from the Pulse archetype (OWL Manchester syntax)

```
DATAPROPERTY: magnitude
       RANGE: integer [>= 0]
```

that the constrained object is mandatory while occurrences ∈ {1..0} indicates that it is optional.

An occurrences{...} statement differs from a cardinality{...} one in the sense that it affects the contained structures themselves instead of the whole collection count. Both occurrences and cardinality are equivalent restrictions only in the case where the container includes a single type of structure. For the rest, the occurrences restriction is stronger than cardinality. There is a rule[44] defined by Beale and Heard (2008b) for the purpose of validating the relation between both restrictions: *the interval represented by <the sum of all occurrences minimum values> .. <the sum of all occurrences maximum values> must be inside the interval of the cardinality.*

Despite the fact that OWL 1.0 lacks of a direct mechanism to simulate the ADL occurrences statement, there is a workaround based on logical class operations that fulfils it. The following procedure takes as example the ITEM_TREE shown in Figure 8.

1. Each occurrences restriction is first considered as if it were the only one inside the container so it can be replaced by a cardinality restriction on the container. For example, the occurrences restriction on the *Rhythm pattern* ELEMENT is substituted by a cardinality restriction on the items property of the ITEM_TREE and expressed in OWL as appears in Figure 9.
2. Then the cardinality restriction is merged with a *universal* restriction to guarantee the correct ITEM_TREE<->ELEMENT link as explained in section 4.1.
3. Repeat the above steps for every other structure belonging to the container (i.e. *Heart_rate*, *Rate* and *Comment* ELEMENTs).

Figure 8. Occurrences restrictions in the Heart rate and rhythm archetype (ADL)

```
ITEM_TREE[at0001] matches {    -- structure
  items cardinality matches {0..*; unordered} matches {
    ELEMENT[at1005] occurrences matches {0..1} matches {          -- Heart rate present
      value matches {...}
    }
    ELEMENT[at0004] occurrences matches {0..1} matches {          -- Rate
      value matches {...}
    }
    ELEMENT[at0005] occurrences matches {0..1} matches {          -- Rhythm pattern
      value matches {...}
    }
    ELEMENT[at0009] occurrences matches {0..1} matches {          -- Comment
      value matches {...}
    }
  }
}
```

Figure 9. A constraint on the items cardinality (OWL XML/RDF syntax)

```
<owl:Restriction>
  <owl:onProperty
  rdf:resource="http://.../Data_Structures_RM.owl#items"/>
  <owl:maxCardinality rdf:datatype="http://www.w3.org/2001/XMLSchema#int"
  >1</owl:maxCardinality>
</owl:Restriction>
```

4. Finally, all universal-cardinality restriction pairs must be joined using an *intersection* closure to create an *anonymous* class[45] that will become a superclass of the container class.

It should be noted that the container cardinality that was originally defined in the ADL code is no longer significant after applying the above mentioned steps.

Nevertheless, the selected solution to capture the semantics of the ADL occurrences restrictions is based on Qualified Cardinality Restrictions (QCRs)[46], provided by the latest version of OWL. QCRs are suitable to represent occurrences because the term qualified indicates that they apply only to a specific type of value rather than to the property overall. Taking as example the ITEM_TREE shown in Figure 8, those occurrences restrictions can be translated using QCRs and represented in the OWL Manchester Syntax as in Figure 10.

Alternative workarounds based on *subproperties* were discarded because they do not enforce the property to be used only through one of its subproperties, thus allowing for the archetype tree-like structure to be invalid. This kind of workaround was discussed by Rector and Schreiber (2005).

4.4 A Reuse Technique Based on Annotation Properties

As every other information model, archetypes need to exploit the advantages of reusing previously defined CLUSTERs, ITEM_TREEs, ELEMENTs, etc. in order to make the entire definition more efficient and less redundant. The use_node ADL keyword has been created for this purpose. It works by referencing an ADL node from the location where it should be repeated. A reliable path that identifies the node in the ADL text (concatenating the [atXXXX] IDs of its containers) serves as internal reference. As explained in section 4.1, those term IDs are mapped in OWL as the annotation property *NodeID* that links the OWL classes with their ADL ID. It is the annotations peculiarity of taking classes as operands instead of instances who led this chapter approach to use them in the implementation of the reusing technique.

A fragment from the *Palpation* archetype that includes an example of a use_node statement and the referenced ELEMENT is shown in Figure 11. The purpose of the archetype is to record data found on examination through palpation. Within the archetype specification, the *Body_site* ELEMENT must be recorded

Figure 10. ADL occurrences statements expressed in OWL Manchester Syntax

```
CLASS Structure
  SUBCLASSOF: items ONLY (Heart_rate_present OR Rate OR Rhythm_pattern OR Comment)
  SUBCLASSOF: items MAX 1 Heart_rate_present
  SUBCLASSOF: items MAX 1 Rate
  SUBCLASSOF: items MAX 1 Rhythm_pattern
  SUBCLASSOF: items MAX 1 Comment
```

twice (i.e. in the *Localised_palpation* CLUSTER and in the *Tenderness* CLUSTER) and therefore the use_node keyword is included to allow a single definition and a double use. When parsing an ADL file, use_node keywords are interpreted as instances of the ArchetypeInternalRef AOM class. This class supports the finding process of the archetype node that is going to be reused. Figure 12 contains the translation into OWL of the *Body_site* ELEMENT (i.e., the referenced object in this case). In order to map the *use_node* statement to OWL, the container structure (i.e. the *Tenderness* CLUSTER) is linked to the referenced node. The OWL fragments in Figure 12 and Figure 13 guarantees such linkage by means of the *owl:allValuesFrom* restriction.

4.5 Constraining Possible Values to a Finite and Small Set

Pieces of data that must be recorded as text fragments are usually instances of DV_TEXT. This RM class is used to contain any amount of legal characters arranged as words, sentences, etc. However, if a controlled vocabulary or terminology is required, then the DV_CODED_TEXT class allows the definition of value

Figure 11. Use_node keyword in the Palpation archetype

```
CLUSTER[at0010] occurrences matches {0..*} matches {     -- Localised palpation
  items cardinality matches {1..*; unordered} matches {
    ELEMENT[at0011] matches { -- Body site
      value matches {
        DV_TEXT matches {*}
      }
  }
}
```

```
CLUSTER[at0019] occurrences matches {0..*} matches {     -- Tenderness
  items cardinality matches {1..*; unordered} matches {
    ELEMENT[at0002] occurrences matches {0..1} matches {...}    -- Depth of palpation
    ELEMENT[at0020] occurrences matches {0..1} matches {...}    -- Degree
    ELEMENT[at0005] occurrences matches {0..1} matches {...}    -- Category
    use_node ELEMENT /items[at0080]/items[at0010]/items[at0011] -- reference to Body_site
  }
}
```

Figure 12. Reusing the Body_site class in the Tenderness CLUSTER (OWL XML/RDF syntax)

```
<owl:Class rdf:about="#Body_site">
  <NodeID rdf:datatype="http://www.w3.org/2001/XMLSchema#string"
  >at0011</NodeID>
  <rdfs:subClassOf rdf:resource="http://.../Data_Structures_RM.owl#ELEMENT"/>
  ...
</owl:Class>
```

```
<owl:Class rdf:ID="Tenderness">
  ...
    <owl:Restriction>
      <owl:onProperty rdf:resource="http://.../Data_Structures_RM.owl#items"/>
        <owl:allValuesFrom>
          <owl:Class>
            <owl:unionOf rdf:parseType="Collection">
              <owl:Class rdf:about="#Depth_of_palpation"/>
              <owl:Class rdf:about="#Degree"/>
              <owl:Class rdf:about="#Category"/>
              <owl:Class rdf:about="#Body_site"/>
            </owl:unionOf>
    ...
  ...
</owl:Class>
```

Figure 13. Reusing the Body_site class in the Tenderness CLUSTER (OWL Manchester syntax)

```
CLASS Tenderness
  SUBCLASSOF: items ONLY (Depth_of_palpation OR Degree OR Category OR Body_site)
  SUBCLASSOF: items MAX 1 Depth_of_palpation
  SUBCLASSOF: items MAX 1 Degree
  SUBCLASSOF: items MAX 1 Category
  SUBCLASSOF: items MAX 1 Body_site
```

sets in groups using codes and rubrics. Codes themselves are contained within the defining code attribute of the class.

Other situations require the recording of symbolic values when exact values are not of interest or they are unknown. The main purpose is usually to classify patients into fuzzy intervals for which different decisions might be made. Take for example the categorization of *Tenderness* as being "Superficial tenderness", "Deep tenderness", "Rebound tenderness", "Tenderness" or "Rigidity". This is what DV_ORDINAL class is designed for.

In both cases the translation process must ensure that instances from the resulting OWL class can only take values among the listed finite set. The procedure is here elucidated working from the *coded text* in Figure 14. We must specialise the OWL version of the ELEMENT class to obtain a *Category_ELEMENT* class that only accepts instances from a given specialisation of DV_CODED_TEXT, which name is automatically generated as *Category_DV_CODED_TEXT*. Such class will in turn be linked to a specialisation of the CODE_PHRASE class that only accepts the codes: at0007, at0008, at0009, at0019 or at0025. To represent all possible values, an *anonymous* class is created using the union closure and it is established to be a superclass of the *Tenderness_Category_CODE_PHRASE* class. This way every instance fulfilling at least one of the restrictions specified in the union may be considered as a member of the *Tenderness_Category_CODE_PHRASE* class. Then the code set is traversed in order to add every possible value to the union closure. Finally, as rubrics are human readable information (i.e. "Deep tenderness", "Rigidity", etc.) they are connected to the class through an annotation comment. Figure 15 and Figure 16 show the resulting OWL definition.

There is another workaround for this translation that is based on the *owl:allValuesFrom*. At first a new Enumerated Datatype[47] is created, including all accepted codes. Then the code_string property is restricted using an *owl:allValuesFrom* so all related data values are within the data range that has been created. This second procedure does not require a union operation. Although both approaches

Figure 14. The category ELEMENT in Palpation archetype

```
ELEMENT[at0005] occurrences matches {0..1} matches {     -- Category
  value matches {
    DV_CODED_TEXT matches {
      defining_code matches {
            [local::
            at0007,  -- Superficial tenderness
            at0008,  -- Deep tenderness
            at0009,  -- Rebound tenderness
            at0019,  -- Tenderness
            at0025]  -- Rigidity
      }
    }
  }
}
```

Figure 15. Specialisation of CODE_PHRASE to represent Tenderness categories (OWL XML/RDF syntax)

```
ELEMENT[at0005] occurrences matches {0..1} matches {     -- Category
  value matches {
    DV_CODED_TEXT matches {
      defining_code matches {
             [local::
             at0007,  -- Superficial tenderness
             at0008,  -- Deep tenderness
             at0009,  -- Rebound tenderness
             at0019,  -- Tenderness
             at0025]  -- Rigidity
      }
    }
  }
}
```

Figure 16. Specialisation of CODE_PHRASE to represent Tenderness categories (OWL Manchester syntax)

```
CLASS Tenderness_Category_CODE_PHRASE
  ANNOTATIONS: rdfs:comment "at0007 -> Superficial tenderness, at0008 -> Deep tenderness,
                            at0009 -> Rebound tenderness, at0019 -> Tenderness,
                            at0025 -> Rigidity"
  SUBCLASSOF: CODE_PHRASE
  SUBCLASSOF: code_string VALUE "at0007" OR code_string VALUE "at0008" OR
              code_string VALUE "at0009" OR code_string VALUE "at0019" OR
```

have the same effect, the first one has been selected for implementation issues.

4.6 Translation Reference

This reference includes a list of the basic translations and mapping rules applied in the translation of leaf data and ADL constraints keywords. As pointed out below, the translation of many common data types from their ADL representation (dADL) to an OWL compatible representation is straightforward. The *W3C XML Schema*[48] and *RDFS Literals*[49] have been chosen for this purpose (Tables 2 and 3).

4.7 The ADL2OWL Translator Implementation

The ADL to OWL translation principles described in Section 4 have been implemented in the *ADL2OWL* translator, which is a Java based and open source project. It includes, on one hand, a translation library composed of two packages (the *adl2owl.parser* and the *adl2owl.translator*), that can be invoked by third party applications to launch the translation process of a provided ADL archetype. On the other hand, the project includes a standalone application with a GUI (i.e. the *adl2owl.gui* package) that allows selecting an ADL file and translating it to an OWL representation. The GUI is based on the Swing toolkit (Loy & Eckstein, 2002), that provides a set of components for building GUIs and adding rich graphics functionality and interactivity to Java applications. The translator project has become part of the *openEHR Java Implementation Project*[53] and its source code is been integrated as a module[54].

The structure chart in Figure 17 shows the breakdown of the ADL2OWL functionality. This kind of chart, which has been typically

Table 2. Data ADL (dADL) to OWL

<table>
<tr><th>ADL Leaf Data</th><th>W3C XML Schema and RDFS Literals</th></tr>
<tr><td>Character Data: 'a'</td><td>xsd:string</td></tr>
<tr><td>String Data: "systolic blood pressure"</td><td>xsd:string</td></tr>
<tr><td>Integer Data: 3456</td><td>xsd:int</td></tr>
<tr><td>Real Data: 3.1415926</td><td>xsd:double</td></tr>
<tr><td>Boolean Data: True, False</td><td>xsd:boolean</td></tr>
<tr><th colspan="2">Complete Date/Times</th></tr>
<tr><td>Date: yyyy-MM-dd</td><td>xsd:date</td></tr>
<tr><td>Time: hh:mm:ss[,sss][Z|+/-hhmm]</td><td>xsd:time</td></tr>
<tr><td>Date/Time: yyyy-MM-ddThh:mm:ss[,sss][Z]</td><td>xsd:dateTime</td></tr>
<tr><th colspan="2">Partial Date/Times</th></tr>
<tr><td>Date with no days:
yyyy-MM and yyyy-MM-??</td><td>xsd:gYearMonth</td></tr>
<tr><td>Time with no seconds:
hh:mm and hh:mm:??</td><td>Translated as single integers[51]</td></tr>
<tr><td>Date/time with no seconds:
yyyy-MM-ddThh:mm</td><td>Translated as single integers</td></tr>
<tr><td>Date/time, no minutes or seconds:
yyyy-MM-ddThh</td><td>Translated as single integers</td></tr>
<tr><td>Date, no month or day:
yyyy-??-?? and yyyy-??-?T??:??:??</td><td>xsd:gYear</td></tr>
<tr><td>Time, no minutes or seconds: hh:??:??</td><td>Translated as a single integer</td></tr>
<tr><td>Date/time with no seconds:
yyyy-MM-ddThh:mm:??</td><td>Translated as single integers</td></tr>
<tr><td>Date/time with no minutes or seconds:
yyyy-MM-ddThh:??:??</td><td>Translated as single integers</td></tr>
<tr><th colspan="2">Intervals and Lists</th></tr>
<tr><td>Intervals of Ordered Primitive Types
Examples:
|0..7| |0.0..5000.0|
|0.0..<5000.0| |02:13..05:10|
|>= 1984-02-05| |10.0 +/-10.0|
|>=0|</td><td>User-Defined Datatypes based on the xsp.owl ontology (see section 4.2)</td></tr>
<tr><td>Lists of Built-in Types
Examples:
{"immobile", "very limited", "reduced", "full"}
{"at0012", "at0013", "at0014"}
{1, 4, 9, 16}</td><td>Two approaches have been studied (see section 4.5):
- Enumerated Datatypes
- owl:hasValue restrictions</td></tr>
</table>

Note: All dADL data eventually devolve to instances of the primitive types String, Integer, Real, Double, String, Character, various date/time types, lists or intervals of these types, and a few special types. The dADL representation do not use type or attribute names for instances of primitive types, only manifest values, making it possible to assume as little as possible about type names and structures of the primitive types.

Table 3. Constraint ADL (cADL) to OWL

Set membership: matches, is_in	*owl:allValuesFrom* and/or *owl:hasValue* restrictions
Container Attributes	
Cardinality constraint: cardinality	*owl:cardinality*
Occurrences constraint: occurrences	*OWL 2.0 Qualified Cardinality Restrictions*[52]
"Any" constraint: {*}	Unrestricted OWL properties
Node Identifiers: [at0123]	*OWL Annotation Property* named NodeID
Internal References: use_node	*owl:allValuesFrom* restriction (see section 4.4)

used in structured programs design (Martin & McClure, 1985), allows understanding the sequence of subtasks that compose the translation mechanism, as well as their objectives.

5. INTEGRATING RULES WITH CLINICAL ARCHETYPES

Archetype definition languages (as the ADL specified by the OpenEHR consortium) currently support neither inference nor rules, so a first recommended step is to represent them as OWL ontologies that can be then enriched with clinical rules. The automatic mechanism of translation explained in sections 4 and 4.7 allows developing and integrating archetypes into decision support and knowledge management software, as the archetype semantics are fully transferred to the ontology representation. Going a step further and incorporating rules to the OWL version of archetypes (e.g. SWRL rules) is an essential task toward the interoperability between heterogeneous systems.

In addition, sharing the knowledge expressed in the form of rules is coherent with the philosophy of open sharing underlying archetypes. While ontologies provide the basic framework for computational semantics, some inferential mechanisms allow reaching new conclusions that expand the boundaries of the declarative knowledge encoded in archetyped data. This is useful, for example, to support the application of knowledge about procedures

Figure 17. Structure chart of the ADL2OWL translator

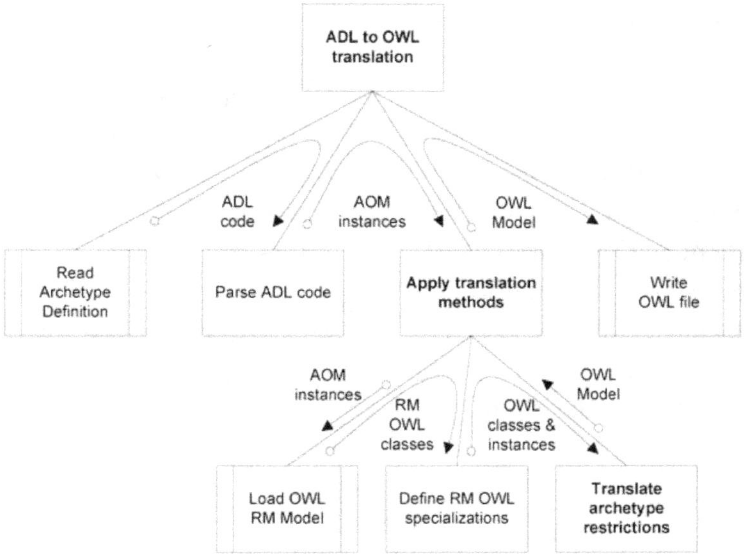

which is typically contained in clinical guidelines. Besides, having inference mechanisms and descriptive knowledge combined under the same syntactic structure provides means for the interoperability of rule systems. As pointed out by Horrocks, Patel-Schneider, Bechhofer, and Tsarkov (2005), the integration of the OWL ontologies and SWRL offers several advantages and goes beyond that of either OWL DL or Horn rules alone.

This section is structured as follows: section 5.1 describes the rationale for sharing SWRL rules in the context of archetype-based ontologies. Then section 5.2 explains in four subsections the *ArchOnt* framework approach to archetype, rules and inference integration. The explanation is illustrated with a case study designed to improve patient safety for a particular situation, i.e. to provide decision support for *Intraoperative Monitoring and Prevention of Complications during Ligation of the Sigmoid or Transverse Sinus*. It should be noted that medical approval must be requested if the clinical guidelines referenced in this chapter to illustrate the representation and inference mechanisms will be used in new real scenarios.

5.1 Sharing and Reusing SWRL Rules

As SWRL rules are defined, the need for a sharing method appears. Rule storage is not a problem because it is already implemented how to represent them as OWL individuals, and they can be stored using Semantic Web frameworks for data management as HP Jena[55]. As explained by O'Connor et al. (2005), SWRL rules are described by the SWRL Ontology[56]. However we must consider the case where the OWL version of an archetype and the SWRL rule associated with it are stored in separated files. This supports archetype translation and rule definition to be carried out at different times or by different groups of experts.

It should be noted that this is only a storage/management issue and it really does not make sense to semantically separate rules from ontologies. Like standard OWL axioms, SWRL rules are not disembodied entities so they can be interpreted only in terms of the ontology that they refer to. In order to preserve the semantic link, the following procedure is accomplished. Every time the same archetype is translated, an identical and unique URI is assigned to its OWL version. The URI generation is based on the archetype name and version. By applying the same generation mechanism, SWRL rules can safely reference to their archetypes. Thereby, whenever they are imported in the same OWL project they will connect properly.

Modelling knowledge by using SWRL rules and then sharing them by means of SWRL repositories can be considered practices consistent with the sharing principles of archetypes. It should be noted that SWRL rules based on openEHR archetypes can be hosted together with archetypes or in their own *Clinical Rules Repository*, as illustrated in Figure 19. Reasons for sharing and reusing SWRL rules include the ones listed in what follows:

- **Interoperable decision support**: The ability of systems to reliably communicate with each other regarding clinical decision support. To encourage the development of interoperable mechanisms for triggering critical aids to decision making like alerts, reminders and monitoring tasks that improve effectiveness and reduce clinical risks.

- **Inheritable compatibility**: Given the archetypes' capability of being defined as specialisations of more general archetypes, a SWRL rule originally designed according to the OWL version of a parent archetype is also applicable to derived archetypes.
- **Fostering semantics for clinical guidelines**: The introduction of SWRL rules and inferential mechanisms together with the archetypes expand the boundaries of the declarative knowledge that can be migrated from clinical guidelines to healthcare information systems. In this manner, a means for standardized representation, reuse and execution of the essential fragments of declarative knowledge contained in clinical guidelines is provided.
- **Specialists' empowerment**: To enable domain rules and guidelines to be modelled in a formal way by domain experts. By defining the declarative knowledge they work with, they can gain direct control over their information systems.
- **Consistency checking**: Rules integration can offer consistency checks to help guaranteeing data correctness in EHR fragments.
- **Archetype validation**: To support archetype validation and inconsistent restrictions detection, according to the RM or the specialised parent archetype.
- **Full semantic interoperability**: For all above mentioned reasons, integrating rules with clinical archetypes and EHR is an essential step towards level 3 of SIOp.

This has the additional potential benefit of being complemented with inferential models defined on some clinical ontologies (not coming from archetype translation) as will be described in the case studies of Section 7.

5.2 Rules Integration and Inference Execution

The four subsections of this section will explain the information and knowledge workflow from archetypes' translation to inference execution. The process is illustrated in Figure 18 and it is essentially a concatenation of the four white boxes that compose the *ArchOnt* Framework.

The first step is to translate the involved openEHR archetypes to OWL by combining their ADL definitions with the RM already expressed in OWL (*ADL2OWL translator* box). Then the resulting ontology is enriched with bindings to SNOMED-CT terms and clinical rules (*Semantic Enrichment* box). Once that all the required clinical knowledge is represented in a common OWL context, the archetypes are instantiated with patients' data coming from hospitals databases (*Instance Mapper* box). Finally, a semantic reasoner is invoked to gather the results from inference and feedback the hospitals' information systems (*Inference* box).

To support the framework explanation, each step will be described by means of an example based on the *Guidelines for the Ligation of the Sigmoid or Transverse Sinus during Large Petroclival Meningioma Surgery* (Hwang et al., 2004), supported by the Seoul National University Hospital the Korea

Figure 18. The ArchOnt framework

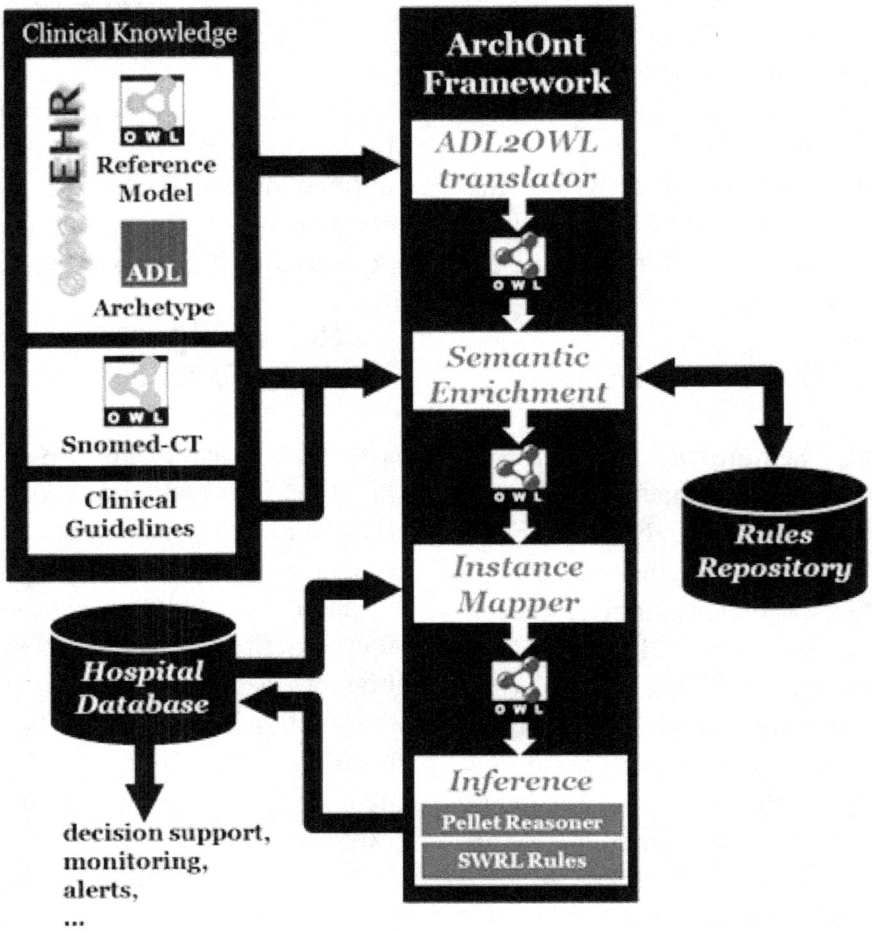

Figure 19. ADL to OWL translation of the Intravascular Pressure archetype

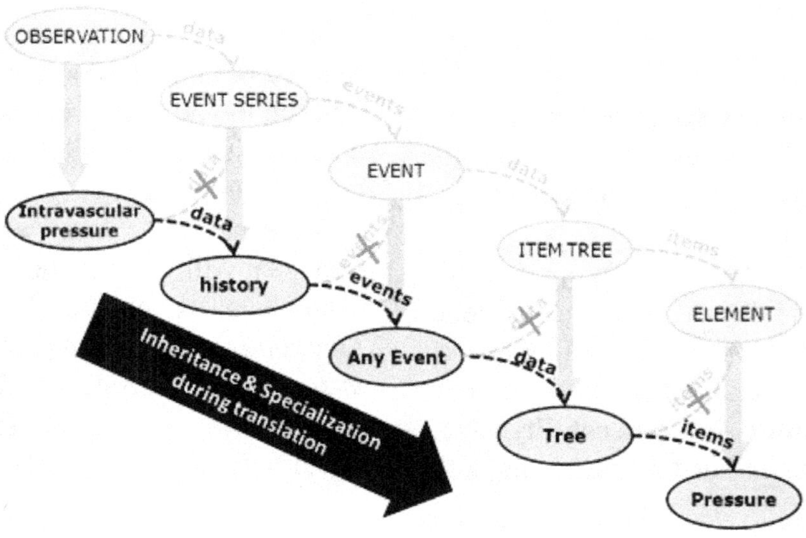

Brain and Spinal Cord Research Foundation. In order to properly understand the role that archetypes and SWRL rules can play in this scenario, a brief description of the guideline and its key concepts is given below.

Transverse Sinuses are two areas within a human head and beneath the brain, which allow blood veins to span the area, from the back of the head towards the nose. *Sigmoid Sinuses* are also two areas beneath the brain, which allow blood veins to span from the centre of the head downward. A *Petroclival Meningioma* is a type of brain tumour located near the skull base, in an area known as the *petroclival junction*. Such tumours are challenging to treat, as they are located deep inside the brain and may be difficult to access surgically. Integral to the surgery application are the manipulation, management, and sacrifice of the transverse or sigmoid sinus, as total resection of large tumours requires ligation and resection of the sinus to obtain a sufficiently wide exposure of the tumour.

So, one of the moments where decision support is quite useful is while assessing whether sinuses can be ligated or not, as ligation under inappropriate circumstances can take to venous complications. The guideline section titled "*Intraoperative Monitoring and Prevention of Complications*" includes two references to straightforward recommendations on how to avoid such complications:

- The first one involves measuring sigmoid sinus pressure after test clamping of the sinus to assess contralateral venous drainage before cutting the sinus (Spetzler, Daspit, & Pappas, 1992). If pressure in the sigmoid sinus increases more than 10 mm Hg by temporary occlusion testing, the sinus should be kept intact.
- The second one is provided by Day, Fukushima, and Giannotta (1997), founding that intravascular pressure no greater than 5 mm H2O was safe during test clamping. It should be noted that different units are used in each case to represent intravascular pressure, mercury (Hg) and water (H2O).

5.2.1 Translating Involved Archetypes

Integrating the above introduced clinical knowledge with a reasoner requires representing intravascular pressure measures before and after temporary occlusion testing of the sinuses. Besides, it should be a widely accepted representation in order to foster rules interoperability between heterogeneous healthcare systems. The *openEHR-EHR-OBSERVATION.intravascular_pressure* serves this purpose as it supports pressure measures, allowing both units (Hg and H2O), as well as related information like location and device. In this case, the SWRL rule will retrieve data from this archetype only, but there is no limit on the number of archetypes that can be accessed from a single rule. In fact, richer results come from processing several sources as illustrated in the case studies of Section 7.

In the first stage, illustrated as the *ADL2OWL translator* box in Figure 18, the *IntravascularPressure* archetype is translated to OWL according to the translation principles in Section 4 and the implementation described in Section 4.7. Some of the translated nodes are shown in Figure 19.

5.2.2 *Defining* Linker Rules *and* Guideline Rules

When the archetype is represented in OWL, SWRL rules with above clinical guidelines recommendations can be attached. Two kinds of rules with different goals can be devised. First, there are rules that search for useful data in the archetype and associate it to the *Patient* class. This kind of rule will be called *linker rule*. Given that archetype tree structures can get very dense and deep when describing some concepts, linker rules help to quickly access relevant information, and therefore make other rules simpler. It should be noted that relevant information depends on the clinical guideline that is been represented in each case. In the *Sinus Ligation* example under study relevant data includes pressure values, location, and units of measure.

Figure 20 and Figure 21 contain two *linker rules* that connect *Patient* instances directly to pressure measures from before and during test clamping. In order to reach data, both rules traverse the archetype from containers to leaf nodes. A brief description about SWRL syntax and operations is given in section 2.3.2. The rule in Figure 20 checks that the measure has been taken in the *Sigmoid Sinus* (represented by it SNOMED code "279264003"), and "BEFORE Test Clamping". Then it sets the direct link *hasBeforeTCpressure* (TC –> Test Clamping) between the patient and the pressure value. The rule in Figure 21 proceeds analogously but checking if the measure has been taken during test clamping and setting the *hasDuringTCpressure* predicate.

Now we are in place to define the SWRL rule that actually captures the Spetzler et al. (1992) recommendation. This kind of rule will be called *guideline rule*. It is shown in Figure 22, where the *subtract* and *greaterThan* mathematical built-ins allow asserting an "inadequate" ligation.

The semantics of the above presented approach to clinical guideline representation heavily relies on the combination of *linker rules* and *guideline rules*. The *Intravascular Pressure* archetype provides significant information like *Location* and *Device*, but they are not enough to completely define the *Sinus Ligation* monitoring context that is needed. Currently, such gap is filled by *linker rules*. However, an alternative approach could benefit from the archetypes' capability to be defined as specialisations of a parent and more general archetype. A solution can

Figure 20. Monitoring Sinus Ligation (SWRL context preparation I)

$$
\begin{array}{rcl}
\mathit{Patient}(?pat) & \wedge & \mathit{IntravascularPressure}(?ipr) \wedge \\
\mathit{tests}(?pat,?ipr) & \wedge & \mathit{List}(?lis) \wedge \\
\mathit{protocol}(?ipr,lis?) & \wedge & \mathit{Device}(?dev) \wedge \\
\mathit{itmes}(?lis,?dev) & \wedge & \mathit{I\_DV\_Text}(?txt) \wedge \\
\mathit{value}(?dev,?txt) & \wedge & \mathit{value}(?txt,\text{"BEFORE Test Clamping"}) \wedge \\
\mathit{History}(?his) & \wedge & \mathit{data}(?ipr,?his) \wedge \\
\mathit{Any\_event}(?evt) & \wedge & \mathit{events}(?his,?evt) \wedge \\
\mathit{Tree}(?tre) & \wedge & \mathit{data}(?evt,?tre) \wedge \\
\mathit{Location}(?loc) & \wedge & \mathit{items}(?tre,?loc) \wedge \\
\mathit{Location\_DV\_CODED\_TEXT}(?ctx) & \wedge & \mathit{defining\_code}(?ctx,\text{"279264003"}) \wedge \\
\mathit{Pressure}(?prs) & \wedge & \mathit{itmes}(?tre,?prs) \wedge \\
\mathit{Pressure\_DV\_QUANTITY}(?iqt) & \wedge & \mathit{value}(?prs,?iqt) \\
\Longrightarrow & & \\
 & & \mathit{hasBeforeTCpressure}(?pat,?iqt)
\end{array}
$$

Figure 21. Monitoring Sinus Ligation (SWRL context preparation II)

$$
\begin{array}{rcl}
Patient(?pat) & \wedge & IntravascularPressure(?ipr) \wedge \\
tests(?pat, ?ipr) & \wedge & List(?lis) \wedge \\
protocol(?ipr, lis?) & \wedge & Device(?dev) \wedge \\
itmes(?lis, ?dev) & \wedge & I\_DV\_Text(?txt) \wedge \\
value(?dev, ?txt) & \wedge & value(?txt, \text{"DURING Test Clamping"}) \wedge \\
History(?his) & \wedge & data(?ipr, ?his) \wedge \\
Any\_event(?evt) & \wedge & events(?his, ?evt) \wedge \\
Tree(?tre) & \wedge & data(?evt, ?tre) \wedge \\
Location(?loc) & \wedge & items(?tre, ?loc) \wedge \\
Location\_DV\_CODED\_TEXT(?ctx) & \wedge & defining\_code(?ctx, \text{"279264003"}) \wedge \\
Pressure(?prs) & \wedge & itmes(?tre, ?prs) \wedge \\
Pressure\_DV\_QUANTITY(?iqt) & \wedge & value(?prs, ?iqt) \\
\Longrightarrow & & \\
 & & hasDuringTCpressure(?pat, ?iqt)
\end{array}
$$

Figure 22. SWRL representation of the assessment of Sinus Ligation

$$
\begin{array}{rcl}
Patient(?pat) & \wedge & Pressure\_DV\_QUANTITY(?btValue) \wedge \\
hasBeforeTCpressure(?pat, ?btValue) & \wedge & units(?btValue, \text{"mm[Hg]"}) \wedge \\
Pressure\_DV\_QUANTITY(?drValue) & \wedge & hasDuringTCpressure(?pat, ?drValue)) \wedge \\
units(?drValue, \text{"mm[Hg]"}) & \wedge & swrlb : subtract(?result, ?drValue, ?btValue) \wedge \\
swrlb : greaterThan(?result, 10) & & \\
\Longrightarrow & & \\
 & & hasLigationAssessment(?pat, \text{"inadequate"})
\end{array}
$$

be then the creation of the *Intravascular Test Clamping* archetype as a specialisation of *Intravascular Pressure* including specific concepts like *Prior to test occlusion pressure* and *During test occlusion pressure.* In this sense, the equilibrium should be found between the specificity of archetypes and the size and complexity of SWRL rules. Then a similar procedure can be carried out for the Day et al. (1997) recommendation.

5.2.3 Mapping Patients' Data to OWL Instances

For the inference to generate results, the OWL version of archetypes must be first provided with patient's data. Concrete clinical data may come from a variety of sources, e.g. relational databases or flat files. Here the general approach of translating scalar data from comma separated value (CSV) files into ontology instances is described. It should be noted that a similar procedure can be followed if the data is provided by a relational database.

Archetype instantiation involves the creation of a set of OWL individuals that conforms the archetype hierarchy. Because upper level instances cannot a priori establish which lower level instances will be supplied, the latter ones should be created first in order to properly fulfil the properties between levels. Thus, instantiation process performs a bottom-up traverse of the archetype.

Leaf nodes instances are concrete clinical values, originally stored outside the boundaries of OWL domain, for example, in a CSV file. For that reason, a mapping between those values and their archetype slots should be provided. Once the source values are transformed into OWL customized Datatypes, they are linked to ELEMENT instances, which are organized by an ITEM_STRUCTURE instance and so on, until the archetype's root instance is created.

The CSV fragment in Figure 23 contains an extract of clinical measures required to instantiate the *Intravascular Pressure* archetype. Each row is parsed and transformed into a set of OWL individuals, assembling an *Intravascular Pressure* instance.

The lowest constraints in the archetype tree structure having a node ID are the ELEMENTs. Therefore, at0005 indicates a *Pressure* ELEMENT value, at0015 a *Relative Pressure* ELEMENT, and so forth. Neither *Patient_ID* nor *Date* fields have mappings to the archetype because such information is not described as a part of *Intravascular Pressure* concept. Actually, it is administrative information that should be captured by other archetypes. Assuming that CSV attributes notation is compatible with archetype slots or that it can be made compatible by an automatic transformation, the above procedure can be generalized to any kind of archetype.

Hospitals and healthcare centres sometimes provide very large files of data like these, including measures and results of thousands of tests and patients. So many rows of data can generate huge ontologies that compromise the efficiency and performance of the semantic reasoner. In fact, analysing and improving the performance and scalability of OWL reasoners is an ongoing challenge (Bail, Parsia, & Sattler, 2010). Under the context described above and considering clinical guidelines particular characteristics, several scalability tests were carried out. It has been found that the best performance is reached when not all patients' records are simultaneously loaded in the knowledge base. Instead, the whole inference cycle is execute over a set of 50 or 100 records, and then executed again over the next 50 or 100 records, until data is over. It should be noted that the fragmentation is feasible because records do not depend on each other. Such straightforward fragmentation approach cannot be done for example when loading the OWL version SNOMED-CT.

Figure 23. CSV fragment

```
Patient_ID | Date | Pressure | Relative | Location | Device
846385 | 09-03-2007 | 0.15 mmHg | normal | 279264003 | BEFORE Test Clamping
846385 | 09-03-2007 | 0.40 mmHg | raised | 279264003 | DURING Test Clamping
973589 | 20-10-2007 | 0.25 mmHg | normal |279264003 | BEFORE Test Clamping
973589 | 20-10-2007 | 10.45 mmHg | markedly increased |279264003 | DURING Test Clamping
123453 | 12-02-2008 | 0.22 mmHg | normal | 279264003 | BEFORE Test Clamping
123453 | 12-02-2008 | 0.30 mmHg | normal | 279264003 | DURING Test Clamping
745385 | 15-05-2010 | 0.19 mmHg | normal | 279264003 | BEFORE Test Clamping
745385 | 15-05-2010 | 13.7 mmHg | markedly increased | 279264003 | DURING Test Clamping
984647 | 03-07-2010 | 0.14 mmHg | normal | 279264003 | BEFORE Test Clamping
984647 | 03-07-2010 | 0.48 mmHg | raised | 279264003 | DURING Test Clamping
```

Mappings are node IDs of the current archetype ordered the same way as CSV fields:

```
|   | at0005 | at0015 |at0006 | at0022
```

5.2.4 SWRL Edition and Execution

Two implementations have been explored that support the edition and execution of above defined clinical rules. Firstly, the capabilities of Protégé 3.4 that includes a SWRL editor have been tested in combination with the Jess[57] engine. The Jess engine is a production rule system with forward chaining to achieve inferred results. Mei and Paslaru (2005) have demonstrated that mappings between SWRL and Jess are possible. An alternative and newer approach is the one provided by Protégé 4 in combination with Pellet[58].

6. BINDINGS TO CLINICAL ONTOLOGIES

The creation of methods for properly binding archetypes and terminologies, and the capacity to do it at a semantic level, is a necessary condition to reach level 3 of SIOp. For the purpose of executing the inference, previous sections has described an approach where archetypes are firstly translated into OWL and then enriched with SWRL rules. The translation allows for the bindings listed in the term binding section of the archetypes to be transformed into a set of equivalence relations between the archetype OWL classes and the SNOMED-CT OWL classes. An example of bindings attached to the *Blood Pressure* archetype is illustrated in Figure 24. SNOMED-CT codes and Physiology ontology URIs are provided for *Systolic* and *Diastolic Blood Pressures*.

An equivalence relation can be stated using the *owl:equivalentClass* built-in[59] property that links a class description A to another class description B. Then we can say that if an individual is a member of the class A then it also satisfies the conditions to be a member of the class B and viceversa. In other words, the two class descriptions involved have the same class extension or contain exactly the same set of individuals. Such symmetry is exemplified in Figure 25 by the arrows indicating two-way

Figure 24. Bindings examples in the blood pressure archetype

```
definition
      OBSERVATION[at0000] matches { -- Blood pressure
            data matches {
                        .
                        .
                        .
                  ELEMENT[at0004] occurrences matches {0..1} matches {  -- systolic
                        .
                        .
                        .
                  ELEMENT[at0005] occurrences matches {0..1} matches {  -- diastolic
            .
            .
            .
term_binding = <
            ["SNOMED-CT"] = <
                  items = <
                        ["at0000"] = <[SNOMED-CT(2003)::163020007]>
                        ["at0003"] = <[SNOMED-CT(2003)::364090009]>
                        ["at0004"] = <[SNOMED-CT(2003)::163030003]>
                        ["at0005"] = <[SNOMED-CT(2003)::163031004]>
                  >
            >
            ["PHYSIOLOGY ontology"] = <
                  items = <
                        ["at0004"] = <[http://www.medicalcomputing.net/owl/physiology.owl#SystolicBloodPressure]>
                        ["at0005"] = <[http://www.medicalcomputing.net/owl/physiology.owl#DiastolicBloodPressure]>
      >
```

Figure 25. Protégé and OWLViz[60] view of archetypes term bindings represented by equivalence relations

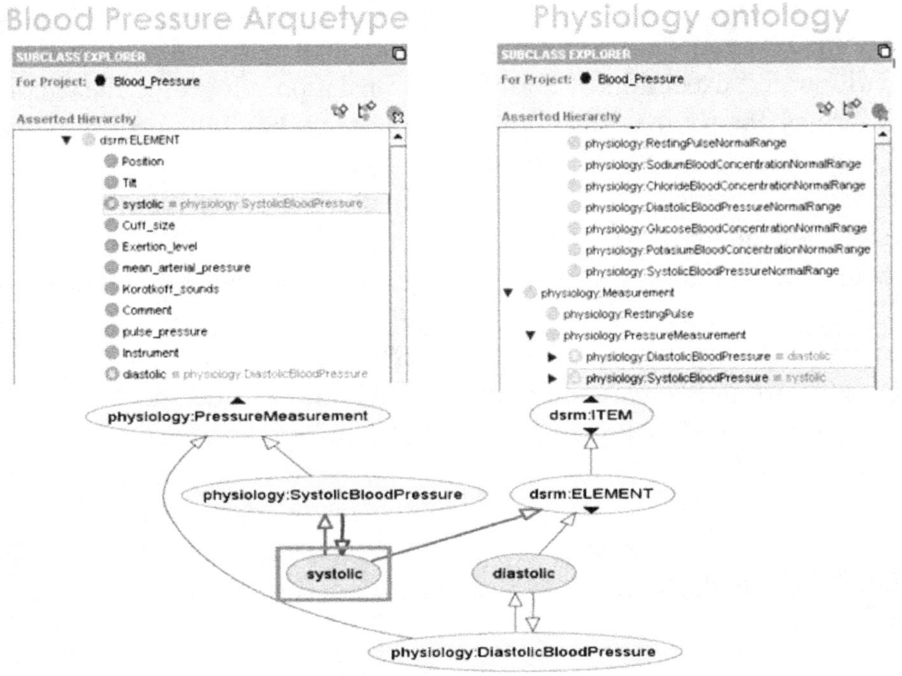

subsumption between *systolic* and *physiolog y:SystolicBloodPressure*.

It is worth mentioning that the establishment of such strong logical binding requires the previous finding and selection of the semantically correct external concept that will be bound to archetype components. This is difficult task that is commonly carried out by clinical experts, spending many time and effort. This issue has been addressed by the *Model Standardisation using Terminology* (MoST) methodology, and its supporting application, that provide a mechanism by which users can quickly find semantically equivalent terminology codes to bind/map to the data model fragments. Although the research focuses on the mapping of archetypes' fragments to SNOMED codes, the methodology is applicable to any other complementary model (Qamar & Rector, 2007). However, the success of this approach depends on the quality and accuracy of data mapping to terminology codes, which is still controversial as stated by Qamar, Kola, and Rector (2007).

The combination of that complementary work with the mapping techniques describe in this section is essential to ensure semantically equivalent coded data to achieve interoperability. This is quite helpful in practice because it encourages the following features to be implemented.

6.1 Ontology Navigability

Equivalence relations allow setting bridges between both ontologies and find paths that link previously unconnected concept. For example, the OpenEHR repository organizes archetypes according to the ENTRY type that they specialise. That makes the *Pregnancy* archetype and the *Movement of the fetus* archetype being classified separately because the former is an EVALUATION while the latter is an OBSERVATION. Consequently the indirect path connecting both concepts through the ENTRY class is the only one that can be found between them.

However, a semantically more significant path is found when mapping the *Pregnancy* archetype to the SNOMED-CT concept with the same name (SNOMED code 289908002) and the *Movement of the fetus* archetype to the SNOMED-CT *Fetal movement feature* (code 364617005). Then the new path can be traced through the next steps as shown in Figure 26:

1. Within the SNOMED ontology, *Fetal movement feature* is a subtype of *Fetal observable*.
2. At the same time, the *Measure of fetus* is also related to the *Fetal observable* concept through the *is-a* SNOMED-CT attribute.
3. Going further, this *Measure of fetus* has the *Number of fetuses* concept as one of its subtypes.
4. Finally the SNOMED-CT *Number of fetuses* can be directly mapped or set as equivalent to the *Number of fetuses* ELEMENT which is part of the *Pregnancy* archetype.

Relating archetypes from different sources supports better management and user navigation in archetype repositories. A computational technique to generate tentative archetype associations by mapping them through terms from the UMLS Metathesaurus is detailed in Lezcano, Sánchez-Alonso, and Sicilia (2010).

6.2 Checking the Mapping Context

The incorporation of SWRL rules into ontologies improves the reasoners' capabilities to maintain the coherence with current knowledge. Besides, the requirements for fulfilling a larger set of logical conditions, because of the equivalence relations, increase the likelihood of data correctness. For example, an archetype ELEMENT like *Herpes simplex* may be misused in some cases because its name accepts two different classifications.

The term "herpes simplex" may be classified as an organism (i.e. the human herpes simplex virus) or it may act as a disorder (i.e. the herpes simplex viral infection)[61]. SNOMED-CT solves this ambiguity by assigning a unique Concept ID to each one of the classifications, the *herpes simplex (organism)* is the 19965007 and the *herpes simplex (disorder)* is the 88594005. If an equivalence relation is established between the ELEMENT OWL class and the SNOMED-CT disorder concept then it has to support a number of SNOMED-CT attributes like *causativeAgent*, *severity*, etc. On the other hand, if it is mapped to the organism concept, then relations through mentioned attributes are not allowed.

6.3 Knowledge Integration

Figure 27 represents the combination of archetypes with the SNOMED-CT contribution in defining the *Drug Prescription* and the *Adverse Reaction* concepts after the establishment of the equivalence relations.

Figure 26. Archetypes connected through the SNOMED-CT ontology

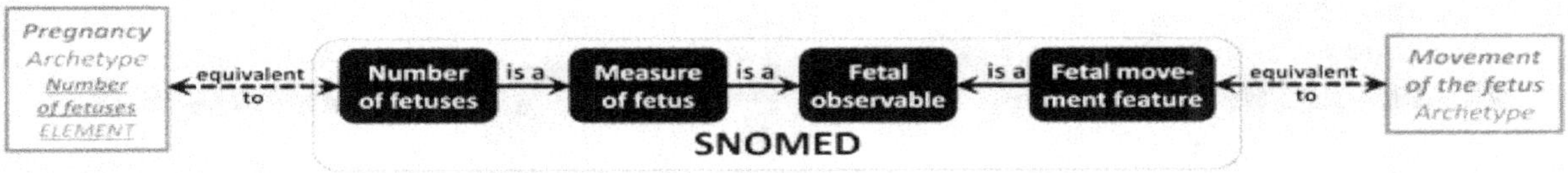

For example, the *Adverse Reaction* concept contains the *Date of Exposure* property that comes from the archetype, while the *severity* attribute comes from SNOMED-CT. It should be noted that properties are automatically available on both sides (archetype ontology and SNOMED-CT ontology) once the equivalence is asserted. This avoids the redefinition of clinical concepts while providing a means for reusing the already existing ones.

Another example of knowledge integration can be appreciated in Figure 28, when defining the *Systolic Blood Pressure* concept with attributes coming from two different sources: a *Physiology* ontology and the openEHR *Blood Pressure* archetype.

As it was explained in the Background Section, the OpenEHR Model is separated in two layers: a variable one described by archetypes and a stable one described by the RM. These models are different in the levels of abstraction from models of reality such as classifications (e.g. ICD), process description (e.g. clinical guidelines), descriptive terminologies (e.g. SNOMED-CT) and ontologies like OGMS (Ontology for General Medical Science). These models describe the real phenomena and therefore they have different types of authors, representations and purposes. However, the integration of both kinds of models is necessary to achieve SIOp and to improve patient safety.

OGMS[62,63] is a small and upper-level ontology for the domain of clinical medicine and research. Following the OBO Foundry principles, OGMS defines general terms in medicine like Disease, Disorder, Sign, Symptom, Finding, etc. It is designed to serve as anchor point for domain ontologies within medication, disease and laboratory test areas, as well as to bridge clinical medicine and basic science. The integration of OGMS and the openEHR AM has been studied as part of this chapter. Concrete benefits of such integration include the prevention of overlappings between archetype definitions as well as the

Figure 27. Archetypes and SNOMED-CT contribution in defining the Drug Prescription and the Adverse Reaction concepts

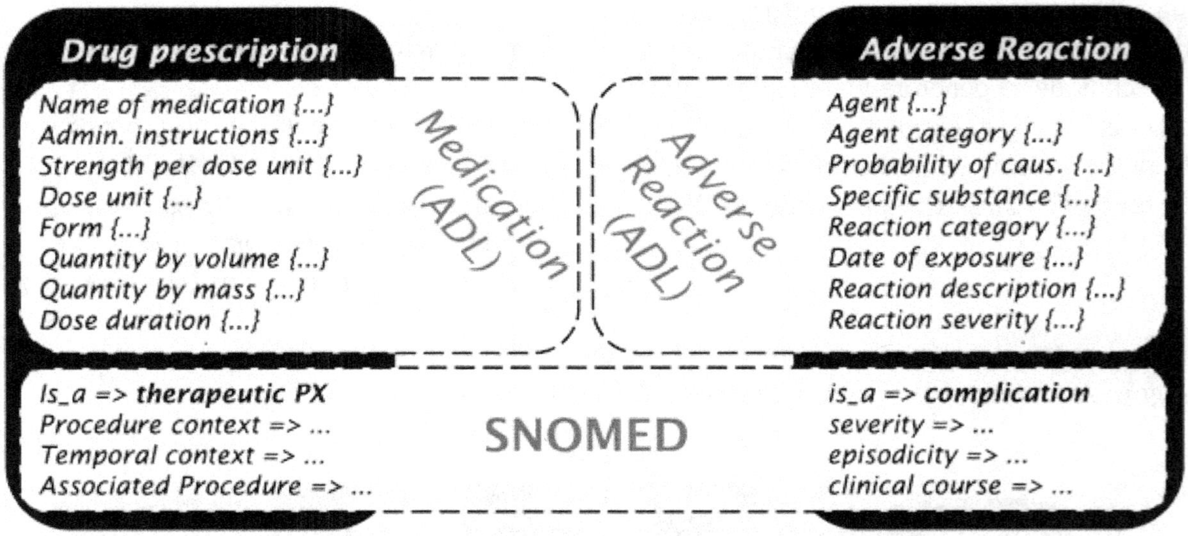

Figure 28. The screenshot shows the contribution of Physiology ontology and Blood Pressure archetype in defining the Systolic Blood Pressure concept. The properties in the bottom are provided by the Physiology ontology while the ones in the top come from the archetype

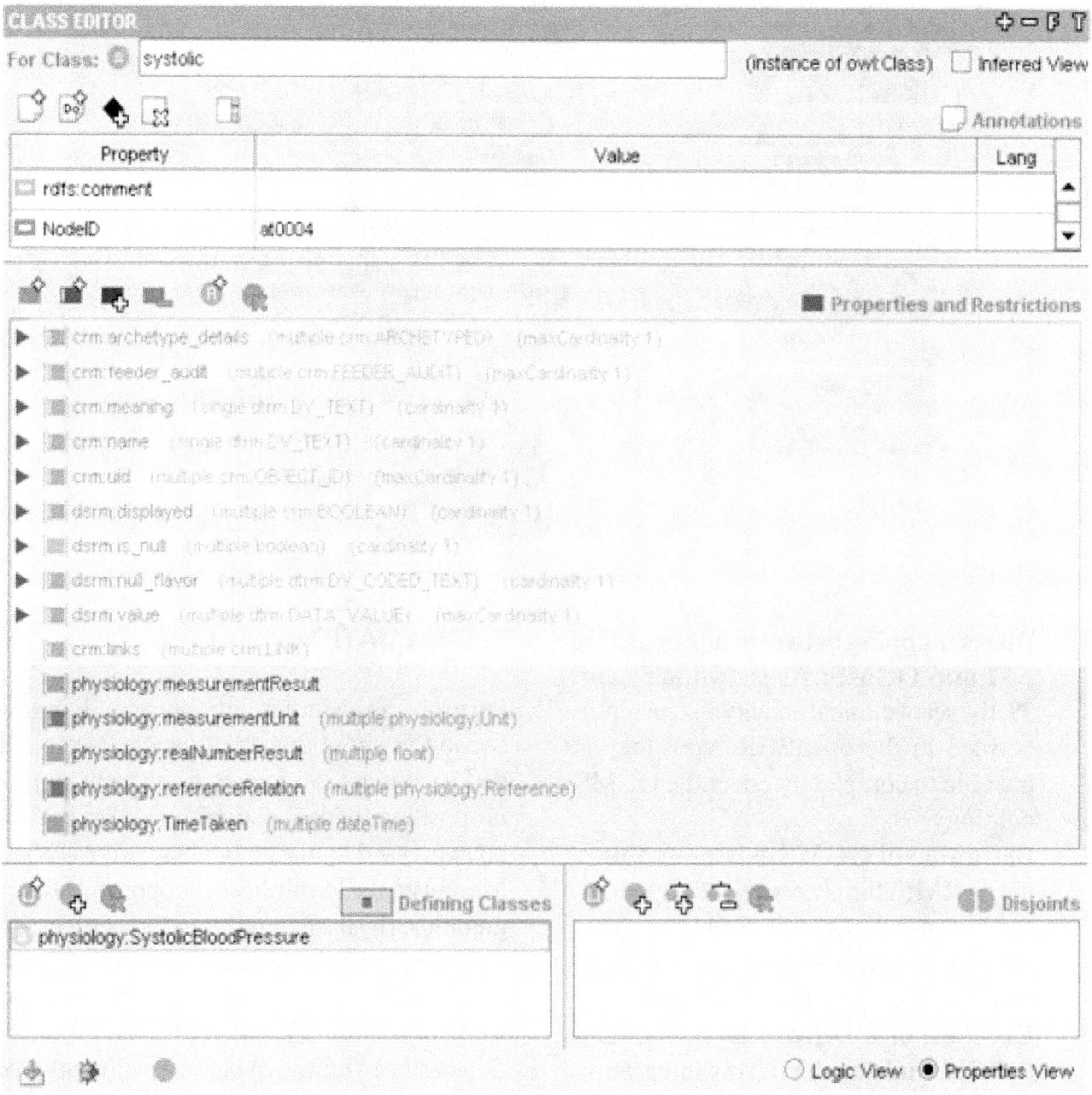

reduction of ambiguities in the AM. Figure 29 illustrates a tentative mapping between OGMS concepts and clinical archetypes from the openEHR repository. Examples of incompleteness (i.e. OGMS concepts without an exact openEHR mapping) and overlapping when covering the OGMS concepts are there revealed. Then, three approaches were considered for the integration of the OGMS ontology in order to solve above mentioned problems:

Figure 29. Tentative mapping between OGMS and openEHR archetypes

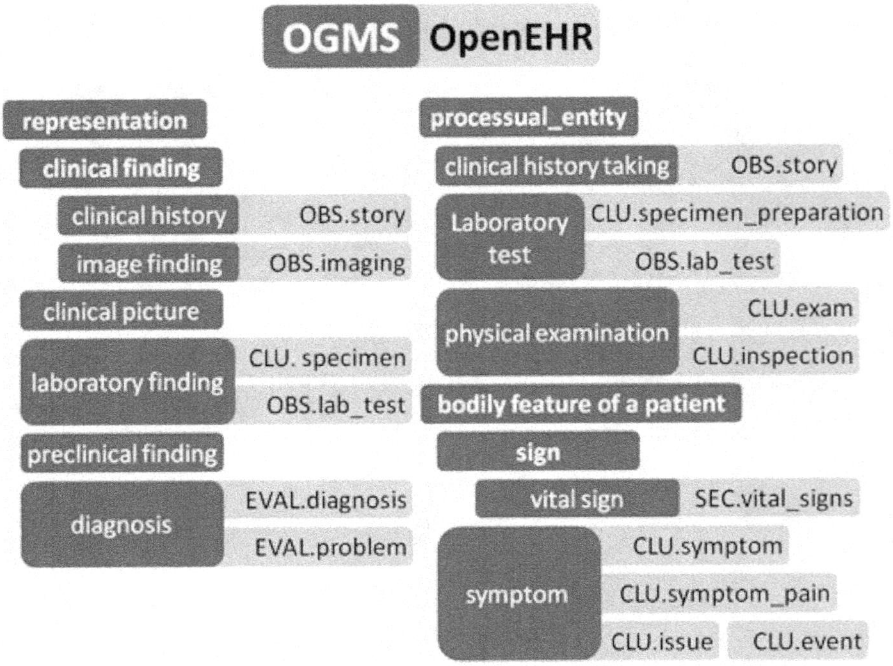

1. **Direct mapping between the openEHR AM and OGMS:** As shown in Figure 29, the set of clinical archetypes currently defined in the openEHR repository is not able to completely cover the OGMS ontology.
2. **Definition of OGMS classes as a part of the RM:** This is not very likely to happen because the openEHR philosophy is to keep the RM as stable as possible and this would clearly affect such stability.
3. **Creation of a *Disease* layer between the RM and the AM:** This integration option is the most feasible because it preserves the RM stability while provides a common set of general concepts about the *Disease* domain to more specific clinical archetypes. It was presented by Lezcano (2009). Figure 30 shows some examples of the elements in each layer.

7. EVALUATION

Several case studies are presented in this section to show that the procedures embedded in clinical guidelines frequently contain propositions of declarative knowledge that can be expressed by a rule language like SWRL. Moreover, the feasibility of supporting clinical guidelines by the integration of archetypes, ontologies, rules and terminologies is analysed.

In addition to the *Sinuses Ligation* case study of section 5.2, the ADL2OWL translation has been employed in three clinical projects described in this section. According to the requirements of the those clinical projects, the implementation introduced in Section 4.7 was first oriented to the translation of OBSERVATION and EVALUATION categories of archetypes, as the *Heart rate and rhythm* archetype and the *Pulse* archetype translated in Section 4, and the *Intravascular Pressure*

Figure 30. OGMS-openEHR integration approach

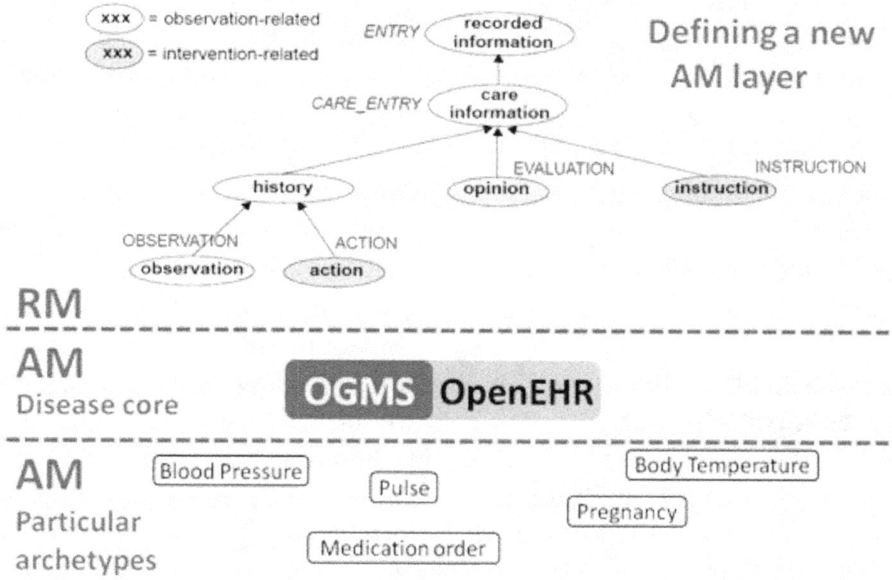

of section 5.2. Currently there are around 250 archetypes definitions in the openEHR repository and 40% of them are OBSERVATIONs and EVALUATIONs. After its integration as a module of the *openEHR Java Implementation Project*[64,65], the implementation is being completed in order to cover all subtypes of archetypes.

These archetypes have been authored by experts and clinicians from all over the world, moderated by the *openEHR Archetype Editorial Group*[66]. The translator has also been tested with an archetype designed by clinicians at the Fuenlabrada Teaching Hospital[67] in Madrid (see section 7.2), as well as with three new archetypes oriented to the *Diabetic Foot* prevention and management (see section 7.3). For the automatic ADL to OWL translation to perform correct parsing and translation of any kind of archetype, the implementation must cover the entire set of RM types and all their possible combinations. In order to avoid the maintenance problems that this approach could provoke, the design process should consider as far as possible all possible constraining mechanisms defined in the AOM. This way, the ease of evolution of the implementation is fostered.

As for integration with SWRL, ten rules have been tested including the ones described in this section. Although the mapping mechanism has not always been the same as the one described in section 5.2.3, it should be noted that SWRL rules are defined in terms of archetype elements, thus they are totally independent of the underlying architecture. In fact, once the SWRL rules are bound to the OWL version of the archetype, their proper execution only depends on the support provided by the selected reasoner (e.g. Pellet, Jess, etc.).

This promotes the reusability and shareability of the knowledge expressed in the form of rules, which is consistent with the philosophy of open sharing of archetypes. Although rules can be executed individually, substantial results come from forward chaining reasoning and rules concatenation as the example illustrated section 7.1. With regard to the limitations of the inference process, there is no specific restriction for this OWL and SWRL integration. Thus, inference boundaries are imposed by the language itself and the reasoner (e.g. the creation of new named individuals and the use of complex mathematical functions, as fractal functions or exponential sums, which are not currently supported by SWRL, see section 2.3.2).

7.1 Decision Support in the IEF-EHRS Research Project

The IEF-EHRS (*Information Exchange Framework for EHR Systems*) is a research project (IMADE-PIE 2009) that is been currently carried out by the Information Engineering Research Unit (*IERU*)[68] at the University of Alcalá, in combination with the *Henares Teaching Hospital*[69] and the *Alamo Consulting*[70] company. The project goals include the application of the research outcomes to clinical practice in order to improve healthcare assistance and patient security. In addition, a full CDSS[71] is being built to automatically reach to conclusions, raise alerts, as well as other monitoring aids that decrease the response time of care tasks and reduce human errors. At the same time, semantic interoperability of this framework is been taken to the highest possible level by defining a set of sharable software components that can be reused by the rest of organizations and research groups in the field. Therefore, clinical concept representation relies on clinical archetypes and the two-level approach proposed by openEHR.

7.1.1 The Antibiotic Prescribing and Allergy Detection Case Study

As pointed out in Section 4 of the European Commission report on Semantic Interoperability (Stroetmann et al., 2009), more complex Electronic Transfer of Prescription is considered among the areas for which reaching full SIOp or level 3 is a crucial trend. Those recommendations guided this chapter search for level 3 to the area of the new medication prescriptions that require comprehensive information on concurrent medication and details of known allergies and conditions.

Concretely, the translation of three fragments of the *Respiratory tract infections - antibiotic prescribing* published by NICE is described. The objective is to automatically recommend antibiotic prescriptions based on three SWRL rules defined according to the NICE guideline[72] and the information retrieved from the OWL version of the *Problem* archetype, downloaded from the openEHR repository[73]. Results are attached to the archetype instance using the *hasInferredAlert* property that can be defined in the same OWL file that stores the SWRL rule. These results provide means for automatically improving decision making and monitoring tasks.

7.1.1.1 Immediate Antibiotic Prescription

The first guideline fragment states that immediate antibiotics should be offered to patients who have symptoms and signs suggestive of "Pneumonia", "Mastoiditis", "Peritonsillar abscess" or "Peritonsillar cellulitis". These disorders are uniquely identified by instances of terminology codes (e.g. the SNOMED-CT code for "Pneumonia" is 233604007). We can reuse them to fill a new class named *ImmediateAI*, that is to say *Immediate Antibiotics Infections*. Hence, the immediate prescribing depends on whether the code of the diagnosed disorder is a member of this class or not. It should be noted that further guideline modifications in the list of disorders requiring immediate prescribing will only force the update of the *ImmediateAI* class while the SWRL rule can stay unmodified.

The diagnostic data is collected from the *Problem* archetype that is designed to record a condition or issue defined by a clinician who is deemed summative of a range of symptoms of the person. The archetype provides the SNOMED-CT codes for the *described condition* and for the *attributed diseases*. If any of them is a member of the *ImmediateAI* class, then the patient is considered to be at risk of developing complications so the rule raises an alert that recommends immediate antibiotic prescribing. Such rule should include a disjunction operator as there are two ELEMENTs to check in the archetype, and the same happens in the other two guideline fragments that are described below. However, SWRL does not support disjunctions of atoms, so they are checked in separated rules[74]. Figure 31 shows the rule that queries the *described condition* according to the guideline's first fragment.

As explained in section 5.2.2, the *hasDescribedCondition* property is previously filled by a *linker rule* in order to rapidly access the *described condition* value in further clinical rules (i.e., first, second and third SWRL fragment representation of the guideline). Linker rules are also used to fill the *hasAgeOnsetELT* property, which is then used in the second fragment representation and with the *hasMedicationSubstance* and *hasReactionSubstance* properties from the allergy detection SWRL rule shown in Figure 34.

Depending on the clinical assessment of severity, the second fragment analyzed here states that an immediate prescribing strategy should be agreed for children younger than 2 years with "Bilateral acute otitis media". There is a single disorder to check in this case so it makes no sense to define a new class; the SNOMED-CT code can be directly used. The patient's age is obtained from the *Age at initial onset* ELEMENT, also included in the OWL version of the *Problem* archetype. The antecedent part of the SWRL rule in Figure 32 considers all these parameters, including the age comparison, while the consequent part is the same as the former rule because the prescribing strategy is also immediate.

7.1.1.2 Delayed Antibiotic Prescribing

The third guideline fragment states that a delayed antibiotic prescribing strategy should be considered for patients with "Acute otitis media", "Acute pharyngitis/Acute tonsillitis", "Common cold", "Acute rhinosinusitis" or "Acute bronchitis". A new class named *DelayedAI* or *Delayed Antibiotics Infections* is defined in an analogous manner with the first fragment translation. Figure 33 illustrates the new rule that attaches SNOMED-CT codes recommending delayed prescribing when one of the above disorders (classified as *DelayedAI*) is detected. The consequent part

Figure 31. Antibiotic prescribing - SWRL rule (1st fragment)

$Problem(?p) \wedge ImmediateAI(?iai) \wedge$
$hasDescribedCondition(?p, ?prob) \wedge value(?prob, ?cod) \wedge$
$hasConceptID(?iai, ?cod)$
$\Longrightarrow$
$hasInferredAlert(?p, \text{"306807008"}) \wedge$
$hasInferredAlert(?p, \text{"255631004"}) \wedge$
$hasInferredAlert(?p, \text{"88694003"})$

SNOMED terms involved:
255631004 - Antibiotic
88694003 - Immediate
306807008 - Recommendation to start drug treatment

Figure 32. Antibiotic prescribing - SWRL rule (2nd fragment)

$$
\begin{array}{rll}
hasAgeOnsetELT(?p, ?a) & \wedge & Problem(?p) \wedge \\
hasDescribedCondition(?p, ?prob) & \wedge & value(?a, ?age) \wedge \\
swrlb : lessThanOrEqual(?age, 2) & \wedge & value(?prob, \text{"194290005"}) \\
\Longrightarrow & & \\
hasInferredAlert(?p, \text{"306807008"}) & \wedge & \\
hasInferredAlert(?p, \text{"255631004"}) & \wedge & \\
hasInferredAlert(?p, \text{"88694003"}) & &
\end{array}
$$

SNOMED terms involved:
255631004 - Antibiotic
88694003 - Immediate
306807008 - Recommendation to start drug treatment
194290005 - Bilateral acute otitis media

is also similar to the one in the first rule. In contrast the priority qualifier has been set to "Delayed".

7.1.1.3 Validating Medical Prescriptions

Working in the context of abnormal reactions and allergies to medications, where decision support can substantially improve support to the medication process, the OWL version of two archetypes (*Medication* and *Adverse Reaction*) and a subset of SNOMED-CT are taken as the point of departure (see section 2.4). The objective is to prevent interactions according to known allergies stored in the patient's EHR.

The *Medication* archetype specifies the description of the medication as part of an INSTRUCTION or ACTION record taken with respect to medication. This will usually occur in response to a medication order or prescription, but may be self administered or supplied by a pharmacy. The archetype provides the SNOMED-CT code that links with the term that represents the *medication substance*. It also includes a *Deferred supply* ELEMENT that is set if the medication supply is delayed, as occurs in the previous mentioned guideline.

In other direction, the *Adverse Reaction* archetype is usually employed for recording anomalous reaction(s) to a particular 'Agent'. The SNOMED-CT code corresponding to the *reaction substance* is provided. Thus, it may be specified that the decision on whether the prescription should be approved or not depends on the *proximity* between both terms, the *medication substance* and the *reaction substance*, inside the SNOMED-CT ontology. Such *proximity* can be traced by following the *causative Agent* relationship that links every allergy with the drugs or substances that caused it. For example, the *Co-fluampicil allergy* is related to *Ampicillin* and *Floxacillin* through the *causative Agent* relationship. Therefore an *Ampicillin* prescription must not be issued to a patient whose EHR stores a sample of the *Adverse Reaction* archetype

Figure 33. Antibiotic prescribing - SWRL rule (3rd fragment)

$$
\begin{array}{rll}
Problem(?p) & \wedge & DelayedAI(?dai) \wedge \\
hasDescribedCondition(?p, ?prob) & \wedge & value(?prob, ?cod) \wedge \\
hasConceptID(?dai, ?cod) & & \\
\Longrightarrow & & \\
hasInferredAlert(?p, \text{"306807008"}) & \wedge & \\
hasInferredAlert(?p, \text{"255631004"}) & \wedge & \\
hasInferredAlert(?p, \text{"75784006"}) & &
\end{array}
$$

SNOMED terms involved:
255631004 - Antibiotic
75784006 - Delayed
306807008 - Recommendation to start drug treatment

containing the code for *Floxacillin* and vice-versa. Once the problem is detected, a new alert is attached to the instance of *Medication* archetype using the *hasInferredAlert* property as explained previously in this section.

In the SNOMED-CT ontology the *causative Agent* is a relationship between the *DrugAllergy* class and the *Drug* class. Thus the SWRL rule in Figure 34 captures the allergy detection algorithm described above. This rule can be invoked independently as an aid to the prescription validation process. Nevertheless, the benefits are more evident when SWRL rules are chained than when they are isolated. In fact, the execution of the antibiotic prescribing rules in this section can be considered as a triggering event for the rule in Figure 34.

The flow chart in Figure 35 describes the control flow for the combined execution of these rules. It should be noted that the process cannot be carried out without human intervention in between the inference execution blocks. For example, a doctor must select the type of antibiotics and the active ingredient that is going to be offered to the patient between the antibiotic prescribing alert, which is raised in the left side of Figure 35, and the moment when the prescription becomes effective in the right side. Still, it is a reliable method that improves patient security during diagnosis and treatment. Also, execution scalability is well supported as newly prescribing guidelines can be concurrently launched in the left side, previously to the prescribing validation stage in the right side.

7.2 Alerts in the CISEP Project

The CISEP (*Intelligent Clinical Records for Patient Safety*) is a finished research project (code FIT-350301-2007-18), that was funded by the Spanish Ministry of Science and Technology. The project was carried out by the *Fuenlabrada Teaching Hospital*[75], the *iSOCO*[76] company and several universities, including the *University of Carlos III*, the *European University of Madrid* and the *University of Alcalá*, specifically the Information Engineering Research Unit (*IERU*).

The main objective of the project was to design, develop and implement a healthcare system based on information processing techniques and semantic modelling. Such system was oriented to offer value added services working from the electronic health records, in order to improve patient safety. A key goal in this project was to guarantee the interoperability of the heterogeneous software components that were functioning in the hospital.

Concrete objectives included supporting alerts and decision making aids within a specific subset of patient security problems like medication, primary and secondary care. Pressure ulcer management is one of those security problems for which monitoring aids are essential in the *Fuenlabrada Hospital*. Following the approach presented in this chapter a pilot service was developed and

Figure 34. Allergy detection - SWRL rule

$$\begin{array}{rcl} Medication(?med) & \wedge & AdverseReaction(?ar) \wedge \\ hasMedicationSubstance(?med, ?x) & \wedge & DrugAllergy(?dga) \wedge \\ hasReactionSubstance(?ar, ?y) & \wedge & causativeAgent(?dga, ?x) \wedge \\ causativeAgent(?dga, ?y) & & \\ \Longrightarrow & & \\ hasInferredAlert(?med, \text{“281647001”}) & & \end{array}$$

SNOMED terms involved:
281647001 - Adverse Reaction

Figure 35. Control flow for the chained execution of SWRL rules as an aid to decision making in antibiotic prescribing and allergy detection

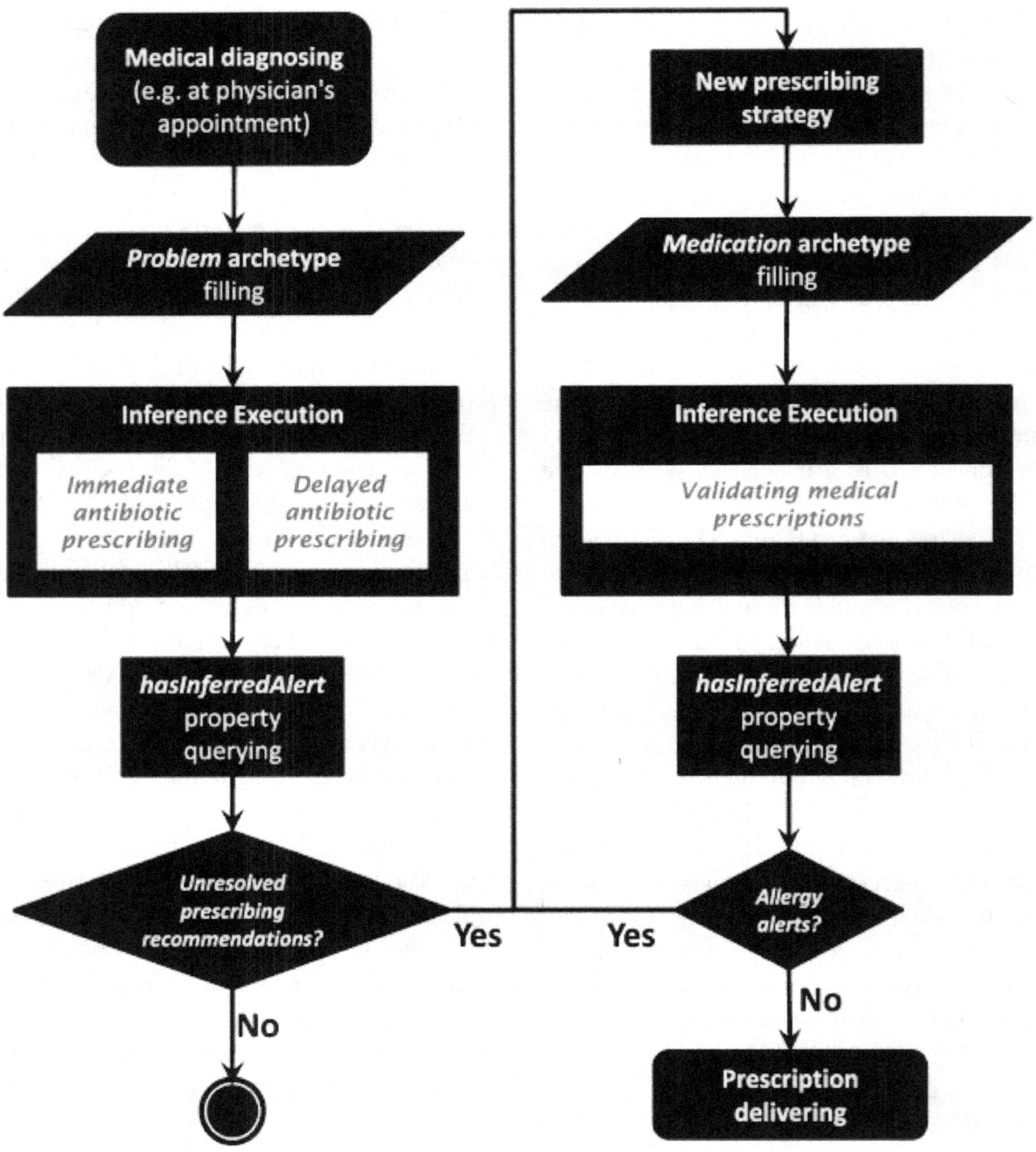

tested for pressure ulcer prevention. Section 7.2.1 describes the archetype and clinical rules integration that was undertaken in such pilot service.

7.2.1 The Pilot Service for Pressure Ulcer Prevention

A clinical guideline for pressure ulcer risk assessment and prevention has been published by NICE[77]. According to the guideline, treatment and care should take into account patients' individual needs and preferences. In addition, a good communication is essential to properly asses several risk factors. The *Fuenlabrada Hospital* has defined the *Norton* archetype as an OBSERVATION, in order to keep track of five risk factors that must be considered when assessing the pressure ulcer risk. The risk factors are: *Activity*, *Incontinence*, *Mobility*, *Mental Condition* and *Physical Condition*. A level of risk (*integer*) is assigned to each one of them in a way that the higher the value, the better the status. It was translated to OWL according to the translation principles described in Section 4 and the implementation in Section 4.7, in order to attach it SWRL rules. In this manner, a significant part of the evaluation of the data contained in the *Norton* archetype is automatically inferred. Satisfactory results were gathered from the first tests, so subsequent goals included the adjustment of the inference execution frequencies in order to maximize patients' safety within an affordable processing power.

The *Total Points* ELEMENT (at0031) in the Norton archetype is a DV_COUNT designed to store the sum of the five risk factors values. The risk assessment rules are based on the value of this ELEMENT. If the archetype instance is completed without filling the *Total Points* ELEMENT, then the linker rule shown in Figure 36 can fill it. Although some approaches could give more weights to some risk factors than others, in the implemented pilot service the weight distribution was homogeneous.

It should be noted that the linker rule in Figure 36 depends in turn on several linker rules that fill each risk factor property (i.e., *hasActivity*, *hasMobility*, etc.). Then three clinical rules are defined to make the automatic assessment of pressure ulcer risk. Allowed values for the risk are: *"none"*, *"high"*, *"very high"*. The SWRL rules representing the guideline are shown in Figure 37. The resulting OWL ontology, enriched with inferred knowledge, provide means for automatically

Figure 36. Linker rule to fill the Total Points ELEMENT

$$
\begin{aligned}
Patient(?pat) \;&\wedge\; hasActivity(?pat, ?act) \wedge \\
hasIncontinence(?pat, ?inc) \;&\wedge\; hasMobility(?pat, ?mob) \wedge \\
hasMentalCond(?pat, ?men) \;&\wedge\; hasPhysicalCond(?pat, ?phy) \wedge \\
add(?subt1, ?act, ?inc) \;&\wedge\; add(?subt2, ?mob, ?men) \wedge \\
add(?subt3, ?subt1, ?subt2) \;&\wedge\; add(?total, ?subt3, ?phy) \\
\Longrightarrow \;& \\
& hasTotalNortonPoints(?pat, ?total)
\end{aligned}
$$

improve decision making and monitoring tasks on the pressure ulcer management field.

7.3 Other Current Projects and Directions

The experiences earned in the previously sketched projects are being applied in the new contexts described in this section, serving as a complement to the Future Work Section.

7.3.1 The Clinical DSS Research and Development Project

The Clinical DSS (Clinical and Social Security Decisions Support System) is a research and development project currently carried out by a consortium of private enterprises and public universities and research organisations. The main objective is to develop a set of applications to support, in first place, the integration and homogenization of the clinical data retrieved from several and heterogeneous healthcare systems. Then the set of applications must be able to react to certain clinical episodes by triggering alerts and/or making recommendations in a way that resembles a doctor's procedure when acceding and assessing current and historical EHRs. It has been structured as a cooperation project, in order to take advantage of the particular technological capabilities offered by each part.

Given that many and heterogeneous technologies and systems will meet in unique context, the highest levels of semantic interoperability (section 2.1) are required to guarantee a fast and proper development of the project. In the context of knowledge representation and inference, such interoperability is being encouraged by the *IERU* by applying the *archetypes-rules* integration approach studied in this chapter.

7.3.2 Diagnosing the Obstructive Chronic Pulmonary Disease

The *IERU* at the University of Alcalá has recently begun to study the representation and automatic inference opportunities when diagnosing the Obstructive Pulmonary Disease (COPD)[78].

Figure 37. SWRL clinical rules for pressure ulcer risk assessment

$$\begin{aligned} Patient(?pat) \quad &\wedge \quad hasTotalNortonPoints(?pat, ?tot) \wedge \\ greaterThan(?tot, 11) \quad &\wedge \quad lessThan(?tot, 15) \\ \Longrightarrow& \\ &\quad hasNortonRisk(?pat, \text{"high"}) \end{aligned}$$

$$\begin{aligned} Patient(?pat) \quad &\wedge \quad hasTotalNortonPoints(?pat, ?tot) \wedge \\ greaterThan(?tot, 4) \quad &\wedge \quad lessThan(?tot, 12) \\ \Longrightarrow& \\ &\quad hasNortonRisk(?pat, \text{"very high"}) \end{aligned}$$

$$\begin{aligned} Patient(?pat) \quad &\wedge \quad hasTotalNortonPoints(?pat, ?tot) \wedge \\ greaterThan(?tot, 14) \quad & \\ \Longrightarrow& \\ &\quad hasNortonRisk(?pat, \text{"none"}) \end{aligned}$$

According to the clinical guideline for *Diagnosis, Management, and Prevention of COPD* published by GOLD[79,80], a diagnosis of COPD should be considered if any of the following indicators are present in an individual over age 40: *Dyspnea, Chronic Cough, Chronic Sputum Production* and/or history of exposure to risk factors (especially cigarette smoking). However, there is incomplete evidence that the individuals who meet these indicators necessarily progress on to develop COPD. Therefore, the diagnosis should be confirmed by a Spirometry test[81] that allows classifying the severity of COPD into four stages: *Stage I - Mild COPD, Stage II – Moderate COPD, Stage III – Severe COPD* and *Stage IV – Very Severe*. At this point, inference execution can automatically deduce such COPD stage in order to trigger the search for underlying causes and to recommend a therapy procedure according to the severity of the stage.

As in previous decision support examples, one or more archetypes are required to homogeneously represent the patient's data that will be used during inference. In this case, the openEHR archetype repository does not provide a Spirometry archetype or any other definition supporting the representation of Spirometry results. Therefore, an OBSERVATION.*spirometry* was created, in collaboration with medical experts at *Henares Teaching Hospital*. The archetype includes the *Forced Expiratory Volume in 1 Second* (FEV_1) and the ratio of FEV_1 to the *Forced Vital Capacity* (FVC), which will be used in the clinical rules in Figure 38 to infer the stage of COPD and attached it to the patient OWL instance.

It should be noted that a Stage 0 or "none" has been added to the four stages defined by GOLD, allowing to fill the *hasStageCOPD* property of every patient, regardless of being healthy or not. It should also be noted that evaluated ranges of FEV_1 have an empty intersection, so any patient can receive two different assessments at the same time. Once the stage is inferred, the appropriate therapy can be followed from the GOLD guideline.

8. CONCLUSION AND FUTURE WORK

Different approaches to support the interoperability between heterogeneous systems are currently being conceived by enterprises and researchers in the Healthcare domain. Along with that, large clinical terminologies like SNOMED-CT and information models like the one proposed by the openEHR Foundation are developed. The objective of present chapter, as stated in the introductory section, was to extend such previous efforts and to enhance the archetype approach to clinical information and knowledge representation by means of ontologies and semantic web languages, in order to support features that correspond to level 3 of SIOp between EHRs. This main objective has been successfully achieved from several angles and perspectives, defined by each one of the concrete objectives.

It has been shown that it is possible to integrate patients' data, clinical knowledge and terminologies in a way that is meaningful to computers, allowing to automatically interpret the evidence and making possible to reach significant clinical conclusions. When provided to healthcare systems, such conclusions are used to trigger alerts as well as to generate monitoring recommendations and decision making aids that considerably improve patient safety.

Concretely, archetypes have been extended with computational semantics by translating

Figure 38. SWRL rules to infer the stage of COPD according to the GOLD guidelines

$$\mathit{Patient(?pat)} \wedge \mathit{hasFEV1\_FVC\_DVQuantity(?pat, ?qratv)} \wedge \mathit{greaterThanOrEqual(?qratv, 70)} \Longrightarrow \mathit{hasStageCOPD(?pat, \text{“}none\text{”})}$$

$$\mathit{Patient(?pat)} \wedge \mathit{hasFEV1\_FVC\_DVQuantity(?pat, ?qratv)} \wedge \mathit{hasFEV1\_DVQuantity(?pat, ?gfevv)} \wedge \mathit{lessThan(?qratv, 70)} \wedge \mathit{greaterThanOrEqual(?gfevv, 80))} \Longrightarrow \mathit{hasStageCOPD(?pat, \text{“}mild\text{”})}$$

$$\mathit{Patient(?pat)} \wedge \mathit{hasFEV1\_FVC\_DVQuantity(?pat, ?qratv)} \wedge \mathit{hasFEV1\_DVQuantity(?pat, ?gfevv)} \wedge \mathit{lessThan(?qratv, 70)} \wedge \mathit{greaterThanOrEqual(?gfevv, 50))} \wedge \mathit{lessThan(?gfevv, 80)} \Longrightarrow \mathit{hasStageCOPD(?pat, \text{“}moderate\text{”})}$$

$$\mathit{Patient(?pat)} \wedge \mathit{hasFEV1\_FVC\_DVQuantity(?pat, ?qratv)} \wedge \mathit{hasFEV1\_DVQuantity(?pat, ?gfevv)} \wedge \mathit{lessThan(?qratv, 70)} \wedge \mathit{greaterThanOrEqual(?gfevv, 30))} \wedge \mathit{lessThan(?gfevv, 50)} \Longrightarrow \mathit{hasStageCOPD(?pat, \text{“}severe\text{”})}$$

$$\mathit{Patient(?pat)} \wedge \mathit{hasFEV1\_FVC\_DVQuantity(?pat, ?qratv)} \wedge \mathit{hasFEV1\_DVQuantity(?pat, ?gfevv)} \wedge \mathit{lessThan(?qratv, 70)} \wedge \mathit{lessThan(?gfevv, 30)} \Longrightarrow \mathit{hasStageCOPD(?pat, \text{“}very\_severe\text{”})}$$

them into OWL. A translation method was devised to accomplish this task automatically. The principles for the ADL to OWL translation were explained in Section 4. They were initially designed considering the expressiveness of OWL 1.o. However, the OWL 2 new features like Qualified Cardinality Restrictions allowed improving the translation method which is now easier to implement as roundabout workarounds are reduced. It should be noted that, apart from being the first step towards clinical rules support and the rest of explained applications, the translation of the ADL semantic and syntactic constraints to OWL restrictions is itself a source of new opportunities for checking logical coherence and validating mechanisms that arises from the inference capabilities of semantic reasoners.

According to the requirements of the clinical research projects described in Section 7, the translations principles were implemented for the first purpose of translating the OBSERVATION and EVALUATION categories of archetypes (currently accounting for roughly 70% of the openEHR repository). After its integration as a module of the *openEHR Java Implementation Project*[82], the translation implementation is being migrated to the new *OWLAPI*[83], which is focused towards OWL 2. At the same time, the remaining subtypes of archetypes are being integrated in the implementation in order to cover the full range of possibilities of ADL. Further details about the translator implementation can be found in Section 4.7.

While archetypes foster a seamless exchange of clinical data, section 2.1 explains why it is essential to extend such effect to clinical decision support in order to achieve SIOp. This chapter proves that sharing the knowledge expressed in the form of rules is consistent with the philosophy of open sharing and decentralized development, encouraged by archetypes. The two-level approach, introduced in section 2.2, offers a great flexibility to archetype model instances without compromising the interoperability of a unique reference model. Analogously, inference rules and particularly SWRL clinical rules can be specified by means of previously agreed archetypes expressed in OWL. The feasibility of taking advantages from such analogy is studied in Section 5, with emphasis on the integration of clinical guidelines.

When translated to OWL, archetypes' definitions can be enriched with SWRL rules and solve the ADL's lack of support for introducing inference content in the definition of archetypes. Any compatible reasoner can then execute the inference and produce data for different purposes. For many years, hospitals and healthcare providers have given very little or no importance at all to interoperability issues when designing their decision support systems. This chapter can be considered as part of a global scale movement towards convincing the entire health community to modify that behaviour. If healthcare systems remain isolated, then the good practice expressed through clinical guidelines and pathways will continue to require up to twenty years to be adopted by the profession as a whole, even when evidence on its favour is unequivocal. The research described in sections 5 and 7 shows that having inference mechanisms and descriptive knowledge combined under the same syntactic structure provides means for the interoperability of rule systems.

The archetypes and SWRL integration has been successfully evaluated in the research projects briefed in Section 7. The collaboration of teaching hospitals like the *Fuenlabrada Hospital* and the *Henares Hospital* has provided the opportunity to test this approach with real clinical data. Technical details of patient's data instantiation and inference execution are given for the *Transverse Sinus Ligation* case study described in section 5.2, and a graphic workflow description of the general *ArchOnt* framework is provided in Figure 19. Although the rest of rules were tested in slightly different environments, it should be noted that they are defined in terms of archetype elements, so they are totally independent of the underlying architecture.

In fact, once the SWRL rules are bound to the OWL version of the archetype, their proper execution only depends on the support provided by the selected reasoner (e.g. Pellet or Jess). Rules can be executed individually, but substantial results come from forward chaining reasoning and rules concatenation as the *Prescription Validation and Allergy Detection* case study illustrated in section 7.1.1. With regard to the limitations of the inference process, there is no specific restriction for this OWL and SWRL integration. Thus, inference boundaries are imposed by the language itself and the reasoner (e.g. the creation of new named individuals and the use of complex mathematical functions, as fractal functions or exponential sums, which are not currently supported by SWRL).

In addition to the value added by the inference capabilities, this research explored a way to have archetypes and SNOMED-CT working together through the OWL interface. The SemanticHEALTH report (Stroetmann et al., 2009) claims that in order to achieve the overall objective of SIOp, it is imperative that both methodologies and tools are developed with the aim of binding terminologies, EHRs and decision support. As a result, Section 6 illustrates a series of benefits from the mappings between archetype concepts and SNOMED-CT terms when establishing semantic OWL connections. This includes improving navigability between clinical ontologies, checking representation correctness and supporting clinical knowledge integration. Nevertheless, offering an OWL environment that provides resources to consistently bind archetypes and clinical terminologies is not enough to guarantee the efficiency of this mapping approach. The success also depends on the quality and accuracy of data mapping to terminology codes, which is still controversial, as stated by Qamar, Kola, and Rector (2008).

A long road is still ahead of us in the way to full semantic interoperability. It involves such a large number of changes at both the technical and use case level that only a gradual emergence can be achieved in the best scenario. This chapter has presented a bottom-up approach that supports further development of concrete applications. They should be first implemented in areas of clinical practice that are known to be of high patient safety risk, as well as in priority areas for which the evidence is strongest for a gap to be bridged between current and good practice. The ADL to OWL translation and the rules integration approach constitute a first step toward several semantic tasks related to clinical archetypes that will be addressed as a continuation of this chapter. In addition to the projects mentioned in section 7.3, the most significant are introduced here below.

8.1 Sharing Archetypes as Linked Data

Linked Data is about using Web technologies to create typed links between data from different sources[84]. The OWL representation of clinical archetypes provides the basic semantic web capabilities which are required to link them with other data sources. For example, every element in an archetype can be expressed as a URI. The benefits of Linked Data for clinical archetypes and SIOp include: reducing redundancy, overlapping detection and enabling network effects to add value to data. Having most important repositories and archetype sources linked by this mechanism provides the means to answer queries like: "Is there any archetype definition in any repository related to *Lung Cancer*?" or "Which overlaps are there between archetype repository A1 and A2?"

The first step in order to meet above mentioned benefits will be the implementation of a mechanism to allow clinical archetypes to fulfil the four rules of Linked Data, defined by Berners-Lee (2006). Then, the overall planned architecture will include a RDF triple store like the one provided by the Jena framework[85] that will be feed by the ADL to OWL translation mechanism presented in this chapter. ADL archetypes can be retrieved by a query client from archetypes stores and repositories. Once in the triple store, the RDF representation of archetypes can be shared by an RDF server like Joseki[86] that provides and HTTP interface that fully support SPARQL querying. Finally, this will allow a linked data frontend like Pubby[87] to provide dereferenceable URIs by rewriting the ones found in the SPARQL exposed dataset into the Pubby server's namespace. Such data can be then accessed by a wide variety of existing RDF browsers like Disco[88] or the OpenLink RDF Browser[89], RDF crawlers (e.g. SWSE[90]) and query agents (e.g. SemWeb Client Library[91], SWIC[92]).

8.2 Implementing Clinical Guidelines and Managing Archetypes

Several process models have been elaborated to provide support for the specifics of processes in healthcare (Fox, Alabassi, Patkar, Rose, & Black, 2006), and particularly to support clinical guidelines (Sutton & Fox, 2003; Mulyar, van der Aalst, & Peleg, 2007). However, Isern and Moreno (2008) offer an analysis and a comparison of eight systems that allow the enactment of clinical guidelines in a (semi) automatic fashion. That analysis concluded that further work is required to integrate such languages in existing healthcare information systems.

Therefore, the research to combine archetypes, ontologies and rules described sections 5, 6 and 7 will continue to study how clinical archetypes can be used to bridge existing process models and integrate process languages like GLIF in order to encourage full integration of clinical guidelines with the existing healthcare information systems. In this sense, the Map of Medicine[93] may be a very useful source of clinical knowledge as it provides a homogeneous and precise representation of many clinical guidelines.

On the other hand, there is an increasing archetype specification activity that raises the need for techniques to associate archetypes looking for better management and user navigation in archetype repositories. Different computational techniques will be explored in order to generate associations between the OWL version of archetypes, for example, by mapping them to clinical ontologies. A first approach based on mappings to term clusters obtained from the UMLS Metathesaurus is already published by Lezcano et al. (2010).

REFERENCES

Argüello, M., & Des, J. J. (2008). Clinical practice guidelines: A case study of combining OWL-S, OWL, and SWRL. *Knowledge-Based Systems*, *21*(3), 247–255. doi:10.1016/j.knosys.2007.11.008

Ashburner, M., Ball, C. A., Blake, J. A., Botstein, D., Butler, H., & Cherry, J. M. etal. (2000). Gene ontology: Tool for the unification of biology. *Nature Genetics*, *25*(1), 25–29. doi:10.1038/75556 PMID:10802651

Aspden, P. (2004). *Patient safety: Achieving a new standard for care. Committee on Data Standards for Patient Safety, Institute of Medicine*. U.S.: National Academies Press.

Baader, F., Calvanese, D., McGuinness, D., Nardi, D., & Patel-Schneider, P. (2003). *The description logic handbook: Theory, implementation, and applications*. New York, NY: Cambridge University Press.

Bail, S., Parsia, B., & Sattler, U. (2010). JustBench: A framework for OWL benchmarking. *The Semantic Web–ISWC*, *2010*, 32–47.

Bangalore, A., Thorn, K. E., Tilley, C., & Peters, L. (2003). The UMLS knowledge source server: An object model for delivering UMLS data. *AMIA Annual Symposium Proceedings 2003* (Vol. 2003, pp. 51-55). Presented at the AMIA Annual Symposium.

Beale, T. (1999). The GEHR software architecture for a reliable EHR. *Toward an Electronic Health Record Europe, 99*, 328–339.

Beale, T. (2002). Archetypes, constraint–based domain models for future–proof information systems. In *Proceedings of the OOPSLA 2002 Conference* (pp. 16–32). Seattle, WA: Northeastern University, Boston.

Beale, T. (2007). *The openEHR archetype object model*. The openEHR Foundation.

Beale, T., & Heard, S. (2007). *Archetype definitions and principles*. The openEHR Foundation. Retrieved from http://www.openehr.org/releases/1.0.2/architecture/am/archetype_principles.pdf

Beale, T., & Heard, S. (2008a). *openEHR architecture overview*. The openEHR Foundation. Retrieved from http://www.openehr.org/releases/1.0.2/architecture/overview.pdf

Beale, T., & Heard, S. (2008b). *The openEHR archetype definition language*. The openEHR Foundation. Retrieved from http://www.openehr.org/releases/1.0.2/architecture/am/adl.pdf

Beale, T., Heard, S., Kalra, D., & Lloyd, D. (2008). *The openEHR EHR information model*. The openEHR Foundation. Retrieved from http://www.openehr.org/releases/1.0.2/architecture/rm/ehr_im.pdf

Beale, T., Heard, S., Kalra, D., Lloyd, D., & Schloeffel, P. (2006). *Introducing openEHR* (No. Technical Report 1.1). The openEHR Foundation.

Berners-Lee, T. B. (2006). *Linked data*. Retrieved February 15, 2011, from http://www.w3.org/DesignIssues/LinkedData.html

Berners-Lee, T. B., Hendler, J., & Lassila, O. (2001). The semantic web. *Scientific American*, *284*(5), 34–43. doi:10.1038/scientificamerican0501-34 PMID:11396337

Bicer, V., Kilic, O., Dogac, A., & Laleci, G. B. (2005). Archetype-based semantic interoperability of web service messages in the health care domain. *International Journal on Semantic Web and Information Systems*, *1*(4), 1–23. doi:10.4018/jswis.2005100101

Bodenreider, O. (2004). The Unified Medical Language System (UMLS), integrating biomedical terminology. *Nucleic Acids Research*, *32*(90001), 267D–270. doi:10.1093/nar/gkh061 PMID:14681409

Carroll, J. J., & Pan, J. Z. (2006). *XML schema datatypes in RDF and OWL (No. Note NOTE-swbp-xsch-datatypes-20060314)*. World Wide Web Consortium.

Chen, C., Chen, K., Hsu, C. Y., & Li, Y. C. (2010). Developing guideline-based decision support systems using protégé and jess. Computer Methods and Programs in Biomedicine. In Press, Corrected Proof. doi: doi:10.1016/j.cmpb.2010.05.010

Chen, R., & Klein, G. (2007). The openEHR Java reference implementation project. *Studies in Health Technology and Informatics*, *129*(1), 58–62. PMID:17911678

Christiaens, S. 2006. Metadata mechanisms: From ontology to folksonomy..., & back. In OTM Workshops (1), 199-207.

Coiera, E. 1997. *Guide to Medical informatics, the Internet and telemedicine* (1st ed.). A Hodder Arnold Publication, January 15.

Collen, M. F., Van Brunt, E. E., & Davis, L. S. (1976). Problems of computerization of large computer medical record systems. *Informatics for Health & Social Care*, *1*(1), 47–53. doi:10.3109/14639237609017803

Cormen, T. H., Leiserson, C. E., Rivest, R. L., & Stein, C. (1990). *Introduction to algorithms*. NEw York: McGraw-Hill Companies.

Day, J. D., Fukushima, T., & Giannotta, S. L. (1997). Cranial base approaches to posterior circulation aneurysms. *Journal of Neurosurgery*, *87*(4), 544–554. doi:10.3171/jns.1997.87.4.0544 PMID:9322845

Dogac, A., Laleci, G. B., Kirbas, S., Kabak, Y., Sinir, S. S., Yildiz, A., & Gurcan, Y. (2006). Artemis: Deploying semantically enriched Web services in the healthcare domain. *Information Systems*, *31*(4-5), 321–339. doi:10.1016/j.is.2005.02.006

Drummond, N., Rector, A. L., Stevens, R., Moulton, G., Horridge, M., Wang, H., & Seidenberg, J. (2006). Putting OWL in order: Patterns for sequences in OWL. In *Proc. 2nd Workshop on OWL: Experiences and Directions*.

Field, M. J., & Lohr, K. N. (1990). Attributes of good practice guidelines. In *Clinical Practice Guidelines: Directions for a New Program* (pp. 53–77). Washington, DC: The National Academy Press.

Forrey, A. W., McDonald, C. J., DeMoor, G., Huff, S. M., Leavelle, D., & Leland, D. etal. (1996). Logical observation identifier names and codes (LOINC) database: A public use set of codes and names for electronic reporting of clinical laboratory test results. *Clinical Chemistry*, *42*(1), 81–90. PMID:8565239

Fox, J., Alabassi, A., Patkar, V., Rose, T., & Black, E. (2006). An ontological approach to modelling tasks and goals. *Computers in Biology and Medicine*, *36*(7-8), 837–856. doi:10.1016/j.compbiomed.2005.04.011 PMID:16169546

Garde, S., Knaup, P., Hovenga, E. J. S., & Heard, S. (2007). Towards semantic interoperability for electronic health records: Domain knowledge governance for openEHR archetypes. *Methods of Information in Medicine*, *46*(3), 332–343. PMID:17492120

Girosi, F., Meili, R., & Scoville, R. P. (2005). *Extrapolating evidence of health information technology savings and costs*. Santa Monica, CA: Rand Corporation.

Golbreich, C., & Imai, A. (2004). Combining SWRL rules and OWL ontologies with Protégé OWL Plugin, Jess, and Racer. In *Proceedings of 7th International Protégé Conference*. Bethesda. Retrieved from http://protege.stanford.edu/conference/2004/abstracts/Golbreich.pdf

Grimson, J., Grimson, W., Berry, D., Stephens, G., Felton, E., Kalra, D., Toussaint, P., et al. (1998). A CORBA-based integration of distributed electronic healthcare records using the synapses approach. *IEEE Transactions on Information Technology in Biomedicine: A Publication of the IEEE Engineering in Medicine and Biology Society, 2*(3), 124-138.

Grimson, W., Berry, D., Grimson, J., Stephens, G., Felton, E., Given, P., & O'Moore, R. (1998). Federated healthcare record server–The Synapses paradigm. *International Journal of Medical Informatics*, *52*(1-3), 3–27. doi:10.1016/S1386-5056(98)00121-X PMID:9848399

Gruber, T. R. (1993). A translation approach to portable ontology specifications. *Knowledge Acquisition*, *5*(2), 199–220. doi:10.1006/knac.1993.1008

Gruber, T. R. (2009). Ontology. In L. Liu & T. Özsu, (Eds.), *Encyclopedia of database systems*. Retrieved from http://tomgruber.org/writing/ontology-definition-2007.htm

Guha, R., McCool, R., & Miller, E. (2003). *Semantic search*. Paper presented at the Twelfth International World Wide Web Conference, Budapest, Hungary.

Heard, S. (2000). The Good electronic health record: Trial of a standard healthcare record in Australian general practice. *British Journal of Healthcare Computing and Information Management, 17*(1), 24–26.

Heiler, S. (1995). Semantic interoperability. *ACM Comput. Surv., 27*(2), 271–273. doi:http://doi.acm.org/10.1145/210376.210392

Horridge, M. (2009). *A practical guide to building OWL ontologies using Protégé 4 and CO-ODE Tools*. The University Of Manchester. Retrieved from http://owl.cs.manchester.ac.uk/tutorials/protegeowltutorial/resources/ProtegeOWLTutorialP4_v1_2.pdf

Horrocks, I., Patel-Schneider, P. F., Bechhofer, S., & Tsarkov, D. (2005). OWL Rules: A Proposal and Prototype Implementation. *Journal of Web Semantics, 3*, 23–40. doi:10.1.1.65.9856

Hwang, S.-K., Gwak, H.-S., Paek, S.-H., Kim, D.-G., & Jung, H.-W. (2004). Guidelines for the Ligation of the sigmoid or transverse sinus during large petroclival meningioma surgery. *Skull Base, 14*(1), 21–28. doi:10.1055/s-2004-821356 PMID:16145581

Isern, D., & Moreno, A. (2008). Computer-based execution of clinical guidelines: A review. *International Journal of Medical Informatics, 77*(12), 787–808. doi:10.1016/j.ijmedinf.2008.05.010 PMID:18639485

Jiang, G., & Chute, C. G. (2009). Auditing the semantic completeness of SNOMED CT using formal concept analysis. *Journal of the American Medical Informatics Association, 16*(1), 89–102. doi:10.1197/jamia.M2541 PMID:18952949

Kalra, D. (2008). Terminologies and EHR systems. In *Toward Semantic Interoperability of EHR systems: A joint effort for Europe. Expert Workshop*. Brussels.

Kalra, D., Blobel, B., & Regensburg, G. (2007). Semantic interoperability of EHR systems. *Medical and Care Compunetics, 4*, 231. PMID:17901615

Kifer, M., Lausen, G., & Wu, J. (1995). Logical foundations of object-oriented and frame-based languages. *Journal of the ACM, 42*(4), 741–843. doi:10.1145/210332.210335

Kilic, O., Bicer, V., & Dogac, A. (2005). *Mapping archetypes to OWL* (Technical Report).

Knublauch, H. (2005). *User-defined datatypes in protégé-owl*. Retrieved from http://protege.stanford.edu/plugins/owl/xsp.html

Kuhn, I. M., Wiederhold, G., Rodnick, J. E., Ramsey-Klee, D. M., Benett, S., & Beck, D. D. (1982). *Automated ambulatory medical record systems in the US* (Report No. STAN-CS-82-928). Retrieved from ftp://reports.stanford.edu/pub/cstr/reports/cs/tr/82/928/CS-TR-82-928.pdf

Lezcano, L. (2009). A model for integrating disease and diagnosis semantics in clinical archetypes. In *Signs, symptoms and findings: Towards an ontology for clinical phenotypes (SSFW09)*. Milan, Italy. Retrieved from http://bimib.disco.unimib.it/index.php/SSFW09_Presentations

Lezcano, L., Sánchez-Alonso, S., & Sicilia, M. A. (2010). (in press). Associating clinical archetypes through UMLS metathesaurus term clusters. *Journal of Medical Systems*. doi: doi:10.1007/s10916-010-9586-9 PMID:20827566

Lezcano, L., Sicilia, M. A., & Rodríguez-Solano, C. (2011). Integrating reasoning and clinical archetypes using OWL ontologies and SWRL rules. *Journal of Biomedical Informatics*, *44*(2), 343–353. doi:10.1016/j.jbi.2010.11.005 PMID:21118725

Lezcano, L., Sicilia, M. A., & Serrano-Balazote, P. (2008). Lecture Notes in Computer Science: Vol. 5288. *Combining OpenEHR archetype definitions with SWRL rules - A translation approach. Emerging Technologies and Information Systems for the Knowledge Society* (pp. 79–87). doi:10.1007/978-3-540-87781-3_9

Lindberg, D. A., Humphreys, B. L., & McCray, A. T. (1993). The unified medical language system. *Methods of Information in Medicine*, *32*(4), 281–291. PMID:8412823

Lowe, H. J., & Barnett, G. O. (1994). Understanding and Using the Medical Subject Headings (MeSH) vocabulary to perform literature searches. *Journal of the American Medical Association*, *271*(14), 1103–1108. doi:10.1001/jama.1994.03510380059038 PMID:8151853

Loy, M., & Eckstein, R. (2002). *Java Swing*. Sebastopol, CA: O'Reilly Media, Inc.

Markwell, D., Sato, L., & Cheetham, E. (2007). Representing clinical information using SNOMED Clinical Terms with different structural information models. *KR-MED*, *2008*, 72.

Martin, J., & McClure, C. L. (1985). *Diagramming techniques for analysts and programmers*. Upper Saddle River, NJ: Prentice-Hall.

Martínez-Costa, C., Menárguez-Tortosa, M., Fernández-Breis, J. T., & Maldonado, J. A. (2009). A model-driven approach for representing clinical archetypes for Semantic Web environments. *Journal of Biomedical Informatics*, *42*(1), 150–164. doi:10.1016/j.jbi.2008.05.005 PMID:18590985

Mei, J., & Paslaru Bontas, E. (2005). Reasoning paradigms for SWRL-enabled ontologies. In *Proceedings of International Workshop on Protege with Rules*. Madrid, Spain.

Mulyar, N., van der Aalst, W. M. P., & Peleg, M. (2007). A pattern-based analysis of clinical computer-interpretable guideline modeling languages. *Journal of the American Medical Informatics Association*, *14*(6), 781–787. doi:10.1197/jamia.M2389 PMID:17712087

Nardon, F. B., & Moura, L. A. (2004). Knowledge sharing and information integration in healthcare using ontologies and deductive databases. In *Medinfo 2004: Proceedings Of THe 11th World Congress On Medical Informatics* (p. 62).

O'Connor, M., Knublauch, H., Tu, S., Grosof, B., Dean, M., Grosso, W., & Musen, M. (2005). supporting rule system interoperability on the Semantic Web with SWRL. *The Semantic Web - ISWC 2005* (pp. 974–986). Retrieved fromhttp://dx.doi.org/10.1007/11574620_69

Pan, J. Z. (2004). *Description logics: Reasoning support for the Semantic Web (PhD chapter)*. School of Computer Science, The University of Manchester.

Pan, J. Z., & Horrocks, I. (2005). OWL-Eu: Adding customised datatypes into OWL. In The Semantic Web: Research and applications (pp. 153–166). Retrieved fromhttp://dx.doi.org/ doi:10.1007/11431053_11

Pedersen, T. B., & Jensen, C. S. (1998). Research issues in clinical data warehousing. In *Proceedings of the 10th International Conference on Scientific and Statistical Database Management* (pp. 43–52).

Preston, H. (2000). Information management and technology strategy in healthcare: Local timescales and national requirements. *Information Research, 5*(3).

Pulido, J. R. G., Ruiz, M. A. G., Herrera, R., Cabello, E., Legrand, S., & Elliman, D. (2006). Ontology languages for the Semantic Web: A never completely updated review. *Knowledge-Based Systems, 19*(7), 489–497. doi:10.1016/j.knosys.2006.04.013

Qamar, R. (2008). *Semantic mapping of clinical model data to biomedical terminologies to facilitate interoperability (PhD chapter).* University of Manchester, Faculty of Engineering and Physical Sciences.

Qamar, R., Kola, J., & Rector, A. L. (2007). Unambiguous data modeling to ensure higher accuracy term binding to clinical terminologies. *AMIA ... Annual Symposium Proceedings / AMIA Symposium. AMIA Symposium, 2007*, 608–613. PMID:18693908

Qamar, R., Kola, J., & Rector, A. L. (2008). Interoperability of data models and terminology models: Issues with using the SNOMED CT terminology. *KR-MED*. Retrieved from http://ceur-ws.org/Vol-410/Paper09.pdf

Qamar, R., & Rector, A. L. (2007). Semantic mapping of clinical model data to biomedical terminologies to facilitate data interoperability. In *Proceedings of Health Care Computing Conference*.

Rector, A. L. (1989). Helping with a humanly impossible task: Integrating knowledge based systems into clinical care. In J. Hanmu, L. Seppo (Eds.), *Proceedings of the Second Scandinavian Conference on Artificial Intelligence SCAI-89, 89*, 560–572.

Rector, A. L. (1999). Clinical terminology: Why is it so hard? *Methods of Information in Medicine, 38*(4/5), 239–252. PMID:10805008

Rector, A. L. (2007). *Barriers, approaches and research priorities for integrating biomedical ontologies* (No. D6.1). EC-supported FP6 SA. Retrieved from http://www.semantichealth.org/DELIVERABLES/SemanticHEALTH_D6_1.pdf

Rector, A. L., Johnson, P., Tu, S., Wroe, C., & Rogers, J. (2001). Interface of Inference models with concept and medical record models. *Artificial Intelligence in Medicine* (pp. 314–323). Retrieved fromhttp://dx.doi.org/10.1007/3-540-48229-6_43

Rector, A. L., Nowlan, W. A., Kay, S., Goble, C. A., & Howkins, T. J. (1993). A framework for modelling the electronic medical record. *Methods of Information in Medicine, 32*(2), 109–119. PMID:8321129

Rector, A. L., Qamar, R., & Marley, T. (2009). Binding ontologies and coding systems to electronic health records and messages. *Applied Ontology, 4*(1), 51–69.

Rector, A. L., Rogers, J. E., Zanstra, P. E., & Van Der Haring, E. (2003). OpenGALEN: Open source medical terminology and tools. In *AMIA Annual Symposium Proceedings 2003* (Vol. 2003). Presented at the AMIA Annual Symposium.

Rector, A. L., & Schreiber, G. (2005). *Qualified cardinality restrictions: Constraining the number of values of a particular type for a property*. Retrieved from http://www.w3.org/2001/sw/BestPractices/OEP/QCR/

Rogne, P. (1984). Use of electronic data processing in primary health care. Experiences and thoughts after 2 years' use of a record system for physicians. *Tidsskrift for Den Norske Lægeforening: Tidsskrift for Praktisk Medicin. Ny Række*, *104*(14), 993–995.

Román, I., Roa, L. M., Reina-Tosina, J., & Madinabeitia, G. (2006). Demographic management in a federated healthcare environment. *International Journal of Medical Informatics*, *75*(9), 671–682. doi:10.1016/j.ijmedinf.2006.04.006 PMID:16766223

Rose, J. S., Fisch, B. J., Hogan, W. R., Levy, B., Marshall, P., Thomas, D. R., & Kirkley, D. (2001). Common medical terminology comes of age, Part One: Standard language improves healthcare quality. *Journal of Healthcare Information Management*, *15*(3), 307–318. PMID:11642147

Rossille, D., Laurent, J., & Burgun, A. (2005). Modelling a decision-support system for oncology using rule-based and case-based reasoning methodologies. *International Journal of Medical Informatics*, *74*(2-4), 299–306. doi:10.1016/j.ijmedinf.2004.06.005 PMID:15694636

Sánchez-Macián, A., Pastor, E., Vergara, J. de L., & López, D. (2007). Extending SWRL to enhance mathematical support. In *Web Reasoning and Rule Systems* (pp. 358–360). Retrieved from. doi:10.1007/978-3-540-72982-2_30

Schloeffel, P., Beale, T., Hayworth, G., Heard, S., & Leslie, H. (2006). The relationship between CEN 13606, HL7, and openEHR. In *Proceedings of HIC 2006 Bridging the Digital Divide: Clinician, consumer and computer*. Seattle, WA.

Schulz, S., & Hahn, U. (2005). Part-whole representation and reasoning in formal biomedical ontologies. *Artificial Intelligence in Medicine*, *34*(3), 179–200. doi:10.1016/j.artmed.2004.11.005 PMID:15993045

Schulz, S., Suntisrivaraporn, B., Baader, F., & Boeker, M. (2009). SNOMED reaching its adolescence: Ontologists and logicians health check. *International Journal of Medical Informatics*, *78*, S86–S94. doi:10.1016/j.ijmedinf.2008.06.004 PMID:18789754

Sheth, A. P. (1999). 0 changing focus on interoperability in information systems: From system, syntax, structure to semantics. In *Interoperating Geographic Information Systems* (pp. 5–29). Norwell, MA: Kluwer. doi:10.1007/978-1-4615-5189-8_2

Sirin, E., Parsia, B., Grau, B. C., Kalyanpur, A., & Katz, Y. (2007). Pellet: A practical owl-dl reasoner. *Web Semantics: Science. Services and Agents on the World Wide Web*, *5*(2), 51–53. doi:10.1016/j.websem.2007.03.004

Smith, B. (2006). From concepts to clinical reality: An essay on the benchmarking of biomedical terminologies. *Journal of Biomedical Informatics*, *39*(3), 288–298. doi:10.1016/j.jbi.2005.09.005 PMID:16293444

Smith, B., & Ceusters, W. (2005). An ontology-based methodology for the migration of biomedical terminologies to electronic health records. *AMIA ... Annual Symposium Proceedings / AMIA Symposium. AMIA Symposium*, *2005*, 704–708. PMID:16779131

Spetzler, R. F., Daspit, C. P., & Pappas, C. T. (1992). The combined supra- and infratentorial approach for lesions of the petrous and clival regions: Experience with 46 cases. *Journal of Neurosurgery*, *76*(4), 588–599. doi:10.3171/jns.1992.76.4.0588 PMID:1545251

Stroetmann, V. N., Kalra, D., Lewalle, P., Rodrigues, J. M., Stroetmann, K. A., & Surjan, G. etal. (2009). *Semantic interoperability for better health and safer healthcare (Project report)*. Luxembourg: Office for Official Publications of the European Communities: European Commission.

Sutton, D. R., & Fox, J. (2003). The syntax and semantics of the PROforma guideline modeling language. *Journal of the American Medical Informatics Association*, *10*(5), 433. doi:10.1197/jamia.M1264 PMID:12807812

Tu, S. W., Bodenreider, O., Çelik, C., Chute, C. G., Heard, S., Jakob, R., et al. (2010). *A content model for the ICD-11 revision* (Technical Report BMIR-2010-1405). Stanford Center for Biomedical Informatics Research.

Tzitzikas, Y. T. (2002, September). *Collaborative ontology-based information indexing and retrieval* (PhD chapter). Department of Computer Science, University of Crete.

Walker, J., Pan, E., Johnston, D., Adler-Milstein, J., Bates, D. W., & Middleton, B. (2005). The value of health care information exchange and interoperability. *Health Affairs*. doi:10.1377/hlthaff.w5.10 PMID:15659453

Wroe, C. (2006). Is Semantic Web technology ready for healthcare? In *3rd European Semantic Web Conference (ESWC'06)*. Budva, Montenegro. Retrieved from http://ftp.informatik.rwth-aachen.de/Publications/CEUR-WS/Vol-194/paper2.pdf

ENDNOTES

1. These concepts are introduced in further sections of the Background.
2. http://www.openehr.org
3. http://www.cen.eu
4. http://www.cen.eu/cen/Sectors/Sectors/ISSS/Committees
5. http://www.iso.org
6. http://openehr.org/knowledge/
7. http://openehr.org/knowledge/
8. http://www.openehr.org/releases/1.0.2/architecture/am/archetype_principles.pdf
9. http://www.uml.org/
10. http://www.openehr.org/projects/java.html
11. http://www.openehr.org/svn/ref_impl_java/SANDBOX/ehr2ont/
12. http://semanticweb.org
13. http://www.obofoundry.org
14. http://bioontology.org
15. http://www.w3.org/TR/owl-overview/
16. http://protege.stanford.edu/
17. http://protege.stanford.edu/plugins/owl/api/
18. http://owlapi.sourceforge.net
19. http://www.w3.org/TR/owl2-overview
20. http://www.w3.org/Submission/SWRL
21. http://www.ruleml.org
22. NICE - National Institute for Health and Clinical Excellence
23. http://guidance.nice.org.uk/CG29/
24. CVD - Cardiovascular disease
25. http://www.nhlbi.nih.gov/guidelines/hypertension/jncintro.htm
26. COPD - Chronic Obstructive Pulmonary Disease
27. http://www.goldcopd.com/guidelinesresources.asp
28. http://www.ihtsdo.org/snomed-ct/
29. http://www.ihtsdo.org/members/spain/

30 http://www.opengalen.org/

31 http://www.who.int/classifications/icd/en/

32 http://www.nlm.nih.gov/research/umls/rxnorm/

33 http://medical.nema.org/

34 http://sig.biostr.washington.edu/projects/fm/

35 http://bioportal.bioontology.org/

36 http://www.radlex.org/

37 http://openehr.org/knowledge/

38 The *Guideline Interchange Format (GLIF)* is a computer-interpretable language for modelling and executing clinical practice guidelines. GLIF supports sharing of computer-interpretable clinical guidelines across different medical institutions and system platforms. GLIF has a formal representation. It defines an ontology for representing guidelines, as well as a medical ontology for representing medical data and concepts. Tools are under development to support guideline authoring and execution. http://mis.hevra.haifa.ac.il/~morpeleg/Intermed/

39 http://www.w3.org/TR/2009/REC-owl2-syntax-20091027/#Annotation_Properties

40 A restriction containing an *owl:cardinality* constraint describes a class of all individuals that have exactly ***N*** semantically distinct values (individuals or data values) for the property concerned, where ***N*** is the value of the cardinality constraint. http://www.w3.org/TR/owl-ref/#cardinality-def

41 A restriction containing an *owl:hasValue* constraint describes a class of all individuals for which the property concerned has at least one value semantically equal to a given *individual* or a *data value* (it may have other values as well). http://www.w3.org/TR/owl-ref/#hasValue-def

42 http://www.w3.org/TR/xmlschema-2/

43 http://www.w3.org/TR/owl2-syntax/#Real_Numbers.2C_Decimal_Numbers.2C_and_Integers

44 The ADL Validity Rules describe formal and checkable semantics of archetypes. It is recommended that parsing tools use the identifiers published here in their error messages, as an aid to archetype designers.

45 *Anonymous* classes or *unnamed* classes are described by a restriction. Hence the anonymous class contains all of the individuals that satisfy that restriction, (Horridge, 2009).

46 While OWL 1 allows for restrictions on the number of instances of a property, e.g., for defining persons that have at least three children, it does not provide a means to restrain the class or data range of the instances to be counted (*qualified cardinality restrictions*), e.g., for specifying the class of persons that have at least three children who are girls. In OWL 2, both qualified and unqualified cardinality restrictions are possible. http://www.w3.org/TR/owl2-new-features/

47 http://www.w3.org/TR/owl-ref/#EnumeratedDatatype

48 http://www.w3.org/TR/xmlschema-2/

49 http://www.w3.org/TR/rdf-schema/#ch_literal

50 http://www.w3.org/TR/rdf-concepts/#section-Literals

51 Not all partial Date/Times are supported by the W3C XML Schema

52 A workaround for OWL 1.0 implementations is described in section 4.3

53 http://www.openehr.org/projects/java.html

54 http://www.openehr.org/svn/ref_impl_java/SANDBOX/ehr2ont/

55 http://jena.sourceforge.net/

56 http://www.w3.org/Submission/SWRL/swrl.owl

57 http://www.jessrules.com/

58 http://clarkparsia.com/pellet/

59 http://www.w3.org/TR/owl-ref/#equivalentClass-def

60 http://www.co-ode.org/downloads/owlviz/

61 In OpenGALEN, there are also two different terms *HerpesSimplexVirus* and *HerpesSimplexInfection*

62 http://code.google.com/p/ogms/

63 The OWL version of OGMS can be downloaded from http://ogms.googlecode.com/svn/releases/2011-02-21/ontology/ogms.owl

64 http://www.openehr.org/projects/java.html

65 http://www.openehr.org/shared-resources/usage/academic.html

66 http://www.openehr.org/clinicalmodels/archedgroup.html

67 http://www.madrid.org/cs/Satellite?pagename=HospitalFuenlabrada/Page/HFLA_home

68 http://www.ieru.org/

69 http://www.madrid.org/cs/Satellite?pagename=HospitalHenares/Page/HHEN_home

70 http://www.alamoconsulting.com/

71 Clinical Decision Support System

72 http://guidance.nice.org.uk/CG69/

73 http://openehr.org/knowledge/

74 The *SWRL-FOL* extends SWRL by adding the standard logical connectives such as negation and disjunction from first order logic in spite of the fact that their addition may complicate the language semantics,http://www.w3.org/Submission/2005/SUBM-SWRL-FOL-20050411/

75 http://www.madrid.org/cs/Satellite?pagename=HospitalFuenlabrada/Page/HFLA_home

76 iSOCO was founded in 1999 as a spin-off by the Spanish National Research Council, with the idea to put academic investigation on the market. http://www.isoco.com/

77 http://guidance.nice.org.uk/CG29/

78 COPD is a preventable and treatable disease with some significant extrapulmonary effects that may contribute to the severity in individual patients. Its pulmonary component is characterized by airflow limitation that is no fully reversible. The airflow limitation is usually progressive and associated with an abnormal inflammatory response of the lung to noxious particles of gases.

79 GOLD - Global Initiative for Chronic Obstructive Lung Disease

80 http://www.goldcopd.com/guidelinesresources.asp

81 The Spirometry test measures the amount of air a person can breathe out, and the amount of time taken to do so.

82 http://www.openehr.org/projects/java.html

83 http://owlapi.sourceforge.net/

84 http://linkeddata.org/

85 http://jena.sourceforge.net/

86 http://www.joseki.org/

87 http://www4.wiwiss.fu-berlin.de/pubby/

88 http://www4.wiwiss.fu-berlin.de/bizer/ng4j/disco/

89 http://linkeddata.uriburner.com/ode/

90 http://www.swse.org/

91 http://www4.wiwiss.fu-berlin.de/bizer/ng4j/semwebclient/

92 http://moustaki.org/swic/

93 The Map of Medicine is a collection of evidence-based, practice-informed care maps which connect all the knowledge and services around a clinical condition. The care maps can be customised to reflect local needs and practices by commissioners looking to devise new care pathways. http://www.mapofmedicine.com/

Chapter 6
A Formal Investigation of Semantic Interoperability of HCLS Systems

Ratnesh Sahay
Digital Enterprise Research Institute (DERI), National University of Ireland (NUI) Galway, Ireland

Antoine Zimmermann
École Nationale Supérieure des Mines, France

Ronan Fox
Avaya, Ireland

Axel Polleres
Vienna University of Economics and Business, Austria

Manfred Hauswirth
Digital Enterprise Research Institute (DERI), National University of Ireland (NUI) Galway, Ireland

ABSTRACT

Semantic interoperability facilitates Health Care and Life Sciences (HCLS) systems in connecting stakeholders at various levels as well as ensuring seamless use of healthcare resources. Their scope ranges from local to regional, national and cross-border. The use of semantics in delivering interoperable solution for HCLS systems is weakened by fact that an Ontology Based Information System (OBIS) has restrictions in modeling, aggregating, and interpreting global knowledge in conjunction with local information (e.g., policy, profiles). This chapter presents an example-scenario that shows such limitations and recognizes that enabling two key features, namely the type and scope of knowledge, within a knowledge base could enhance the overall effectiveness of an OBIS. This chapter provides the idea of separating knowledge bases in types with scope (e.g., global or local) of applicability. Then, it proposes two concrete solutions on this general notion. Finally, the chapter describes open research issues that may be of interest to knowledge system developers and broader research community.

DOI: 10.4018/978-1-4666-3000-0.ch006

INTRODUCTION

Nowadays, Health Care and Life Sciences (HCLS) systems are facing challenges to bring healthcare stakeholders together, such that healthcare resources (e.g., data, schema, and applications) are seamlessly accessed across all related domains. Knowledge and HCLS specialists have advocated the use of semantics to (1) create interlinked networks of HCLS resources and (2) overall management and integration of HCLS resources. Ontology Based Information Systems (OBISs) have recently received attention for their flexibility and automation in maintaining, updating, exchanging schemas and underlying data. This strength is due to the fact that schema and data are loosely-coupled (as compared to cohesively-weak schema and data in traditional databases) and both represented and integrated in a logical fashion. However, OBIS in its current form has limitations in dealing with the requirements imposed by heterogeneous information systems. One major limitation is its inability to distinguish between various types of knowledge used or exchanged between information systems. Additionally, knowledge expressed within any typical information system are generally tied to a context (e.g., place, event, time) and their appropriate interpretation is scoped or limited to that context.

Semantics and the reasoning mechanism behind ontological knowledge bases are centralized in the way data and schemas are accumulated and processed. Therefore, when an OBIS experience the use-cases where data, schema, and applications are heterogenous and distributed then that impedes the expected results. This limitation has roots in formalism and corresponding reasoning mechanism underlying ontology-based knowledge bases. Ontology as the symbolic layer is closest to concepts in the real world. An ontology may be defined as the specification of a representational vocabulary for a shared domain of discourse which may include definitions of classes, relations, functions and other objects (Gruber, 1993). Ontologies are good in describing general invariant concepts and mappings or relation among those concepts. When ontologies are applied for information systems, then they describe information which is attached to multiple parameters, for example, information that is local and specific to some domain, time-dependent, constraints applicable to certain domain of discourse.

This chapter discusses how to formally represent information in use in electronic health records (EHR) and related knowledge bases, where the data are distributed, heterogeneous and multi-contextual. We especially explore how existing formalisms are able to deal with the difficult issues provoked by heterogeneity in a globalized information system. To do this, we present in a plausible use case scenario where two hospitals in different countries are involved, as well as labs and clinics. This serves to identify essential issues arising in such environment. We then show that Semantic Web technologies can help solving these issues and consolidate interoperability. Yet, these technologies fail at several levels in this multi-scoped situation. Therefore, we investigate formal approaches that have been proposed on top of Semantic Web technologies to deal with these crucial aspects of world-wide knowledge base systems. As a result of this investigation, we classify the approaches according to five essential features that are meaningful to dealing with our example scenario. We conclude that no approach fully solve the issues but some can be combined to improve the overall formalism. Especially, we notice that those issues eventually amount to delimiting the *scope* and *type* of a knowledge base or its subparts. Subsequently, we detail how to define an extension of existing work to treat more appropriately the identified features. Finally, we discuss the remaining foundational problems that are still not addressed by the presented approaches but are critical to the interoperability of these systems. This way we hope to offer a roadmap and directions for future research in semantic-enabled HCLS system at Web-scale.

We start the chapter with background information about semantics in HCLS systems (Section: Semantics for HCLS). We then describe our use-case scenario (Section: Use-Case Scenario: Lab-Test Order). We show how to apply various formalisms to this scenario in four sections overviewing the state of the arts: first, we present two general theories of reasoning with context (Section: State of the Art - 1: Context Formalisms); second, we detail some instantiation of one of the model of context (Section: State of the Art - 2: Context and Constraint for OBIS); third, we present more concrete formalisms for the description of context on the Semantic Web (Section: State of the Art: 3 - Context in Semantic Web technologies); fourth, we provide other formal approaches built on top of semantic technologies that deals with the identified problems of our scenario (Section: State of the Art - 4: Other formal handling of heterogeneity). After this extensive state of the art, we provide a summary and analysis of the studied approaches (Section: Comparison of formal approaches). Then, we present our proposal for combining existing approaches to better deal with scopes and types of knowledge (Section: Towards a framework for handling context and heterogeneity). Finally, we discuss the remaining open research issues that we deem crucial to enable interoperability (Section: Towards fully interoperable HCLS systems).

BACKGROUND

Semantics for HCLS

An overwhelming amount of HCLS knowledge is represented in natural language, information models, clinical repositories (databases), ontologies for terminologies, vocabularies, etc. Additionally, the involvement of various stakeholders, such as hospitals, healthcare standards, pharmacy, patients, multiplies the integration complexity of this domain. Intelligent processing, logical aggregation of information, synthesis and analysis, and the development of knowledge systems that can serve purposeful ends are needed. HCLS has been one of the primary field of application for knowledge representation and reasoning systems. In the past researchers have tried to formalize and integrate the knowledge bases in HCLS systems and many of the successful systems in earlier times were centralized and limited to sub domain or particular application of a HCLS domain (Szolovits, 1982; Kashyap & Sheth, 1996). Current HCLS systems are much more open and available to global society where stakeholders mobility and seamless use of the overall system is of prime concern.

As discuss above, ontology based information systems (OBISs) offer greater flexibility and automation for the management and integration of very complex intertwined HCLS data and schemas. HCLS specialists increasingly argue in favor of Semantic Web technologies for representing medical and clinical knowledge (Rector, Qamar, & Marley, 2006) in a well formalized way. However, current Semantic Web technologies alone are still too limited to provide a unified framework for all the varieties of applications and sub-domains of life sciences. Also, they show their limits when integrating and exchanging data between different systems. The W3C HCLS Interest Group (IG) (W3CHCLSIG, 2005) and various research projects have taken initiatives for the ontological representation of healthcare information models and their integration with HCLS terminologies and vocabularies (Bicer, Laleci, Dogac, & Kabak, 2005; Rector, 2006; Sahay, Akhtar, & Fox, 2008; Fox, Sahay, & Hauswirth, 2008).

This integration is crucial to effectively achieve a unified-view of electronic health records (EHR). However, this approach is still facing core integration issues such as ontological heterogeneity, ambiguous separation between global and local healthcare knowledge (Jahnke, Bychkov, Dahlem, & Kawasme, 2005). For example, high level ontologies that are shared by all systems cannot describe all possible sub-domains (Berners-Lee & Kagal, 2008) that may be needed by local clinics. Therefore, they must extend common knowledge with domain ontologies, as well as define internal policies, rules and vocabularies that are specific to their context.

In conclusion, HCLS is a complex domain and any data integration system which connects healthcare institutes must facilitate heterogeneous systems at two levels (1) information model specific data, and (2) domain and/or institute specific terminologies or vocabularies. These two levels must interoperate to aggregate and exchange medical records from disparate healthcare systems. In this section we describe these two levels and explain how regional and/or local clinical practices influence the modeling of clinical data.

HCLS Information Models

An information model allows modeling of domain and/or institute specific message requirements. Health Level Seven (HL7) standard Version 3 (HL7V3, 2005) develops information model specific data standards for storing and exchanging information in the healthcare industry. HL7 is the most widely used healthcare standard and shares many semantic equivalences with other influential standards such as openEHR (Beale, 2000).

The HL7 (Version 3) information modeling process recognizes three interrelated types of information models: Reference Information Model (RIM), Domain Message Information Model (DMIM), and Refined Message Information Model (RMIM). The RIM is a unified model which covers all domains in healthcare and defines data structures, data types and vocabularies, as well as the relationships between them. DMIM is a refined subset of the RIM and is used to create messages for a particular domain (*e.g.*, Lab, Hospital Admin). RMIM is a subset of a DMIM and is used to express the information content for a message or set of messages (*e.g.*, Lab-Test Order Message). All three interrelated models use the same notation and have the same basic structure but differ from each other in their information content, scope, and intended use.

In the example scenario presented in Section: Use-Case Scenario: Lab-Test Order, Galway University Hospital (GUH) uses the ontological representation of RIM and creates local ontology using DMIM and RMIM models.

HCLS Terminologies and Vocabularies

HCLS terminologies and vocabularies (e.g., *SNOMED* [Spackman, 2008], *LOINC* [Forrey, McDonald, DeMoor, Huff, Leavelle, Leland, 1996]) describe medical concepts. When these concepts are placed in a clinical record they become associated with an observation (e.g., lab test), time (e.g., effective time), policy and profile (e.g., drug policy, patient profile), and relationships with other records. These associations influence the interpretation of the concepts (Rector & Brandt, 2008). For example, (1) a clinical observation concept (e.g., blood sugar test) has an effective time during which it is valid, and (2) a diabetic concept placed in a "family history" segment of a patient record does not imply that the individual patient is a diabetic patient.

Standard compliant patient records are constructed from the combination of messages derived from an information model and several terminologies or vocabularies referring to message attributes. On the other hand, many healthcare institutes do not use the standard specific information model, rather their messages are constructed using general models. The presence of different healthcare standards, large scale applicability, and limitations of syntactic integration solutions, motivated the healthcare specialists to apply Semantic Web technologies to resolve heterogeneity in a formal and consistent way.

HCLS information models, terminologies and vocabularies can be expressed as a set of RDF (Hayes, 2004), RDFS (Brickley & Guha, 2004) and OWL (Hitzler, Krötzsch, Parsia, Patel-Schneider & Rudolph, 2009) propositions. RDF is best for expressing medical or patient data and OWL allows more expressive propositions to be expressed, like those that represent general knowledge rather than specific patient data elements. The relationships between heterogeneous healthcare data and knowledge can be formally expressed in OWL constructs. The reasoner underlying an expressive Web language like OWL can be used to entail consistent sets of inferred knowledge about the healthcare Web resources.

Figure 1 shows the predicates (*i.e.*, RDF triples) describing relationship between information model (HL7 RIM) specific data and general *LOINC* vocabularies. The upper (HL7 RIM) RDF triple describes the lab observation (*e.g.*, blood test) for a participating patient, and lower triple (*LOINC*) is used to describe the blood pressure (BP) and physical position (*e.g.*, sitting, standing) of the patient while measuring the BP.

USE-CASE SCENARIO: LAB-TEST ORDER

The scenario describes clinical events in course of primary medical care provided to a patient suffering from acute chronic diabetes. Clinical events are recorded as a part of patient medical history where two healthcare providers, namely, hospitals, use different healthcare standards to model the electronic health records (EHRs). The scenario highlights the interoperability issues between HCLS systems due to (1) heterogeneity of data, information models, terminologies and vocabularies, and (2) inability to model and execute local, *i.e.*, context-specific, policy and profiles on a more general framework like the Semantic Web.

Background

In Galway, Ireland community clinic, Dr. Paul Smith is a primary care physician. Galway University Hospital (GUH) has a pathologi-

Figure 1. Ontologies for information model and terminologies

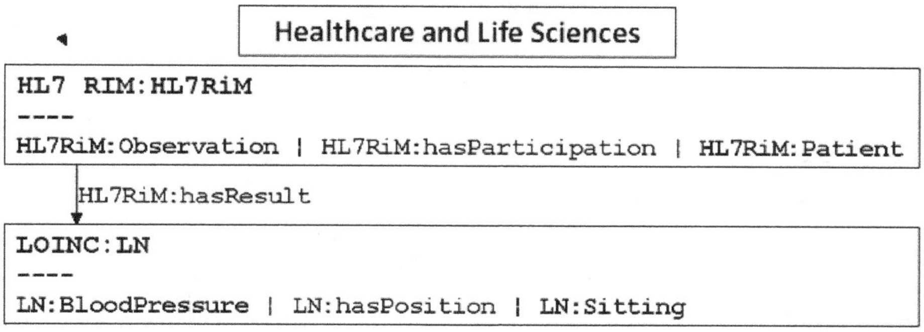

cal laboratory, which is directed by Dr. John Colleen who is responsible for approving and releasing all test results. The information system of the GUH laboratory is standard (i.e., HL7 Version 3), compliant and able to receive orders and return result reports electronically. Dr. Gustav Roth is an internal medicine physician in the City hospital, Göttingen, Germany (GOET). City hospital laboratory is directed by Dr. David Hahn and the only pathological laboratory available in Göttingen. GOET laboratory information systems use general vocabularies and terminologies for information modeling such as *GALEN* (Rector, Nowlan & Consortium, 1994), *Friend of A Friend* (*FOAF*) (Brickley & Miller, 2007), and able to send and receive lab test orders electronically.

Patient Case History 1

Dr. Paul Smith has a patient, Sean Murphy, who is examined on the 16th of July 2007 because of a poor wound healing, weight loss, and increase in urine production. Dr. Paul draws a blood sample, labels it with a bar code, and sends it to Galway University Hospital laboratory, GUH. Sean Murphy has been identified based on his Irish PPS number: 678970W. The blood sample is identified as 7854698. Dr. Paul fills out the electronic order form in his office system for a Glycosylated hemoglobin (HbA1c) test and sends it to Galway University Hospital Laboratory (GUH). Table 1 shows the summary of the lab order data.

GUH received the electronic order and returned a message accepting the order with intent to fulfill it on a routine basis. GUH Lab performs the requested HbA1c test on the 18th of July 2007, after receiving the sample. The result of the HbA1c test is 9%. The LOINC code for the hæmoglobin count is 4548-4. Dr. John reviewed the results of the HbA1c test and noticed that the blood sugar is abnormally high (normal reference range 4%-5.9%).

Dr. John authorized the results of the HbA1c lab tests with an indication that Sean's blood sugar level is abnormal high. The order was complete so a notification is sent to Dr. Paul Smith. It is important to mention that, even though GUH Lab system is HL7 Version 3 compliant and can electronically exchange information, it requires manual effort and paper work to integrate the patient observations.

Sean has been diagnosed as an acute chronic diabetic (Type 2) and that requires him to frequently test his blood sugar level. GUH has special drug-policy for diabetics (Type 2) where patients are treated with either Insulin

Table 1. Sean's lab test orders dated 16/07/2007 (GUH) and 22/12/2008 (GOET)

Items	Lab Value (GUH)	Lab Value (GOET)
Lab order requisition number	6560-89	7779-78
Specimen identifier	7854698	89756
The ordering physician	Dr. Paul Smith	Dr. Gustav Roth
Physician health identifier	68374532	6837-4532
Patient	Sean Murphy	Sean Murphy
Patient health identifier	678970W:IrishPPSId	345678IE:Drivinglicence
Patient birth date	15/07/1974	15-07-1974
Date of Lab test Order	16/07/2007	22-12-2008
Lab Test ordered	Glycosylated hemoglobin	hæmoglobin A1c
LOINC/SNOMED Lab Test Code	4548-4 (LC)	43396009 (SD)
Priority of Lab Test	Routine	Urgent

or Avandia (an insulin equivalent drug), but not both. Sean receives the Insulin therapy and any future abnormal blood sugar level will require immediate and appropriate insulin treatment for him. His nature of job demands frequent travels within Ireland and his travel constraints bring complexities whenever he is in an emergency situation. Every emergency situation requires him to visit a nearby clinic or hospital, and each clinical visit requires repetitive lab tests that may have been performed earlier. Sean original medical records are with GUH lab information system and immediate availability of Sean's medical records is crucial in emergency situation.

Patient Case History 2

On Christmas holidays, Sean went to Göttingen, Germany for a week to meet his friends. On his way back to home he had a major car accident and doctors need to operate him as soon as possible. Sean is identified based on his international driving licence number 345678IE. He had a year of medical history as an acute chronic diabetic patient and his current medical records are in Galway University Hospital (GUH) Lab and other Irish hospitals where Sean visited frequently. Coincidentally, Galway University Hospital (GUH) Lab and City hospital, Göttingen, collaborate as a part of common EU healthcare framework and they can share information. In emergency situations like this, where time is critical, the automated integration of patient data can really improve the overall quality of primary healthcare services. In this scenario, GUH and GOET lab systems are able to send and receive patient's records electronically but require manual intervention, paper work, and phone calls to make sensible understanding of medical records and Sean was running out of time. City hospital, Göttingen has decided to perform all kinds of test locally without depending on his medical history. Sean was able to speak and provided an informal description of his medical history. Dr. Gustav Roth has ordered a similar test dated back on 16/07/2007 to examine his current blood sugar level before going into any surgical treatment. GOET drug policy on type 2 diabetics does not suggest any restrictions for Avandia and Insulin treatments, and thus Dr. Roth decides to prescribe Avandia in complement of Sean's insulin treatment. Table 1 show the summary of the lab order data.

In this scenario, GUH and GOET lab systems are Semantic-Web-enabled and able to send and receive patient's records electronically. But, due to differences in their domain-specific models (local models), terminology schemes, local policy, etc. information between Galway and Göttingen hospitals cannot be integrated in automated way. Figure 2 shows a snippet of the ontologies used in GUH (left) and GOET (right). Figure 3 shows the Table 1 equivalent data described semantically, *i.e.*, RDF triples. GUH is using ontologies that are strongly influenced by HCLS current standards (*e.g.*, HL7) while GOET is using more Semantic Web oriented ontologies (*e.g.*, *GALEN*, *FOAF*) which better ensures interoperability with other Linked Data (*e.g.*, other administrative systems may take advantage of *FOAF* data). They model medical, clinical and patient knowledge using OWL, reusing well established ontologies such as *SNOMED* and *GALEN*. They extend them to represent local domain knowledge, internal policies, etc. The data, *e.g.*, the patient records, are represented in RDF. This presents a realistic situation since GUH has already been involved in a project where Semantic Web technologies were used (Sahay, Fox, & Hauswirth, 2009).

Context and Constraint for OBIS

As a mechanism for representing information, RDF (Hayes, 2004), RDFS (Brickley & Guha, 2004) and OWL (Hitzler, Krötzsch, Parsia, Patel-Schneider & Rudolph, 2009) are very general and primitive (Klyne, 2001). As discussed above, ontologies are monotonic and make an Open World Assumption (OWA). Therefore, they are good at describing general high-level invariant concepts and their mappings. In ontology-based information

Figure 2. Extract of GUH (left) and GOET (Right) ontologies. Correspondences are informally represented by dotted lines. The rectangle shows the local policy axiom.

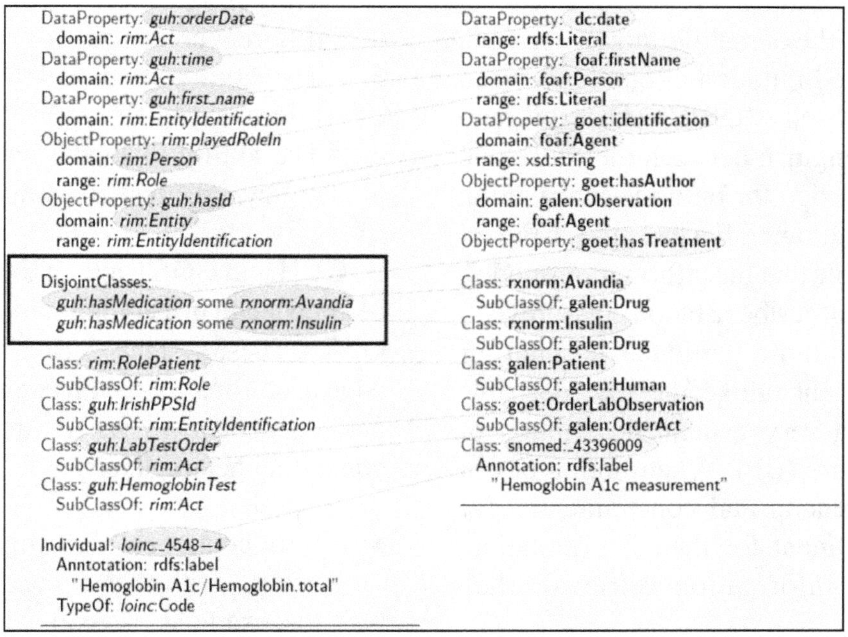

Figure 3. Extract of lab-test orders at GUH (left) and GOET (right)

```
:sean a rim:Person ;
  rim:playedRoleIn [a rim:RolePatient] ;
  guh:hasID :678970W .
:678970W a guh:IrishPPSId ;
  rdfs:label "Sean Murphy's Irish PPS number" ;
  guh:first_name "Sean" ;
  guh:last_name "Murphy" ;
  guh:hasMedication [a rxnorm:Insulin] .
:paul a rim:Person ;
  rim:playedRoleIn [a rim:RolePhysician] ;
  guh:hasID :68374532 .
:68374532 a guh:PID ;
  rdfs:label "Paul Smith's professional Id" ;
:6560-89 a guh:LabTestOrder ;
  guh:orderedBy :paul ;
  guh:hasPatient :sean ;
  guh:orderDate "2007-07-16" ;
  guh:time "13:07:07" ;
  guh:orders :Test743890 .
:Test743890 a guh:HemoglobinTest ;
  rim:effectiveTime "M0717173034" ;
  guh:specimen :7854698 ;
  guh:hasCode loinc:_4548-4 .
```

```
:345678IE a galen:Patient ;
  goet:identification "Irish Driving licence" ;
  foaf:family_name "Murphy" ;
  foaf:firstName "Sean" ;
  goet:hasTreatment [a rxnorm:Avandia] .
:6837-4532 a galen:Doctor ;
  goet:identification "Professional Id" ;
  foaf:family_name "Roth" ;
  foaf:firstName "Gustav" .
:7779-78 a goet:OrderLabObservation ;
  goet:hasAuthor :6837-4532 ;
  goet:hasPatient :345678IE ;
  galen:orders :Test777767 .
:Test777767 a galen:BloodSugarTest ;
  dc:date "2008-12-22T00:30:00" ;
  goet:hasMeasurement [a snomed:_408254005] ;
  goet:hasSpecimen :89756 .
:s89756 a galen:Specimen .
```

systems (OBIS) the knowledge engineers often encounters a situation when describing detailed relationships between physical-world objects and their mappings becomes impossible or tedious task. In traditional ontology modeling and integration approaches, it is assumed that everything is global and the local perspective of the domain is largely ignored. This shows the limitation of ontology-based information systems (OBIS) where it is necessary to distinguish between the *scope* and type of knowledge for both the information models and ontologies. For example, in Figure 1, it is noticeable that the information-model-specific triple describes a blood pressure (BP) observation within a particular hospital for a specific patient unlike the LOINC triple that provide a very general description of a blood pressure (BP). When both types of knowledge, general and constraint, receive a similar treatment for their interpretation, aggregation, information retrieval, then conflicts and inconsistency arises. From the information modeling perspective the major issues in OBIS are:

1. The ability to distinguish local and global information;
2. The ability to deal with informing from different contexts;
3. The ability to model time-dependent information;
4. The ability to model constraints (*e.g.*, policy, profiles) and validation.

GUH and GOET model the same domain of knowledge in a common format (RDF and OWL). These systems define medical knowledge according to two different contexts in a heterogeneous way. There are two levels of contextual heterogeneity:

- Intra-contextual heterogeneity, which occurs within a context. As seen in the example, several vocabularies are used for describing different types of information (*e.g.*, *RxNorm* vocabulary for drugs, *LOINC* for types of tests). Multiple terminologies must be integrated in a modular way. Local systems also have to deal with knowledge of differing natures, *e.g.*, axioms about a domain of discourse (*e.g.*, an hemoglobine test is a kind of act) and internal policy (a patient cannot be treated with both Insulin and Avandia).

- Inter-contextual heterogeneity occurs between contexts. If the terminologies are different, the systems cannot interoperate unless some relations are asserted between the domain ontologies or a translation mechanism exists. Correspondences between local ontologies are informally presented in Figure 2 using dotted lines. Besides, corresponding concepts of distinct ontologies can be modeled in very different ways. For instance, GUH here uses an object property for patient's identification, while GOET is using a datatype. Thus, systems should be able to tolerate such heterogeneity. Finally, we can see that identifying context is crucial, notably to see which policy belongs to which context.

OUTLINE OF THE STATE OF THE ART

The following sections detail the existing formal approaches that were devised to deal with the problem of heterogeneity in multi-contextual knowledge systems. In Section: State of the Art - 1: Context Formalisms, we described foundational work on modeling context, especially focusing on McCarthy's and Guha's approach on the one hand, and Giunchiglia *et al.*on the other hand. The later approach have been more successful in its adoption and led to several instantiation of the approach, that we discuss in Section: State of the Art - 2: Context and Constraint for OBIS. While these formalisms essentially focus on reasoning accross contexts or modularity, they offer a limited infrastructure for "reifying" the notion of context, describing it and constraining it. These aspects are better covered by development of Guha *et al.*'s work that we present in Section: State of the Art: 3 - Context in Semantic Web technologies. Finally, we show that other essential concerns of interoperable HCLS systems, such as modeling constraints, policies, rules, are also tackled by proposed extensions of semantic formalisms that are quite independent of the handling of heterogeneity and context.

State of the Art 1: Context Formalisms

Logic for Context

In artificial intelligence, the notion of context generally concerns the representation and use of information. The notion is used to account for phenomena such as the context of validity of information (Kleer, 1986) and the efficiency of reasoning in narrower contexts (Guha, 1991). An influential but sketchy attempt to formalize context dependency was made by John McCarthy (McCarthy, 1987). The idea was to mark the dependency of propositions on context and track this dependency through changes of context and stages of reasoning. The basic step was to move from a (simple) proposition to the (meta) proposition that the proposition in question is true in a context. The syntax for such meta-propositions was *ist(c,p)* for proposition *p* and context *c*. Contexts thus entered the theory as objects, enabling the theory to express changes of context and the effects of such changes on propositions. Changes of context typically involve making or dropping assumptions, so the syntax also allows compound, functional terms for contexts such as assuming(p, c) (the context obtained from c by assuming p). With such terms, the theory can cover logically interesting consequences of context change, expressed as ist(c, p) ⇒ ist(d, q) and similar formulas, called lifting axioms. McCarthy's ideas were later developed by others, and found their way into a working AI system (Cyc, in the form of micro-theories applied for medical domain (Lenat, 1995)). McCarthy's work made contexts as first class objects in the domain that can be quantified, be the range of functions, and so on. All this allows one to write very expressive formulae that lift axioms from one context to another. While this is very convenient, it also makes it quite difficult to provide an adequate model theory and extremely difficult to compute with (Akman & Surav, 1996).

Contextual Reasoning: Local Model Semantics

In the early nineties, a different line of thought (compared to McCarthy's and Guha's works on context) was proposed—Local Model Semantics (LMS)—by Fausto Giunchiglia (Giunchiglia, 1993; Ghidini & Giunchiglia, 2001), who argued that people do not use all of the knowledge in an attempt to solve a problem instead they construct a "local theory" where each independent theory (or context) is related to some particular domain knowledge. Giunchiglia's formalization of context is motivated by the problem of locality where the reasoning process uses only a subset of the world knowledge. Therefore, in LMS, context is a theory of the world that encodes an agent's perspective of it and that subset is used during a given reasoning process. While reasoning, the user can switch from one context to another in case the original context is not adequate to solve the problem. Giunchiglia's approach is more towards formalizing contextual reasoning than McCarthy's work of formalizing context as a first class object.

Serafini *et al.* then proposed refinements of LMS to concretely realize a distributed reasoning framework, in Section: Distributed Description Logics (DDL), we discuss those refinements, namely Distributed Description Logics (DDL) (Borgida & Serafini, 2003) and a contextualized form of OWL, called C-OWL (Bouquet, Giunchiglia, van Harmelen, Serafini, & Stuckenschmidt, 2003). For instance, DDL is an underlying formalism behind the Contextualized Web Ontology Language (C-OWL) that allows separate ontological models for a domain and correspondences between entities of different models are formalized via domain relations which are in turn used to interpret the bridge rules. Reasoning will then be carried out locally with respect to a single context and is shared only via explicitly specified connections, following the principle of locality and compatibility. Similar authors (Bouquet, Giunchiglia, van Harmelen, Serafini, & Stuckenschmidt, 2004) have attempted to align and map medical ontologies (e.g., *GALEN*, *UMLS* (Lindberg, Humphreys & McCray, 1993)) using three proposed features of contextual ontologies, *i.e.*, directionality of information, local domain, and context based ontology mappings.

State of the Art 2: Context and Constraint for OBIS

Standard Approach: OWL

The representation and reasoning of contextual knowledge is outside the scope of OWL semantics (Motik, Patel-Schneider, & Cuenca-Grau, 2009; Schneider, 2009). When reasoning is performed across different ontologies, then these ontologies share a single and global interpretation domain. The mappings between two ontologies become part of the overall model which is interpreted globally. In OWL, the ability to combine ontologies is restricted to the import of the complete ontology and to the use of the imported elements by direct reference. Thus, a set of local ontologies is globalized in a unique shared model, via the import mechanism. OWL also supports mappings constructs that implicitly exist in terms of the mutual use of statements across ontologies (*e.g.*, *subClass*, *sameAs*, *equivalentClass*, *equivalentProperty*, *differentFrom*, and *AllDifferent* axioms).

Although we have already raised some doubts in the informal discussion above on the suitability of current Semantic Web technologies with respect to heterogeneity and context, we can explore what OWL can offer to overcome these problems. This language partially addresses modularity and expressing correspondences between various ontologies.

OWL Solution

In the example scenario, several well identified terminologies are reused. OWL provides an import feature thanks to the property *owl:imports* which helps to modularly integrate several domain ontologies. By stating that the GUH ontology imports RIM and LOINC, the axioms of these ontologies are automatically made part of the GUH ontology.

In the example scenario, concepts and properties of the two hospitals are modeled differently, but correspondences can be identified and expressed in OWL. In Figure 4, we present the axioms that should be added to make the two systems interoperate. Notice that these mappings relating terms in two different contexts cannot be distinguished from mappings between terms of imported ontologies within one context.

Figure 4. Extract of OWL supported mapping definitions

Class: (**foaf:Person**) SubClassOf: (*rim:Entity*)
Class: (**galen:OrderAct**) SubClassOf: (*rim:Act*)
Class: (*rim:playedRoleIn* some *rim:RolePatient*) EquivalentTo: (**galen:Patient**)
Class: (*guh:LabTestOrder*) EquivalentTo: (**goet:OrderLabObservation**)
Class: (*guh:HemoglobinTest* and (*rim:measures* some *loinc:_4548−4*))
EquivalentTo: (**galen:BloodSugarTest** and (**goet:hasCode** some {**snomed:**_43396009}))

EquivalentProperties: (*guh:first_name*) (**foaf:firstName**)
EquivalentProperties: (*guh:hasMedication*) (**goet:hasTreatment**)

Instance: (*guh:*sean) sameAs: (**goet:**345678IE)

This approach is the only possible way of dealing with heterogeneity which fully complies with established Semantic Web standards. It has been argued that it improves interoperability of HCLS systems (Rector, 2006), when compared to previous standards in this field, such as HL7. However, these standards are clearly not enough to solve the important issues presented in Section:Use-Case Scenario.

OWL Limitations

First, while a form of modularity is offered by OWL, its import statement can only handle the reuse of full ontologies without being able to specify subparts of them. This is particularly problematic with large ontologies like *SNOMED*, which have to be fully integrated, even when only a small subdomain is needed.

Second, not all relevant mappings can be expressed in OWL. For example, (1) the *ObjectProperty* guh:hasId and the *DatatypeProperty* goet:identification are designed for a similar purpose (identify the person) but OWL semantics does not allow to map between *ObjectProperty* and *DatatypeProperty*; (2) OWL does not support operations on attributes, *e.g.*, the concatenation of two *DatatypeProperties* (*e.g.*, guh:orderDate, guh:time) into a single *DatatypeProperty* (*e.g.*, dc:date). Other examples include unit or currency conversion.

Third, OWL does not include any feature for distinguishing between universal facts (*e.g.*, a patient is a person) and local policy or profile (*e.g.*, people should not be treated with both Insulin and Avandia). Additionally, OWL does not permit identifying the context of an axiom or term. The implication of these two limitations is that policies have to be represented as DL axioms, and these axioms are affecting all contexts identically. In our scenario, according to GUH, Sean is treated with Insulin. When he goes to GOET, the record indicates that he has been given Avandia. Thanks to the aforementioned mappings, the terms *hasMedication* and *hasTreatment* can be interpreted interchangeably, so that GOET can understand GUH record automatically. But it leads to a contradiction with the GUH policy because Sean has now both treatments. Yet, it should not be the case because GOET does not have this policy, and therefore should not detect an inconsistency. Note that undesired interactions can be reduced by using subsumption instead of equivalence in mappings, but the problem remains.

Fourth, OWL is not tolerant of diverging modeling of a knowledge domain. Different points of view can equally well describe a domain of interest, while being partially incompatible. Interpreting all axioms and assertions as equally true, in all contexts, may easily lead to inconsistency or nonsensical entailments.

Distributed Description Logics (DDL)

Distributed Description Logics (DDL) (Borgida & Serafini, 2003) is a formalism which was developed to formalize contextual reasoning with Description Logic ontologies. Indices $i \in I$ are used to determine from which context an ontology or an axiom comes from. Given, for instance, an axiom $C \sqsubseteq D$ from an ontology O_i, DDL uses the prefixed notation $i{:}C \sqsubseteq D$ to highlight the context of the axiom. Moreover, cross-context formulas can be defined to relate different terminologies. These particular formulas are called bridge rules and written either $i{:}C \xrightarrow{\sqsubseteq} j{:}D$ or $i{:}C \xrightarrow{\sqsupseteq} j{:}D$ where i and j are two different contexts, and C and D are terms from the contextual ontologies O_i and

O_j respectively. A bridge rule (resp. $i{:}C \sqsupseteq,\!\rightarrow j{:}D$) should be understood as follows: from the point of view of O_j (*i.e.*, in the context j), C is a subclass (resp. superclass) of D.

In terms of model-theoretic semantics, this is formalized by assigning a distinct Description Logic interpretation I_i to each contextual ontology O_i, instead of having one single global interpretation. Thus, there is as many domains of interpretation as there are contexts.

Additionally, cross-context relations are made explicit by so-called domain relations, that is set-theoretic binary relations between each pairs of contexts (formally, $r_{ij} \subseteq \Delta^{I}_{i} \times \Delta^{I}_{j}$). Two contextual interpretations I_i and I_j satisfy a bridge rule $i{:}C \sqsubseteq,\!\rightarrow j{:}D$ (resp. $i{:}C \sqsupseteq,\!\rightarrow j{:}D$) iff $r_{ij}(C^{I}_{i}) \subseteq D^{I}_{j}$ (resp. $r_{ij}(C^{I}_{i}) \supseteq D^{I}_{j}$). The advantage of this approach is the identification of context, a better robustness with respect to heterogeneity, improved modularity. However, it still misses some of the requirements that were identified in the example-scenario.

Solution in DDL

In the scenario, ontologies would be related thanks to C-OWL (Bouquet et al., 2003) bridge rules, which instantiates DDL for the Description Logic of OWL. A P2P reasoning system called Drago (Serafini & Tamilin, 2005) implements a fragment of C-OWL and could be used in each hospital. Each peer manages its own context by reasoning with its internal ontology and "incoming" bridge rules. Messages are sent to neighbour peers according to a distributed algorithm involving bridge rules in order to take advantage of knowledge from other contexts.

In our healthcare use case, GUH and GOET may implement a Drago reasoner. GOET expresses the correspondences by way of bridge rules, as shown with a few examples in Figure 5.

Because of the semantics of bridge rules, no inconsistency can be derived in this case. So DDL reduces the problem of diverging policies. In fact, DDL dicreases interactions between different ontologies, which in turn decrease the chance of inconsistency.

Limitations

Bridge rules are not able to represent mappings between object and datatype properties, nor can they express operations on datatypes. Besides, C-OWL uses the same import mechanism as OWL. Additionally, the non-standard semantics of DDL may be counter intuitive, sometimes. Neither disjointness nor cardinality constraints are "transferred" from an ontology to the other via bridge rules. That is, if Insulin and Avandia are disjoint in

Figure 5. Extract of DDL bridge rules

guh:(*rxnorm:Insulin*) $\xrightarrow{\equiv}$ **goet**:(*rxnorm:Insulin*)

guh:(*rxnorm:Avandia*) $\xrightarrow{\equiv}$ **goet**:(*rxnorm:Avandia*)

guh:(*rim:playedRoleIn* some *rim:RolePatient*) $\xrightarrow{\equiv}$ **goet**:(**galen:Patient**)

guh:(*guh:hasMedication*) $\xrightarrow{\equiv}$ **goet**:(**goet:hasTreatment**)

guh:(*guh:sean*) $\overset{\equiv}{\longmapsto}$ **goet**:(**goet:345678IE**)

GUH, and there are the bridge rules above, it cannot be inferred that Insulin and Avandia are disjoint in GOET. However, a variant of DDL has been defined to treat this specific problem (Homola, 2007). Finally, the problem of policy is not completely solved. By adding the bridge rules of Figure 6, the GOET system can infer that a patient must not be treated with both Avandia and Insulin, which is what we tried to avoid.

While this example may seem a bit artificial, it shows that some restriction would have to be made on bridge rules to avoid undesired inferences. These restrictions are not, by themselves, supported by the formalism.

Other Contextual Reasoning Formalisms

Contextual reasoning formalisms are characterized by a non-standard semantics where several ontologies are assigned distinct interpretations. Apart from DDL, this family of formalisms includes *E*-connections, Package-based Description Logics and Integrated Distributed Description Logics.

Package-Based Description Logics

In package-based Description Logics (P-DL) (Bao, Caragea, & Honavar, 2006), each ontological axiom is associated with an identifier of the ontology, similarly to DDL. Moreover, as in other contextual formalisms, a distinct interpretation is assigned to each ontology in a network of ontologies. However, cross-ontology knowledge can only take the form of *semantic imports* of ontological terms. The reason behind this is that this formalism was essentially designed to compensate the drawbacks of the OWL import mechanism and improve modularity of Web ontologies.

As an example, the GOET ontology only uses a few terms from the *GALEN* ontology. Since the *GALEN* ontology is extremely big and highly expressive, its complete import would result in a very complex, hard to manage ontology. However, while this helps building local ontologies in a modular way, it does not very much help expressing cross-context knowledge such as the correspondences that needed to bridge GUH and GOET. As an ontology alignment formalism, semantic imports have a very limited expressiveness. To express a complex correspondence such as, for instance, the one of Figure 7 one would have to first import the terms *guh:HemoglobinTest*, *rim:measures* and *loinc:_4548-4*, then add a *local* axiom in standard DL using the same approach as in Section: Standard Approach-OWL.

Integrated Distributed Description Logics

Integrated Distributed Description Logics (IDDL) (Zimmermann, 2007) is a formalism that address similar issues as DDL but take

Figure 6. Other possible bridge rules

guh:(*guh:hasMedication* some *rxnorm:Insulin*) $\xrightarrow{\equiv}$ **goet**:(**goet**:**hasTreatment** some *rxnorm:Insulin*)

guh:(not *guh:hasMedication* some *rxnorm:Avandia*) $\xrightarrow{\equiv}$ **goet**:(not **goet**: **hasTreatment** some *rxnorm:Avandia*)

Figure 7. An example of correspondence that cannot be represented with semantic imports

Class: (*guh:HemoglobinTest* and (*rim:measures* some *loinc:_4548−4*))
EquivalentTo: (**galen:BloodSugarTest** and (**goet:hasCode** some {**snomed:_43396009**}))

a different paradigm than other contextual frameworks. Usually, cross-ontology assertions (*e.g.*, bridge rules in DDL, links in *E*-connections, semantic imports in P-DL) define knowledge from the point of view of one ontology. That is to say that the correspondences are expressing the relations "as witnessed" by a local ontology. On the contrary, IDDL asserts correspondences from a "third party"'s point of view which encompasses both the ontologies in relation. One consequence of this approach is that correspondences can be manipulated and reasoned with independently of the ontologies, allowing operations like inversing or composing ontology alignments, as first class objects.

In terms of model theory, this is represented by using an additional domain of interpretation to the whole network of ontologies, as if it was a single ontology. The local domains of interpretation, assigned to all ontologies, are then related to the global domain by way of the so-called *equalizing functions* (ε_j). These functions map the elements of local domains to elements of the global domain. Formally, a correspondence $i{:}C \sqsubseteq,\leftrightarrow j{:}D$ from a concept C of ontology O_i to concept D of ontology O_j is satisfied whenever $\varepsilon_i(C^I_i) \subseteq \varepsilon_j(D^I_j)$.

Furthermore, a reasoning procedure for this formalism has been defined (Zimmermann & Le Duc, 2008), where a central system detaining the correspondences can determine global consistency of a network of ontologies, by communicating with local reasoners of arbitrary complexity. This formalism is useful for federated reasoning systems, while the interactions between local ontologies are rather weak. By separating local reasoning and global reasoning, it better prevents interactions between contexts, thus being quite robust to heterogeneity.

In our example, let us assume that the correspondences of Figure 8 are defined to make the two systems interoperate.

Figure 8. Extract of IDDL correspondences

guh:(*rxnorm:Insulin*) $\xleftrightarrow{\equiv}$ **goet**:(*rxnorm:Insulin*)
guh:(*rxnorm:Avandia*) $\xleftrightarrow{\equiv}$ **goet**:(*rxnorm:Avandia*)
guh:(*rxnorm:Avandia*) $\xleftrightarrow{\perp}$ **goet**:(*rxnorm*:Insuline)
guh:(*rim:playedRoleIn* some *rim:RolePatient*) $\xleftrightarrow{\equiv}$ **goet**:(**galen:Patient**)
guh:(*guh:hasMedication*) $\xleftrightarrow{\equiv}$ **goet**:(**goet:hasTreatment**)
guh:(*guh*:sean) $\xleftrightarrow{=}$ **goet**:(**goet**:345678IE)
guh:(*guh:hasMedication* some *rxnorm:Insulin*) $\xrightarrow{\equiv}$ **goet**:(**goet:hasTreatment** some *rxnorm:Insulin*)
guh:(not *guh:hasMedication* some *rxnorm:Avandia*) $\xrightarrow{\equiv}$ **goet**:(not **goet:hasTreatment** some *rxnorm:Avandia*)

Policy of the form $C \sqsubseteq \neg D$ would only influence another ontology if a disjointness is asserted at the alignment level, *e.g.*, One can see the similarity of these correspondences and bridge rules. Yet the resulting inferences differ. No inconsistency will arise from these correspondences. However, thanks to the third correspondence, the system would detect an inconsistency of a medicine is asserted to be Avandia and Insuline at the time. While this formalism decreases undesired interaction of knowledge, especially with respect to policies, its drawback is the possible missing inferences at the local level. Moreover, correspondences are not more expressive than in DDL.

E-Connections

E-connections is another formalism for reasoning with heterogeneous ontologies (Kutz, Lutz, Wolter, & Zakharyaschev, 2004). Again, different ontologies are interpreted distinctly but formally related using particular assertions. Instead of expressing correspondences of ontological terms, an ontology can connect to another by using special terms (called *links*) which can be combined in conjunction with terms from another ontology. The semantics of links is very similar to the semantics of roles in Description Logics, except that instead of relating elements from the same domain of interpretation, they relate two different domains. In principle, *E*-connections serve to relate ontologies about very different domains of interest. For instance, an ontology of laboratories in GUH could be connected to an ontology of medical staff used in GOET. To do this, one can define the link ‹*hasDirector*› and use it in GUH ontology as in Figure 9.

Thus, *E*-connections are particularly useful for ontology design by modularly reusing and connecting existing blocks. However, one of the main focus of this chapter is on relating existing ontology systems on overlapping domains. So, although *E*-connections is a relevant formalism for the management of heterogeneity, its applicability to the type of scenario we are interested in is weak.

State of the Art 3: Context in Semantic Web Technologies

Models of Provenance

RDF model-theory (Hayes, 2004) provides reification as a mechanism for making statements about statements. There are significant differences between reification and contexts both in what they are intended for and in their structure. Reification is intended to enable statements about potential statements (which may or may not be true). They can be useful for making statements about provenance (Watkins & Nicole, 2006; Stoermer, Bouquet, Palmisano, & Redavid, 2007). Named graphs are also used for making statement about provenance (Carroll, Bizer, Hayes, & Stickler, 2007). In named graphs triples become quadruples where the fourth element is ID (URI), *i.e.*, origin of the graph. In addition to the reification mechanism, named graphs, and quadruples in RDF, the system/language

Figure 9. An axiom of an ontology using a link in the e-connections formalism

$$\mathit{guh}{:}\mathrm{Laboratory} \sqsubseteq \exists\langle \mathrm{hasDirector} \rangle \mathbf{goet}{:}\mathrm{StaffMember}$$

Closed World Machine (CWM)/ Notation 3 (N3) supports a construct called contexts. This notion of context is not substantially different from reification. Since these approaches to include additional information about the graph have no coupling with the truth of the triple that has been reified, they cannot be used to relate the truth of a triple in one graph to its truth in another graph. Consequently, it is hard to see how reification, named graphs, quadruples can be used to mediate data aggregation as far as "truth of a triple" is concerned.

Contextual RDF(S)

The author of (Guha, McCool, & Fikes, 2004) proposed an extension of RDF(S)—Context Mechanism—to incorporate contextual knowledge within RDF model theory. A simpler version of OWL is assumed to be interoperable with the proposed context mechanism. The most basic change in RDFS model-theory introduced—by the addition of contexts—is that the denotation of a resource is not just a function of the term and the interpretation (or structure), but also of the context in which that term occurs. Most importantly, the proposed context mechanism allows RDF statements to be true only in their context. The goal of this RDFS extension is to aggregate triples that are true in the graphs being aggregated, and because of the close coupling between truth and contexts, they cannot be a posteriori introduced at the RDF Vocabulary level (Lutz & Sattler, 2000; Donini, Nardi, & Rosati, 2002; Wagner, 2003; Analyti, Antoniou, Damasio, & Wagner, 2004). They appear in the internals of the model theory, in the definition of an interpretation and satisfaction.

In a standard RDF(S) entailment a vocabulary is interpreted as a tuple $V=\{U,PL,TL\}$ that consists of a set U of URI references, a set PL of plain literals, and a set TL of typed literals where U, PL, TL are mutually disjoint. An interpretation I of vocabulary (V) is a tuple $I=\{IR,IP,LV,IS,IL,IEXT\}$, where IR is a non-empty and finite set, called the domain or universe of I, IP is a finite set of properties, $LV \subseteq IR$ is a finite set of literal values with $PL \subseteq LV$, IS is a mapping $IS{:}U \rightarrow IR \cup IP$, IL is a mapping $IL{:}TL \rightarrow IR$ and $IEXT$ is an extension function $IEXT{:}IP \rightarrow 2^{(IR \times IR)}$. In the proposed context mechanism, minor changes in the definitions of standard RDF(S) interpretation (Hayes, 2004) are as follows:

1. Vocabulary $V=\{U,CU,PL,TL\}$ contains set CU of contextual URIs;
2. A set $C \subseteq IR$, is introduced to denote context (C);
3. A mapping IS from power set $2^{(U \times CU)}$ in V into $IR \cup IP$, the power set $2^{(U \times CU)}$ corresponds to resource-context pairs (U,CU).

The context mechanism updates the standard RDF(S) satisfaction by allowing set of context-dependent graphs instead of a single graph, for example, if E is a ground triple (s,p,o) in the context c then $I(E,c)=true$ if c, s, p and o are in V, $IS(p,c)$ is in IP and $(IS(s,c),IS(o,c))$ is in $IEXT(IS(p,c))$. Otherwise $I(E,c)=false$. Considering the updates within standard RDF(S) interpretation and satisfaction, now graphs will be merged with regard to where they occur. It means that, the definition of entailment is updated so that a ground graph G_1 in a context C_1 is entailed by a set of graph-context pairs (G_i,C_i) if G_1 is true under every interpretation under which (G_i,C_i) is true. The proposed context mechanism may lead to non-monotonic aggregation—depending on the expressivity of *lifting rules* suggested by the authors of (Guha, 2004) — in the following sense. A graph G_1 might imply α but the aggregation of this graph (including lifting rules) with other graphs might not imply α.

In our example-scenario, if the contents at URLs galway.hospital/guh.rdf and Gottingen.hospital/goet.rdf are available as RDF then we can have a context corresponding to these URLs and the contents of an URL is said to be true in that context. Furthermore, lifting rules can be defined to import all or part of the contents from data sources. For example, if we assume that an extended version of RDFS could express the *disjoint* axiom in GUH drug policy as below, then the truth of this axiom in Figure 10 can be scoped to the context galway.hospital/guh.rdf.

In GOET, Sean medical treatment record showed that he has been given Insulin therapy at GUH and Avandia treatment is forbidden in conjunction with Insulin therapy. The truth of GUH drug policy is applicable only within GUH context and when GUH and GOET records will be aggregated then GUH drug policy could be easily ignored (thus avoiding inconsistency) by using appropriate lifting rule. Similarly, when Sean is back to Galway, GOET drug policy would not influence his further treatment in Galway or any other places.

State of the Art 4: Other Formal Handling of Heterogeneity

Database-Style Integrity Constraints for OWL

This approach is motivated by data-centric problems in DL/OWL based applications. The authors of (Motik, Horrocks, & Sattler, 2007) have established the relationship between the role of Integrity Constraints (IC) in databases, *i.e.*, (1) data reasoning (*e.g.*, in checking the integrity of a database) and schema reasoning (*e.g.*, in computing query subsumption), and (2) DL/OWL knowledge bases (*e.g.*, schema (*TBox*) reasoning and data (*ABox*) reasoning). In this approach an additional *TBox* is introduced to model constraint axioms, which results in the knowledge base containing two *TBoxes* and an *ABox*. In *TBox* reasoning, constraints behave like normal *TBox* axioms, and for *ABox* reasoning they are interpreted as constraints in relational databases. This approach is very relevant in solving profile and policy issues of our example scenario. For example, to avoid inconsistency due to hospital specific drug policy in Figure 10, can be placed in *TBox* for constraints and when *TBox* reasoning is performed only standard axioms could be taken into account. In case of *ABox* reasoning, constraints axioms can act

Figure 10. GUH drug policy

$$\exists \text{guh:hasMedication.rxnorm:Avandia} \sqsubseteq \neg \text{guh:hasMedication.rxnorm:Insulin}$$

as Integrity Constraints. To some extent, it helps formalizing policies but since it does not identify the context of these constraints, their utility for this purpose is limited. Moreover, as a standard OWL, robustness to heterogeneity is poor.

Modular Web Rule Bases

Although this approach is not based on current Semantic Web standards, it is relevant to this survey. The framework proposed in (Analyti, Antoniou, & Damasio, 2008) makes the distinction between global knowledge, local knowledge and internal knowledge. The framework is based on a rule-based language rather than Description Logics and provides an approach to express and reason with modularity on top of Semantic Web. In this framework each predicate in a rule base is constrained with "uses" and "scope", which in turn determine the reasoning process. The framework also treats different forms of negation (weak or strong) to include Open-World Assumption (OWA) as well as Closed-World Assumption (CWA) (Analyti, Antoniou, & Damasio, 2008). This rule-based framework provides a model-theoretic compatible semantics and allow certain predicates to be monotonic and reasoning is possible with inconsistent knowledge bases. This framework addresses a few issues of our example scenario because rules can express some DL axioms and can be exchanged with certain restrictions (private, global or local). For example in Figure 11, the drug policy rule of our example scenario can be expressed and treated appropriately. However, the major problem we observe is how DL-based ontologies (as majority of HCLS ontologies are DL ontologies) and rules can work together. The integration of DL with rules is still an open research problem (Eiter, Ianni, Krennwallner, & Polleres, 2008). Moreover, this framework is not concerned about the heterogeneity of the knowledge model, and does not provide an expressive way of relating contextual ontologies.

Query-Based Data Translation

The query-based approach translates data from one knowledge source to another, and is close to the problem of expressing complex correspondences of the example-scenario presented in this chapter. In this approach mappings between ontologies are first expressed in expressive alignment language (Euzenat, Scharffe, & Zimmermann, 2007) and then grounded and executed to a combined query language and engine, SPARQL++ and PSPARQL, called PSPARQL++ (Euzenat, Polleres, & Schare, 2008). Figure 12, show how (a) two ontology entities (guh:orderDate, guh:time) could be concatenated to a single entity (dc:date) and (b) a conversion is possible between an object property and a datatype property by using proposed cast-function that converts *xsd:string* to RDF resource. Expressive correspondences between ontology instances can be constructed using "SPARQL CONSTRUCT" to create additional dataset and query upon them.

Figure 11. Drug policy in rule

$$\mathcal{F} \leftarrow hasMedication(?x,?y),\ Avandia(?y),\ hasMedication(?x,?z), Insulin(?z)$$

Figure 12. Mappings expressed as a SPARQL CONSTRUCT query

```
(a) CONSTRUCT { ?X dc:date fn:concat(?Date,"T",?Time). }
    WHERE { ?X guh:orderDate ?Date . ?X guh:time ?Time . }

(b) CONSTRUCT { ?X guh:hasId rdf:Resource(fn:encode-for-uri(?Id)) . }
    WHERE { ?X goet:identification ?Id . }
```

This approach allows one to express complex correspondences like concatenating attributes or even datatype to object properties and one can avoid some undesired interactions between knowledge of various sources. However, one major limitation is that the query result depends on how the correspondences are written and the knowledge in the domain ontologies are largely unexploited. Similarly, complex correspondences can be expressed in Rule Interchange Format (RIF), which offers a rich set of built-in functions (*e.g., string* manipulations), as well as a formal semantics for interoperating with RDF and OWL knowledge bases. RIF has been recently approved as W3C's standard recommendation and we consider it as a prominent candidate to express rules (like our use-case) over OWL knowledge bases.

Reasoning with Inconsistencies

Robustness to heterogeneity is an important aspect in healthcare integration scenarios. One of the most problematic consequences of heterogeneity is the occurrence of undesired inconsistencies. Therefore, we believe it useful to investigate formal approaches for handling inconsistencies. There are two main ways to deal with inconsistent ontologies. One is to simply accept the inconsistency and to apply a non-standard reasoning method to obtain meaningful answers in the presence of inconsistencies. An alternative approach is to resolve the error, that is, to repair the ontology, whenever an inconsistency is encountered.

Repairing or revising inconsistent ontology is, in principle, a possible solution for handling inconsistency. However, one major pragmatic issue we observe is that healthcare institutes may not expose and/or allow repair of their knowledge bases due to various legal constraints. Also, in a typical Semantic Web setting, importing ontologies from other sources makes it impossible to repair them, and if the scale of the combined ontologies is too large as in the case of HCLS ontologies then repair might appear ineffective. Other work focus on revising mappings only (Meilicke, Stuckenschmidt, & Tamilin, 2008), but they are meant to be used at alignment discovery time, which we are not discussing in this chapter.

Reasoning with inconsistencies is also possible without revision of the ontology. One effective way of tolerating inconsistencies consist of using paraconsistent logics (Beziau, Carnielli, & Gabbay, 2007). Paraconsistent logics use a "weaker" inference system that entails less formulas than in classical logics. This way, reasoning can be done in the presence of inconsistency. A paraconsistent extension of OWL was proposed in (Huang, van Harmelen, & ten Teije, 2005). Alternatively, defeasible argumentation (Chesnevar, Maguitman, & Loui, 2000) and its implementation Defeasible Logic Programs (DeLP [Garcia & Simari, 2004]) have been introduced to reason and resolve inconsistencies. In this case, the TBox is separated into 2 subsets, one being *strict*, which means that it must always be used in reasoning, the other being *defeatable*, which means that an argumentation process may defeat them and nullify them for a particular reasoning task.

While we want to tolerate inconsistency when reasoning with an ontology defined in another context, it is not desirable to tolerate local inconsistencies in a HCLS system. The system should have a strict logical framework when it only treats local data, that are existing in a unique and well understood context. Unfortunately, the approaches mentioned here are not able to distinguish local knowledge and external knowledge. They do not allow specification of the types of mappings we need, and are not capable of treating policies.

Comparison of Formal Approaches

While the previous sections described the state of the art horizontally by merely describing approaches one by one, the present section analyzes the features of formal approaches vertically, that is, each characteristic is compared separately throughout the extent of formal approaches.

Table 2 shows a brief, synthetic summary of what is detailed here. The columns can be seen either as a feature of a formal approach or as an issue related to heterogeneity. Consequently, the content of a cell can be read as "this formal approach possess this feature" (if a + is present) or not (if a – is present) or it can be read as "this issue is addressed by this formal approach" (+) or not (–). In the case of the last two columns, the issue defines a continuum between "this issue is not addressed at all" and "this issue is fully addressed", but all approaches are only partially addressing them. Thereby, we order the extent to which they address the issue in the following way:

Very limited < Limited < Medium < Good < Very good < Excellent

The first column represents *context awareness* (C.A. in the table) which is the ability or possibility to identify the context in which some information or knowledge is described. The second column shows the possibility of *modularizing* ontologies (M. in the table). This is considered fully addressed if subparts of ontologies can be reused rather than reuse of complete ontologies. The third column (P.&P.M. in the table) shows whether the formalism can be used to *manage profiles and policies*. The fourth column gives an indication of *correspondence expressiveness* (C.E. in the table), relatively to the other formalisms. We use here a loose notion of "expressiveness" and our classification is partly based on informal arguments rather than an authentic logical proof. Finally, the fifth column shows the *robustness with respect to heterogeneity* (R.H. in the table). This corresponds to the capability to exploit knowledge from independently designed sources while keeping coherence and relevance of inferences.

Context awareness can be enabled by clearly separating the axioms and facts asserted in distinct ontologies or from distinct provenance. Such formalisms as DDL, P-DL, *E*-connections and IDDL assign an identifier to each of the ontologies such that an axiom $i{:}C \sqsubseteq D$ can be associated with an ontology O_i. This also ensures the distinction between local axioms and cross-ontology correspondences, such as bridge rules $i{:}C \xrightarrow{\sqsubseteq} j{:}D$. However, these formalisms do not allow one to describe or give a type to contexts. The contextual *RDF* framework of (Guha et al., 2004) improves on this by treating context identifiers as any other RDF resource identifiers: they are URIs that can be dealt with as first class objects. The case of query-based transformations is a bit particular because the transformation must say from which and to what datasets the translation occurs, but the transformation could actually be used independently of the context. This explains the +/− sign for this formal approach. Modular rule bases uses a mechanism similar to the one of DDL etc but the underlying formalism is not based on Semantic Web languages.

Modularity is almost always associated with context awareness. This is because in order to reuse modules, one must be able to identify them, that is, have a mean of identifying the provenance of knowledge. Moreover, formalisms such as DDL, *E*-connections, P-DL, IDDL are designed to enable the reuse of external knowledge through the use of cross-context assertions like imports, bridge rules, links, correspondences. Therefore, what identifies a context can be thought of as a module. To a lesser extent, OWL allows some modularisation but is limited the full import of complete ontologies which results—from a logical point of view—in the same ontology as a complete merge of all imported knowledge. OWL/IC has the same behavior as OWL in terms of modularity. Finally, the contextual RDF approach allows to identify contexts and relate them, it is harder to separate knowledge into modular blocks since contexts can overlap and, as first class objects, contexts themselves can be part of a context. These intertwined elements make modularization in contextual RDF(S) more difficult.

Policies and profiles has not been often addressed as a knowledge representation issue. Most of the solutions to this problem are using ad hoc implementations or algorithm that are not explicitly tackled by the underlying formalism. Of course, it is possible to use existing languages—such as RDF and OWL as in (Kolovski, Parsia, Katz, & Hendler, 2005) — to represent policies but OWL cannot formally distinguish between ontological axioms and policy axioms. This is true for most of the formalisms presented here. Notable exceptions are Defeasible Logic Programs for which there is a distinction between "strict" knowledge, which is always true, and "defeatable" knowledge which can be canceled by way of an automatic argumentation process. Policies are typically defeatable by stronger policies (*e.g.*, from GUH's point of view, GOET's policy axioms would be defeated by contradicting local policies). As an alternative, OWL/IC offers a way to separate the usual ontological knowledge from database-style constraints. Unfortunately, both approaches are unable to distinguish the context in which appear the axioms or policies. Thereby, they can only separate the totality of the ontological axioms from the totality of the policy constraints. Finally, Web Rule bases has a similar aptitude to distinguish different types of knowledge by assigning different reasoning scheme to different sets of rules. Additionally, it separates knowledge from different sources in a similar way as contextual formalisms do. However, it is not complying to Semantic Web technologies and it would hardly be possible to integrate it with description logics systems.

Correspondence expressiveness varies a lot depending on the formalism being used. Most of the correspondences given in the example scenario are directly expressible in OWL due to its high expressiveness. However, OWL constructs still have some limitations which appear in practical cases. In formalisms that allow delimiting contextual knowledge, the expressiveness of correspondences is defined by the types of relations that can be asserted between contexts. The case of the query-based approach to transforming data is notable. This approach allows for defining very fine grained correspondences in the form of a data transformation. Basing the approach on queries decreases the exploitation of reasoning but enables all kinds of structural and functional transformations.

Robustness to heterogeneity is the ability to make consistent and useful inferences in spite of the variations of points of view, modeling approaches and contexts. There are two extreme cases: one is the classical logic approach, the other is the context separation approach. In classical logic, all statements are treated equally in a theory and can equally interfere with any other statement. Therefore, incompatible views are very likely to produce inconstencies or nonsense. This results in a formalism very vulnerable to heterogeneous knowledge. On the opposite side, it is possible to simply separate all conclusions drawn from a context from any other context. This is very robust to heterogeneity since, granted that each context is self consistent, it cannot produce incompatible inferences. However, this way, no context can take advantage of information coming from a different context. Context aware formalisms can be ordered in their ability to tolerate heterogeneity: P-DL < modular rule bases < DDL revisited < DDL < IDDL < *E*-connection < Query-based. The reason why the query-based approach is so robust is that it does not actually reason with a source ontology to produce new data according to the target knowledge base. Moreover, the transformation can be designed in such a way that it conform to the destination ontology.

Conclusion of the State of the Art

Although the presented formalisms are significantly different from each others, there are common aspects to them and some of them are not incompatible. First, in all these approaches, we can recognize the need to delimit parts of the knowledge to assign them either provenance information, a type (policy, ontological knowledge) or a distinct reasoning scheme (OWA, CWA). Thereby, a better solution to the problem of heterogeneity

Table 2. Formal approaches towards heterogeneity and context

	C.A.	M.	P.& P.M.	C.E.	R.H.
DL/OWL	-	+/-	-	Good	Very limited
DDL/C-OWL	+	+	-	Very good	Good
P-DL	+	+	-	Very limited	Limited
DDL Revisited	+	+	-	Very good	Medium
E-connections	+	+	-	Medium	Excellent
IDDL	+	+	-	Good	Very good
RDFS-C	+	+/-	-	Good	Good
DeLP/Paraconsistent	-	-	+/-	Good	Good
Query-based	+/-	-	-	Very good	Very good
Modular Rule bases	+	+	+/-	Limited	Limited
OWL/IC	-	+/-	+/-	Good	Limited

Note: C.A. (Context-awareness); M. (Modularity); P.& P.M.(Profile and policy management); C.E. (Correspondence expressiveness); R.H.(Robustness to heterogeneity).

should possess this ability to identify subparts of the knowledge and apply different status to them. Second, context-aware formalisms are usually adequate approaches to modularization thanks to their ability to relate distinct ontologies. Additionally, the separation of knowledge makes them more tolerant to heterogeneous modeling. However, these approaches have very little addressed issues of policies and profiles. Yet, handling constraint-like information differently from ontological knowledge is critical to the management of electronic patient records. Improving the so-called modular ontology languages with policies, or making policy-aware formalisms more context sensitive is an important aspect to achieve interoperability of HCLS systems. For this reason, we will present two possible directions for handling policies within context-aware formalisms in the next section. Since this is by no mean a complete solution to the vast problem of heterogeneity, we thereafter discuss more briefly the other critical issues that should be covered by a semantic formalism to represent the knowledge involved in this type of systems.

TOWARDS A FRAMEWORK FOR HANDLING CONTEXT AND HETEROGENEITY

In this section, we propose a general framework for adding constraint-like axioms to a context-aware formalism such as DDL, P-DL, IDDL. While a semantics must be chosen to allow context aware reasoning, they can be extended with other non-monotonic approaches. There are many possible combinations, too many to compare them all, so we only show possible paths that we think are best suited for the scenarios we consider.

Adding Constraints to Context-Aware Formalisms 1: DL-Based

We propose to combine the formalisms that are identifying the context of axioms with a mechanism for handling policies that do not lead to undesired interactions. This approach is partly inspired by (Motik et al., 2007), where axioms are separated into two T-Boxes, one for ontological axioms, the other for integrity constraints. Figure 13 depicts the general idea behind our framework. This way, we define a local T-Box as a pair (D,P) where D describes a domain ontology, and P represents the internal policies. If several local ontologies and policies exist, the overall knowledge is a distributed system (D_i,P_i). To ensure interoperability, ontology alignments (A_{ij}) are added to the system to bridge the gap between different terminologies. Note that these alignments could be simple DL axioms, DDL bridge rules, P-DL semantic imports, or IDDL correspondences. The resulting system is a pair of tuples $((D_i,P_i),(A_{ij}))$.

To simplify the presentation, consider a simple pair of OBIS as in our example scenario, that is, the system in consideration is $\Omega = (\{(D_{guh},P_{guh}),(D_{goet},P_{goet})\},A_{guh,goet})$.

The semantics of such a system depends on the type of alignments in place, which defines the type of context-aware formalism used. Let us write $\models_d$ the distributed entailment relation of the considered formalism. Thereby, $((O_i),(A_{ij})) \models_d k{:}C \sqsubseteq D$ means that the system of ontologies (O_i) and alignment (Aij) distributively entails the axiom $C \sqsubseteq D$ in ontology O_k.

A policy-enabled distributed entailment $\models_d$ is defined over distributed ontologies Ω as follows. For a given local OWL axiom α = guh: $C \sqsubseteq D$ in the terminology of the ontology of GUH, $\Omega \models_P \alpha$ if and only if α is distributively

Figure 13. Enabling context specific policies-DL based

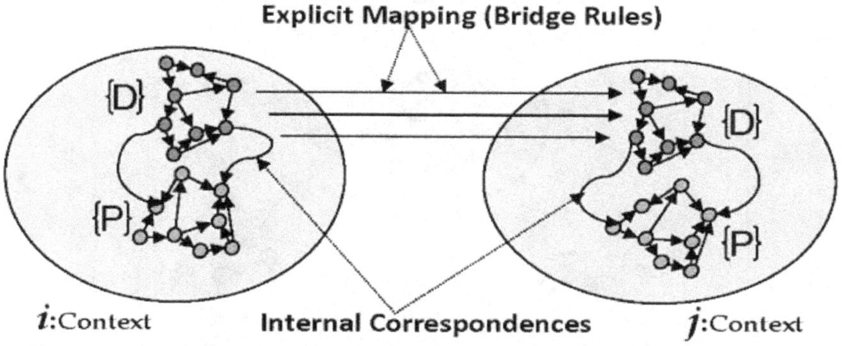

entailed by the system composed of $D_{guh} \cup P_{guh}$, D_{goet} and $A_{guh,goet}$ (and vice versa if the axiom belong to the ontology of GOET).

In other words, only the policy axioms of the ontology which is asking for an entailment is used. In our scenario, it means that if GUH is reasoning, it will take its drug policy into account but not the one of GOET, while GOET would not consider the Avandia-Insulin counter indication of GUH. The very same approach can be easily adapted to DDL, P-DL or IDDL.

Adding Constraints to Context-Aware Formalisms 2: Rule-Based

As discussed above, DL-based solutions are adhering to the Open World Assumption (OWA), that is, conclusions which cannot be derived from an ontology are treated agnostically. The approach presented in last section enables separate context spaces allocated for the special treatment of the context-specific policies. However the intrinsic nature of a DL-based solution may expose limitations when one expects certain rational conclusions, which are reasonable to infer even under incomplete knowledge. To overcome this limitation and to deal with the conservative stance of the DL-based solution, we propose a rule-based approach that will allow the appropriate treatment of context-specific policies by treating them with Closed World Assumption (CWA). Use cases that require data integration from heterogenous information systems are suitable candidates for combining both the formalisms, that is, OWA and CWA (Eiter et al., 2008). In this approach, the knowledge base is split into two parts similar to the DL-based solution, but a separate treatment is provided for each knowledge type (OWA for normal axioms and CWA for policy axioms, see Figure 14).

This rule-based approach is inspired by (Guha et al., 2004) and (Horst, 2005b, 2005a) where authors in (Guha et al., 2004) proposed that the denotation of a resource is not just a function of the term and the interpretation, but also of the context in which that term occurs, that is, ontology axioms are interpreted within certain contexts. The authors suggested an RDFS extension by introducing context within RDFS-Model theory. The extension enables the "Context-Awareness" but the constraints (drug policy) in our example scenario demands expressive semantics (higher expressivity than RDFS), such as *disjointness*. To overcome this issue, Horst (Horst, 2005b, 2005a) proposed a sound and complete rule-based extension of RDFS (called R-entailment) that involves

Figure 14. Enabling context specific policies-rule based

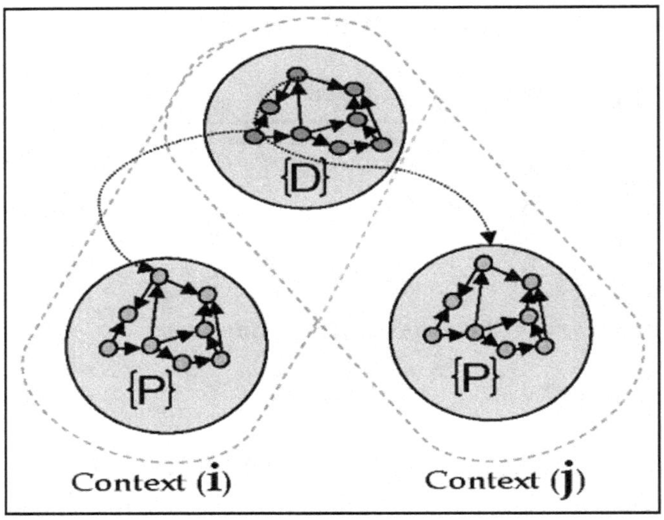

datatypes (useful for modeling HCLS information systems) and a subset of the OWL-vocabulary that includes the property-related vocabulary (*e.g.*, *FunctionalProperty*), the comparisons (*e.g.*, *sameAs*, *differentFrom*, *disjointWith*) and the value restrictions (*e.g.*, *allValuesFrom*). These semantic extensions are in line with the if-semantics of RDFS.

We suggest to combine both the approaches (Horst, 2005a; Guha et al., 2004), calling it RDFS-CR, and providing further extension to this combination by (1) including *Type* and/or *Status* of the knowledge base (normal axioms, constraint axioms), and (2) defining the *scope* of the knowledge bases (global or local). For example, domain ontology (D) (normal axioms and global scope) and context-dependent policies (P) (constraint axioms and local scope). We have combined both the approaches intuitively and requires futher proofs for the formal justificatons. This approach will allow the reuse of existing DL-based HCLS ontologies as normal axioms and define context specific constraints.

Figure 14 defines the knowledge base as a pair (*D*,*P*), where *D* describes a domain ontology and *P* represents the internal policy. Domain ontologies (*D*) will be treated normally by standard RDFS-entailment whereas context-specific policies (*P*) will have RDFS-CR entailment. Policy axioms within a context will share domain ontologies.

One major advantage of this approach is its closeness to the standard semantics. Lightweight extensions of RDFS allows both (1) context-awareness and (2) the ability to model information constraints (IC). Combining integration approaches imposes additional constraints on knowledge-base systems (Eiter et al., 2008), *i.e.*, highly expressive knowledge bases are hard to integrate with less expressive knowledge bases. For example, translating DL-axioms to rules (vice-versa) and faithful preservation of semantics while translation is a known problem.

FUTURE DIRECTIONS: TOWARDS FULLY INTEROPERABLE HCLS SYSTEMS

This section presents critical issues of semantic-enabled HCLS systems that have not been addressed by this paper. Since the breadth of this domain is so wide, this section can only discuss those problems succinctly, but we hope to provide directions for future research on the key obstacles to better interoperability.

Temporal Aspects of HCLS Systems

Temporal information is everywhere in patient records. For example, Lab observations (*e.g.*, blood test, bloop pressure (BP)) have a duration of validity, vaccines must be renewed after some time, medicines have an effect on the body for a certain time (thus, counter-indications are valid beyond the duration of the treatment). One aspect of implicit, contextual information is its temporal component. The ability to identify, represent and reason about time-dependent information is important for various applications, especially for HCLS systems. With respect to temporal information one is often faced with the problem of implicit time (Moldovan, Clark, & Harabagiu, 2005). Sites often publish a piece of data that is true at the time of publication, with the temporal qualification left implicit. Equally often, this data does not get updated when it no longer holds. Even worse, such implicitly temporally qualified data is often mixed with data that is not temporally qualified. In this chapter, we have not directly addressed the time-dependency issue but we assume that framework that enables the two key features (Type and Scope) within the knowledge bases can act as a ground work for enabling and processing such a temporal information in any OBIS.

Efficiency of Reasoning with Non-Standard Logics

Relying on information systems may be great but in many occasions, practitioners must make quick decisions in order to act as soon as possible, especially in emergency situation such as our case study at Göttingen. Thereby, the efficiency of information systems is crucial in many HCLS environment. We did not take this into account in our survey. We simply looked at the possibility to logical represent and models various aspects of common HCLS systems, especially with respect to EHRs. It may be needed to have different approach depending on the type of system or department. Emergency hospitals would sacrifice expressiveness for the sake of faster feedback, while a clinic which only operates when scheduled a long time before would be more favourable to a systems that takes the most precise, most thorough description of all parameters to avoid any potential mistake. Beyond efficiency, simply having an algorithm may be difficult. Undecidability easily occur when throwing in together rules, standard logic axioms, context, policies, time and so on.

Healthcare and Social Networks

There is great perceived value in being able to integrate and use EHR and social network data across clinical and social domains. Healthcare stakeholders belongs to various social ecosystems (or networks), and the vision of patient-centric healthcare seems deemed unrealistic without providing a linkage between a patient and surrounding social networks. The idea is very simple and basic, for example, a semantically described patient data can also have a semantic description of his/her social existence (e.g., friends, family, and location). In situations where both of the networks (i.e., healthcare and social) have mutual correspondences, patient primary care (i.e., treatment of patient) and other secondary care (e.g., home-care, remote monitoring, emergency assistance, etc.) could be easily deployed on top such a linked patient related networks. In Figure 15, we can observe that an HL7 and *FOAF* artifacts are mapped, such correspondences are link between two networks.

Although correspondences between networks can be easily designed but it triggers various challenges with respect to protection, access, policy, etc. of patient and social data. We discussed in the example scenario that each healthcare related stakeholders are open to define their constraints and it is important to interpret and process these context-dependent constraints in a sensible way. The two solutions sketched in Section: Towards a framework for handling context and heterogeneity, can act as an enabler for such interlinked and heterogeneous networks.

Practicality of Formal Approaches

This chapter have presented theoretical or abstract solutions to semantic interoperability, detailing how they are, in theory, able to represent relevant information. However, it must not be forgotten that these approach have to be implemented in practical applications. The implementation itself would lead to even further research issues that are at least equally important and challenging than what we focused on.

First, the more expressive and powerful the formalism is, the more difficult it is to use and to model knowledge with. This can be overcome by building intuitive interfaces that help the user in these tasks. The problem occurs on both the side of the knowledge engineer building ontologies and for the practitioner who needs to understand what the system is telling. Ontology engineering is in itself a whole research field which gained momentum with the development of the Semantic Web. Yet, extending the ontology formalisms would also require updating the engineering methods that are mostly developed specifically for OWL (Cristani & Cuel, 2005). For practitioners, explaining inference results is required.

Second, it can be hypothesised that not all systems will ever use a unique data model. It is thus important to rely on data conversion. For instance, the transformation of syntactic to semantic data format (and vice-versa) is the first basic step in exploring implicit semantics within syntactic data. Initiatives like RDB2RDF (W3CRDB2RDF, 2009), GRDDL (W3CGRDDL, 2007), are improving this transformation and help taking advantage of legacy-database within the framework of the Semantic Web.

Third, the actual distribution of systems leads to many practical consideration such as latency, connectivity, routing and parallelising the algorithms in an efficient way. While hospital computers are all interconnected, they cannot provide any amount of information, or answer any amount of queries from the outside. Yet, to ensure distributed reasoning, the computing power must be shared over the network. These problems relate to other topics such as the Grid and Cloud computing.

Figure 15. HL7 RIM and FOAF correspondences

Class: (**foaf:Person**) SubClassOf: (*rim:Entity*)
EquivalentProperties: (*guh:first_name*) (**foaf:firstName**)

CONCLUSION

In this chapter, we presented how HCLS systems can benefit from semantic technologies to improve interoperability. We focused on formal aspects of knowledge representation formalisms, assessing their ability to effectively model the information commonly needed in electronic health records (EHR). While the discussion was essentially on theoretical aspects, we showed what are the concrete consequences of applying these formalisms to a real-world scenario. The strength and limitation identified for each formalism became the motivation for proposing a framework that identifies the *type* and *scope* of a knowledge base. We argued that an approach to the problem of heterogeneity—or in general interoperability of HCLS systems—relies on the combination of several integration models. However, complexities of different magnitude may arise from this combination. By this approach, we theoretically address an important problem of our example scenario. Nonetheless, the diversity of the field is so vast that we did not cover some relevant issues that we only sketched to provide a roadmap for further research. We believe that these open research issues also requires attention of a broader research community.

ACKNOWLEDGMENT

This chapter is based on a conference paper discussed at ODBASE (Zimmermann, Sahay, Fox, & Polleres, 2009). We thank the anonymous reviewers for their useful comments. This work is partly funded by Science Foundation Ireland (SFI) project Lion-2 (SFI/08/CE/I1380).

The work presented in this article was done while employed in DERI, NUI Galway, Ireland.

REFERENCES

Akman, V., & Surav, M. (1996). Steps toward formalizing context. *AI Magazine*, *17*(3), 55–72.

Analyti, A., Antoniou, G., & Damasio, C. V. (2008). A principled framework for modular Web rule bases and its semantics. In G. Brewka & J. Lang (Eds.), *Principles of Knowledge Representation and Reasoning: Proceedings of the Eleventh International Conference, KR 2008.* Sydney, Australia, (pp. 390–400). AAAI Press.

Analyti, A., Antoniou, G., Damasio, C. V., & Wagner, G. (2004). Negation and negative information in the W3C resource description framework. *Annals of Mathematics. Computing and Teleinformatics*, *2*, 25–34.

Analyti, A., Antoniou, G., Damasio, C. V., & Wagner, G. (2008). Extended RDF as a semantic foundation of rule markup languages. *Journal of Artificial Intelligence Research*, *32*, 37–94.

Beale, T. (2000). Archetypes: Constraint-based domain models for future-proof information systems. In The openEHR archetype object model (openEHR).

Berners-Lee, T., & Kagal, L. (2008). On the semantics of linking and importing in modular ontologies. In I. F. Cruz, S. Decker, D. Allemang, C. Preist, D.Schwabe, P. Mika, M. Uschold, & L. Aroyo (Eds.), *The Semantic Web - ISWC 2006, 5th International Semantic Web Conference, ISWC 2006. Athens, GA, Proceedings (Lecture Notes in Computer Science, 4273).* (pp. 72–86). Germany: Springer-Verlag.

Béziau, J.-Y., Carnielli, W., & Gabbay, D. M. (2007). *Handbook of paraconsistency*. College Publications.

Bicer, V., Laleci, G. B., Dogac, A., & Kabak, Y. (2005). Artemis message exchange framework: Semantic interoperability of exchanged messages in the healthcare domain. [ACM Special Interest Group on Management of Data]. *SIGMOD Record*, *34*(3), 71–76. doi:10.1145/1084805.1084819

Borgida, A., & Serafini, L. (2003). Distributed description logics: Assimilating information from peer sources. *Journal on Data Semantics*, *1*, 153–184.

Bouquet, P., Giunchiglia, F., van Harmelen, F., Serafini, L., & Stuckenschmidt, H. (2003). C-OWL: contextualizing ontologies. In D. Fensel, K. P. Sycara, & J. Mylopoulos (Eds.), *The Semantic Web - ISWC 2003, Second International Semantic Web Conference, Sanibel Island, FL. Proceedings (Lecture Notes in Computer Science, 2870)*. (pp. 164–179). Germany: Springer-Verlag.

Bouquet, P., Giunchiglia, F., van Harmelen, F., Serafini, L., & Stuckenschmidt, H. (2004). Contextualizing ontologies. *Journal of Web Semantics*, *1*(4), 325–343. doi:10.1016/j.websem.2004.07.001

Brickley, D., & Guha, R. V. (2004*). Description Language 1.0: RDF Schema, W3C Recommendation*. Paper presented at the World Wide Web Consortium (W3C).

Brickley, D., & Miller, L. (2007). *The Friend Of A Friend (FOAF) vocabulary specification*. Retrieved from http://xmlns.com/foaf/spec/ http://xmlns.com/foaf/spec/

Calvanese, D., Franconi, E., Haarslev, V., Lembo, D., Motik, B., Tessaris, S., & Turhan, A.-Y. (Eds.). (2007). *Proceedings of the 20th International Workshop on Description Logics DL'07*. Brixen/Bressanone, Italy: Bolzano University Press.

Carroll, J. J., Bizer, C., Hayes, P. J., & Stickler, P. (2007). Named graphs, provenance and trust. In A. Ellis & T. Hagino (Eds.), *Proceedings of the 14th International Conference on World Wide Web, WWW 2005,* (pp. 613–622). ACM Press.

Chesnevar, C. I., Maguitman, A. G., & Loui, R. P. (2000). Logical models of argument. *ACM Computing Surveys*, *32*(4), 337–383. doi:10.1145/371578.371581

Cristani, M., & Cuel, R. (2005). A survey on ontology creation methodologies. *International Journal on Semantic Web and Information Systems*, *1*(2), 49–69. doi:10.4018/jswis.2005040103

Donini, F. M., Nardi, D., & Rosati, R. (2002). Description logics of minimal knowledge and negation as failure. *ACM Transactions on Computational Logic*, *3*(2), 177–225. doi:10.1145/505372.505373

Eiter, T., Ianni, G., Krennwallner, T., & Polleres, A. (2008). Rules and ontologies for the Semantic Web. In C. Baroglio, P. A. Bonatti, J. Maluszynski, M.Marchiori, A. Polleres, & S. Schaffert (Eds.), Reasoning Web, 4th International Summer School 2008, Venice, Italy, Tutorial Lectures (Lecture Notes in Computer Science, 5224). (pp., 1–53). Germany: Springer-Verlag.

Euzenat, J., Polleres, A., & Scharffe, F. (2008). SPARQL extensions for processing alignments. *IEEE Intelligent Systems*, *23*(6), 82–84.

Euzenat, J., Scharffe, F., & Zimmermann, A. (2007). *Expressive alignment language and implementation (Deliverable D2.2.10)*. Knowledge Web NoE.

Forrey, A. W., McDonald, C. J., DeMoor, G., Huff, S. M., Leavelle, D., & Leland, D. et al. (1996). Logical observation identifier names and codes (LOINC) database: A public use set of codes and names for electronic reporting of clinical laboratory test results. *Clinical Chemistry*, *1*, 81–90. PMID:8565239

Fox, R., Sahay, R., & Hauswirth, M. (2008). PPEPR for enterprise healthcare integration. In D. Weerasinghe (Ed.), *Electronic Healthcare, First International Conference, eHealth 2008, London, UK. Revised Selected Papers (Lecture Notes of the Institute for Computer Sciences, Social Informatics and Telecommunications Engineering, 1).* (pp. 130–137). Germany: Springer-Verlag.

Garcia, A. J., & Simari, G. R. (2004). Defeasible logic programming: An argumentative approach. *Theory and Practice of Logic Programming*, *4*(1–2), 95–138. doi:10.1017/S1471068403001674

Ghidini, C., & Giunchiglia, F. (2001). Local models semantics, or contextual reasoning =locality+compatibility. *Artificial Intelligence*, *127*(2), 221–259. doi:10.1016/S0004-3702(01)00064-9

Gil, Y., Motta, E., Benjamins, V. R., & Musen, M. A. (Eds.). (2005). *The Semantic Web - ISWC 2005: 4th International Semantic Web Conference, Galway, Ireland, Proceedings (Lecture Notes in Computer Science 3729).* Germany: Springer-Verlag.

Giunchiglia, F. (1993). Contextual reasoning. *Epistemologica*, *16*, 345–364.

Gruber, T. R. (1993). Towards principles for the design of ontologies used for knowledge sharing. *International Journal of Human-Computer Studies*, *43*(5-6), 907–928. doi:10.1006/ijhc.1995.1081

Guha, R. V. (1991). *Contexts: A formalization and some applications* (Ph.D. thesis). Stanford University, Stanford, CA.

Guha, R. V., McCool, R., & Fikes, R. (2004). Contexts for the Semantic Web. In F. van Harmelen, S. McIlraith, & D. Plexousakis (Eds.), *The Semantic Web - ISWC 2004: Third International Semantic Web Conference, Hiroshima, Japan. Proceedings (Lecture Notes in Computer Science, 3298).* (pp. 32–46). Germany: Springer-Verlag.

HL7V3 (2005). *HL7 version 3 message development framework*. Retrieved from http://www.hl7.org/ library/mdf99/mdf99.pdf

Hayes, P. J. (2004). *RDF Semantics*, (W3C Recommendation 10 February 2004). World Wide Web Consortium (W3C).

Hitzler, P., Krötzsch, M., Parsia, B., Patel-Schneider, P. F., & Rudolph, S. (2009). *OWL 2 Web ontology language primer, (W3C Recommendation)*. World Wide Web Consortium.

Homola, M. (2007). Distributed Description Logics Revisited. In Calvanese et al. (Eds.), *Proceedings of the 20th International Workshop on Description Logics DL'07*. Brixen/Bressanone, Italy: Bolzano University Press.

Horridge, M., & Patel-Schneider, P. F. (2009). OWL 2 Web ontology language Manchester syntax (W3C Working Group Note 27 October 2009). World Wide Web Consortium (W3C).

Horst, H. J. T. (2005a). Combining RDF and Part of OWL with rules: Semantics, decidability, complexity. In Gil et al., (Eds.), *The Semantic Web - ISWC 2005: 4th International Semantic Web Conference, Galway, Ireland, Proceedings (Lecture Notes in Computer Science 3729)* (pp. 668–684). Germany: Springer-Verlag.

Horst, H. J. T. (2005b). Completeness, decidability and complexity of entailment for RDF Schema and a semantic extension involving the OWL vocabulary. *Journal of Web Semantics*, *3*(2–3), 79–115. doi:10.1016/j.websem.2005.06.001

Huang, Z., van Harmelen, F., & ten Teije, A. (2005). *Reasoning with inconsistent ontologies*. In L. P. Kaelbling & A. Saffiotti (Eds.), *IJCAI-05, Proceedings of the Nineteenth International Joint Conference on Artifical Intelligence, Edinburgh, Scotland.* (pp. 454–459). Professional Book Center.

Jahnke, J. H., Bychkov, Y., Dahlem, D., & Kawasme, L. (2005). Context-aware information services for health care. *Revue d'Intelligence Artificielle*, *19*(3), 459–478. doi:10.3166/ria.19.459-478

Kashyap, V., & Sheth, A. (1996). Semantic and schematic similarities between database objects: A context-based approach. *The Very Large Data Base Journal*, *5*, 276–304.

Kleer, J. D. (1986). An assumption-based TMS. *Artificial Intelligence*, *28*(2), 127–162. doi:10.1016/0004-3702(86)90080-9

Klyne, G. (2001). *Information modelling using RDF: Constructs for modular description of complex systems.* Retrieved from http:// xml.coverpages.org/Klyne-RDFInfoModelling.pdf

Kolovski, V., Parsia, B., Katz, Y., & Hendler, J. A. (2005). Representing Web service policies in OWL-DL. In Gil et al., (Eds.), *The Semantic Web - ISWC 2005: 4th International Semantic Web Conference, Galway, Ireland, Proceedings (Lecture Notes in Computer Science 3729)* (pp461–475).Germany: Springer-Verlag.

Kutz, O., Lutz, C., Wolter, F., & Zakharyaschev, M. (2004). *E*-connections of abstract description systems. *Artificial Intelligence*, *156*(1), 1–73. doi:10.1016/j.artint.2004.02.002

Lenat, D. B. (1995). CYC: A large-scale investment in knowledge infrastructure. *Communications of the ACM*, *38*(11), 33–38. doi:10.1145/219717.219745

Lindberg, D., Humphreys, B., & McCray, A. (1993). The unified medical language system (UMLS). *Methods of Information in Medicine*, *32*(4), 281–291. PMID:8412823

Lutz, C., & Sattler, U. (2000). Mary likes all cats. In F. Baader & U. Sattler (Eds.), *Proceedings of the 2000 International Workshop on Description Logics (DL2000), Aachen, Germany (CEUR Workshop Proceedings, 33)* (pp.213–226). Sun SITE Central Europe (CEUR).

McCarthy, J. L. (1987). Generality in artificial intelligence. *Communications of the ACM*, *30*(12), 1029–1035. doi:10.1145/33447.33448

Meilicke, C., Stuckenschmidt, H., & Tamilin, A. (2008). Supporting manual mapping revision using logical reasoning. In D. Fox & C. P. Gomes (Eds.), *Proceedings of the Twenty-Third AAAI Conference on Artificial Intelligence, AAAI 2008, Chicago, Illinois,* (pp. 1213–1218). AAAI Press.

Moldovan, D. I., Clark, C., & Harabagiu, S. M. (2005). Temporal context representation and reasoning. In L. P. Kaelbling & A. Saffiotti (Eds.), *IJCAI-05, Proceedings of the Nineteenth International Joint Conference on Artifical Intelligence, Edinburgh, Scotland.* (pp. 1099–1104). Professional Book Center.

Motik, B., Horrocks, I., & Sattler, U. (2007). Adding integrity constraints to OWL. In C. Golbreich, A. Kalyanpur, & B. Parsia, *Proceedings of the OWLED 2007 Workshop on OWL: Experiences and Directions, Innsbruck, Austria, (CEUR Workshop Proceedings 258).* Sun SITE Central Europe (CEUR).

Motik, B., Patel-Schneider, P. F., & Cuenca-Grau, B. (2009). *OWL 2 Web ontology language direct semantics* (W3C Recommendation 27 October 2009). World Wide Web Consortium (W3C).

Rector, A. L., & Brandt, S. (2008). Why do it the hard way? The case for an expressive description logic for SNOMED. *Journal of the American Medical Informatics Association, 15*(6), 744. doi:10.1197/jamia.M2797 PMID:18755993

Rector, A. L., Nowlan, W. A., & Consortium, G. (1994). The galen project. *Computer Methods and Programs in Biomedicine, 45*(1-2), 75–78. doi:10.1016/0169-2607(94)90020-5 PMID:7889770

Rector, A. L., Qamar, R., & Marley, T. (2006). Binding ontologies & coding systems to electronic health records and messages. In O. Bodenreider (Ed.), *KR-MED 2006, Formal Biomedical Knowledge Representation, Proceedings of the Second International Workshop on Formal Biomedical Knowledge Representation: Biomedical Ontology in Action (KR-MED 2006).* Sun SITE Central Europe (CEUR).

Sahay, R., Akhtar, W., & Fox, R. (2008). PPEPR: Plug and play electronic patient records. In R. L. Wainwright & H. Haddad (Ed.), *Proceedings of the 2008 ACM Symposium on Applied Computing (SAC), Fortaleza, Ceara, Brazil,* (pp. 2298–2304). ACM Press.

Sahay, R., Fox, R., & Hauswirth, M. (2009). Semantic service-oriented design and development methodology for enterprise healthcare integration In J. Filipe & J. Cordeiro (Eds.), *WEBIST 2009 - Proceedings of the Fifth International Conference on Web Information Systems and Technologies, Lisbon, Portugal,* (pp. 159–166). INSTICC Press.

Schneider, M. (2009). *OWL 2 Web ontology language RDF-based semantics* (W3C Recommendation 27 October 2009). World Wide Web Consortium (W3C).

Serafini, L., & Tamilin, A. (2005). DRAGO: Distributed reasoning architecture for the Semantic Web. In A. Gomez-Perez & J. Euzenat (Eds.), *The Semantic Web: Research and Applications, Second European Semantic Web Conference, ESWC 2005, Heraklion, Crete, Greece, Proceedings, (Lecture Notes in Computer Science 3532)* (pp. 361–376). Germany: Springer-Verlag.

Spackman, K. A. (2008). *SNOMED CT style guide: Situations with explicit context. Style Guide 14 January 2008, Version 1.03.* SNOMED CT.

Stoermer, H., Bouquet, P., Palmisano, I., & Redavid, D. (2007). A context-based architecture for RDF knowledge bases: Approach, implementation and preliminary results. In M. Marchiori, J. Z. Pan, & C. de Sainte Marie (Eds.), *Web Reasoning and Rule Systems, First International Conference, RR 2007, Innsbruck, Austria, Proceedings, (Lecture Notes in Computer Science,4524)* (pp. 209–218). Germany: Springer-Verlag.

Szolovits, P. (1982). *Artificial intelligence in medicine*. Boulder, CO: Westview Press, Inc.

W3CGRDDL. (2007). *Gleaning resource descriptions from dialects of languages (GRDDL) working group*. World Wide Web Consortium (W3C).

W3CHCLSIG. (2005). *Semantic Web health care and life sciences (HCLS) interest group*. World Wide Web Consortium (W3C).

W3CRDB2RDF. (2009). *RDB2RDF working group*. World Wide Web Consortium (W3C).

Wagner, G. (2003). Web rules need two kinds of negation. In F. Bry, N. Henze, & J. Maluszynski (Eds.), *Principles and Practice of Semantic Web Reasoning, International Workshop, PPSWR 2003, Mumbai, India, Proceedings, (Lecture Notes in Computer Science 2901)* (pp. 33–50). Germany: Springer-Verlag.

Watkins, E. R., & Nicole, D. A. (2006). Named graphs as a mechanism for reasoning about provenance. In X. Zhou, J. Li, H. T. Shen, M. Kitsuregawa, & Y. Zhang (Eds.), *Frontiers of WWW Research and Development - APWeb 2006, 8th Asia-Pacific Web Conference, Harbin, China, Proceedings, (Lecture Notes in Computer Science 3841)* (pp. 943–948). Germany: Springer-Verlag.

Zimmermann, A. (2007). Integrated distributed description logics. In Calvanese et al. *Proceedings of the 20th International Workshop on Description Logics DL'07, June 8 - 10, 2007, Brixen/Bressanone, Italy* (pp. 507-514). Bolzano University Press.

Zimmermann, A., & Duc, C. L. (2008). Reasoning on a network of aligned ontologies. In D. Calvanese & H. Lausen (Eds.), *Web Reasoning and Rule Systems, Second International Conference, RR 2008, Karlsruhe, Germany, Proceedings, (Lecture Notes in Computer Science 5341)* (pp. 43–57). Germany: Springer-Verlag.

Zimmermann, A., Sahay, R., Fox, R., & Polleres, A. (2009). Lecture Notes in Computer Science: Vol. 5871. *Heterogeneity and Context in Semantic-Web-enabled HCLS systems* (pp. 1165–1182). Germany: Springer-Verlag. doi:10.1007/978-3-642-05151-7_30

KEY TERMS AND DEFINITIONS

Electronic Health Records (EHR): Patient health records including treatment history, medical test reports, and images stored in an electronic format that can be accessed by healthcare providers on a computer network.

Healthcare: Care, services, and supplies related to the health of an individual. Healthcare includes preventive, diagnostic, therapeutic, rehabilitative, maintenance, or palliative care, and counseling, among other services.

HL7 (Health Level Seven): One of the American National Standards Institute (ANSI) accredited.

Life Science: Life Science is a collective term for all sciences concerned with life in all its variations, especially Biology and Medicine and their sub-disciplines.

Provenance: Information about the source and history for an object, entity, or knowledge.

Semantic Web: The Semantic Web (SW) is the architecture, technologies, and implementation of the vision of the Web of data which enables data to be shared and reused across application, enterprise, and community boundaries as a hyperlinked collection of data and metadata represented as Web resources.

Standard Developing Organization (SDO): Health Level 7 domain is the standards for electronic interchange of clinical, financial and administrative info among healthcare oriented computer systems. It is a non-profit volunteer organization. It develops specifications, most widely used is the messaging standard that enables disparate healthcare applications to exchange key sets of clinical and administrative data.

Chapter 7
Sensor Grid Enhancement with Data Management System for Ubiquitous Healthcare Computing

Nikolaos Preve
NTUA, Greece

ABSTRACT

A Wireless Sensor Network (WSN) can be deployed to monitor the health of patients suffering from critical diseases. A wireless network consisting of biomedical sensors can also be implanted into the patient's body and can monitor the patients' conditions. These sensor devices, apart from having an enormous capability of collecting data from their physical surroundings, are also resource constraint in nature with a limited processing and communication ability. Therefore, it is necessary to integrate them with the Grid technology in order to process and store the collected data by the sensor nodes. This chapter proposes the SEnsor Grid Enhancement Data Management system, called SEGEDMA, ensuring the integration of different network technologies and the continuous data access to system users. The main contribution of this work is to achieve the interoperability of both technologies through a novel network architecture ensuring also the interoperability of Open Geospatial Consortium (OGC) and HL7 standards. According to the results SEGEDMA can be applied successfully in a decentralized healthcare environment.

1. INTRODUCTION

Wireless Sensor Network (WSN) is a widely used technology for applications that collect and process data from the physical world (Akyildiz, Weilian, Sankarasubramaniam, & Cayirci, 2002). They allow the physical environment to be measured at high resolutions and greatly increase the quantity and quality of real world data and information for applications. Important applications of wireless sensor networks include environmental and habitat monitoring, healthcare monitoring of patients, weather monitoring and forecasting, military

DOI: 10.4018/978-1-4666-3000-0.ch007

and homeland security surveillance, tracking of goods and manufacturing processes, safety monitoring of physical structures and construction sites, smart homes and offices and many other uses that we do not yet imagine. Sensor devices in a wireless sensor network are resource constrained since they have limited sensing capability, processing power and communication bandwidth. However, with a large number of such devices being deployed and aggregated over a wide area, a wireless sensor network has substantial data acquisition and processing capability. Thus, WSNs are important distributed computing resources that can be shared by different users and applications.

There are many platforms on which the WSN technology has been used and healthcare monitoring being one among them. As suggested by many researchers and scientist across the world, this technology has a potential to create great impact on many aspects of emergency medical care. Sensor devices have been used to capture continuous, real time vital signs from a large number of patients, relaying the data to handheld computers carried by Emergency Medical Technicians (EMTs), physicians and nurses. Moreover due to their small size and energy efficiency it is easy to integrate them into the location of a patient.

Grid Computing was coined in middle 1990s in order to denote a proposed distributed computing infrastructure for advanced science and engineering by Foster, Kesselman, and Tuecke (2001). The unified definition of the term "Grid" and the definitions often address different application areas. In recent years Grid computing has raised interest worldwide in the academic world, industry, and government with fast development cycles. In particular, a variety of applications ranging from aerospace, astronomy, bioinformatics, chemistry, environment, finance, physics and healthcare have been identified. The current technological achievement aims at the definition of a global infrastructure able to share geographically distributed resources such as data, storage, computers, software, tools, applications, instruments and networks with a secure manner at anytime and anywhere. Major efforts, huge resources and funds have been put into research and development (R&D) of core Grid computing technologies, Grid infrastructures and Grid applications in a variety of science fields including healthcare and life science. The Grid software layers are shown in Figure 1. The integration of Grid and HealthCare (HC) has created a new area called HealthGrid by Breton, Dean, and Solomonides (2005), who showed the great impact on almost every aspect of healthcare, from diagnosis, treatment, primary-acute care to social services.

Recently, Breton et al. (2005), and Abbas (2003) have introduced Grid technologies in many healthcare areas including medical applications. The Grid builds an infrastructure that provides resources to medical personnel who access them following the necessary policies in HC. These resources may include computational resources, storage, equipment, and human resources specialists. The access to a medical resource could be given to the clinicians when entering into the Grid system. A healthcare information system can specify certain policies such as authentication, authorization and auditing which are enforced according to a service level agreement.

From the integration of the above technologies the emerging research area which includes the extended Grid computing in the wireless networks is the Sensor Grid. At this process we can have a WSN which is connected with the conventional wired Grid fabric. Sensor Grid

Figure 1. Layers of grid concept

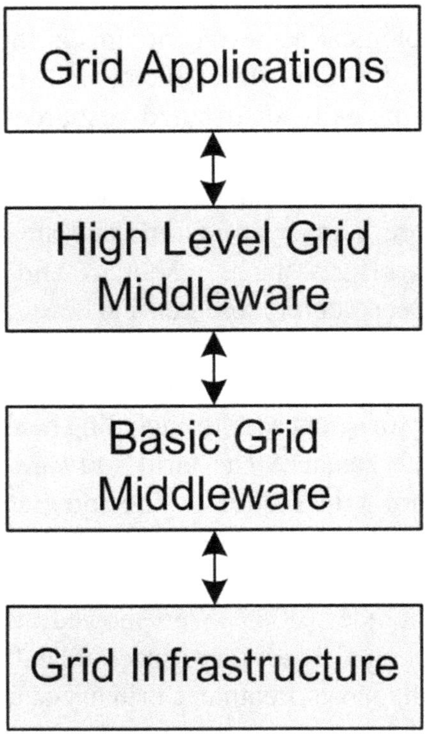

is a relatively new area of research. Thus, the design of Sensor Grids is not well understood yet, unlike that of compute and data Grids. Wireless sensor networks are usually based on proprietary designs and protocols and so it is challenging to integrate them with the standard Grid architecture and protocols. We can categorize Sensor Grids according to several characteristics. First, we have the Data Sensor Grid where the enormous amount of data is collected by the sensors and it can be processed, analyzed and stored using the computational and data storage resources of the Grid. Second, the Sharing Sensor Grid is shared and used between users who can access a subset of the sensors during a particular time period to run a specific application and to collect the desired type of sensor data. Third, the Computational Sensor Grid is used by the sensor devices in order to be more computationally powerful for certain applications. Fourth, the Pervasive Sensor Grid provides access to a wide variety of resources such as data fusion, data mining, and distributed database processing which can be applied to make sense of the sensor data and generate new knowledge of the environment.

The goal of this chapter is to solve issues and challenges of Grid Storage and the important problems which can occur by the integration of Wireless Sensor Networks with the Grid technology in healthcare. SEGEDMA was based on Open Geospatial Consortium (OGC) and HL7 standards in order to ensure the interoperability of our decentralized Health Information System (HIS). So we propose a developed architecture, called the SEnsor Grid Enhancement Data MAnagement model (SEGEDMA) to address these issues. The proposed model tries to integrate Wireless sensor networks with a Grid network via a proxy-based approach and a data management model in order to solve the occurred design issues. Moreover, we developed a decentralized HL7 based system providing healthcare support in real-time. Finally, we develop a testbed to define the usability of the proposed model. According to the results, we can find out that SEGEDMA model is capable of achieving interoperability of the integration of both technologies according to the above standards and it manages data successfully.

The chapter is organized as follows. Section 1 is the introduction to the problem. In Section 2, we report on related work and discuss our contribution. In Section 3, the necessity and the requirements of Grid technology in healthcare is described. Section 4 presents an approach for Grid storage. In Section 5, the implementation and the data management model of the proposed Sensor Grid for healthcare are detailed. Section 6 validates the proposed methodology within the Sensor Grid testbed. Finally, Section 7 concludes the chapter.

2. RELATED WORK

The main idea of Healthcare Grid begun in EU, USA and Asia in order to give an overview of the worldwide efforts in Grid research and development. The European Community funded projects specifically in the healthcare field like MammoGrid which was presented by Warren et al. (2007) and GEMSS (2013). The UK e-Science program invested funding on HealthGrid applications such as eDiaMonND (2013), CLEF (2013), and CareGrid by Liu, Bacon, and Wilson-Hinds (2007).. The MammoGrid project aimed in developing a pan-European distributed database of mammography images with the usage of the Grid technologies. This project was consistent with the development of the European Grid infrastructure from the EDG (2013) to the EGEE (2013). The goal of the Grid-Enabled Medical Simulation Services (GEMSS) project was to create an innovative Grid middleware to support several medical service applications, including maxillofacial surgery simulation, neurosurgery support, radio-surgery simulation, inhaled drug delivery simulation, cardiovascular system simulation and advanced medical image reconstruction.

These simulation tools can assist medical practitioners in diagnosis, pre-operative planning and near real-time surgery support. The Digital Mammography (eDiaMoND) project aimed at delivering a prototype which could support breast screening in the UK through screening, computer based training, epidemiology study and computer aided detection of breast cancer. It gave patients, physicians and hospitals fast access to a vast database of digital mammogram images. The database was also used for image analysis algorithms, searching mechanisms for data mining and imaging standardization techniques. The Clinical E-science Framework (CLEF) project has created a scalable generic architecture based on Grid technology for capturing, integrating, interpreting and using clinical data with genomic data and images within practical clinical systems. The CareGrid project has developed software for supporting decisions based on trust, privacy, security and context models in the healthcare application domain.

Up to now there has been much effort in the development of Healthcare Grid. But the same efforts of development are also presented in the area of software platforms for Grid Computing. The Globus Toolkit (Foster & Kesselman, 1997) became the standard for Grid middleware. It provides tools and libraries for communications, resource management, data management, security, and information services. The Global Grid Forum developed the specifications for the Open Grid Services Architecture (OGSA) based on the concept of Grid services and obtained by Foster, Kesselman, Nick, and Tuecke (2002). The Grid services architecture enables resources to be dynamically discovered and shared. The Open Grid Services Infrastructure (OGSI) is showed by Tuecke, Czajkowski, Foster, Frey, Graham, Kesselman, Maquire, Sandholm, Snelling, and Vanderbilt (2003) and it is the first specification to implement the OGSA framework, and the Globus Toolkit 3 is the first implementation of the OGSI specifications. Recently, the Web Services Resource Framework (WSRF) (Czajkowski, Ferguson, Foster, Frey, Graham, Maquire, Snelling, & Tuecke, 2004) was developed to address some limitations of OGSI. The Globus Toolkit 4 implements the WSRF specifications.

The research community began efforts in the integration area of WSN and Grid computing. Researchers in the UK are already studying how sensors can be integrated into e-Science Grid computing applications (Syed, Ghanem & Guo, 2006). The Discovery Net project is building a Grid based framework for developing and deploying knowledge discovery services to analyze data collected from distributed high throughput sensors. The applications include life sciences, environmental monitoring, and geo-hazard modeling. However, these application driven projects tend to use Sensor Grid architectures that are custom built for specific applications. Although these architectures are efficient and can deliver good performance for the targeted applications, they are neither flexible nor scalable. There are also efforts to define the middleware architecture for sensor devices to facilitate the integration with the Grid. The Common Instrument Middleware Architecture (CIMA) project (Bramley, Chiu, Huffman, Huffman, & McMullen, 2003) aims to Grid enable instruments and sensors as real-time data sources to facilitate their integration with the Grid. The CIMA middleware is based on current Grid standards such as OGSA. Such middleware architecture uses a standard instrument representation format and software stack. The main problem with this approach is the complexity of the middleware architecture in order to be implemented on simple sensor devices with low computational and processing capability.

This chapter tries with SEGEDMA framework to integrate the area of Sensor Grid by using some characteristics from the computing tools in order to meet the requirements of specific target applications. The result of our architecture focuses on scalability which adds a new approach in the analyzed research area and leverages the integration process in heterogeneous wireless sensor networks with the Grid network and the storage services.

3. NECESSITY OF AN INTEGRATED NETWORK

This section provides several parameters of healthcare cases where Grid computing can be used to help speed up a diagnosis or perform tasks. Because the innovative use of HealthGrid aims at the support of broad access to rapid, cost effective and high quality healthcare which has been introduced by Breton et al.(2004). The vision of HealthGrid is based on Grid technologies in order to create an environment where the information can be associated to provide individualized healthcare. HealthGrid has many applications in biomedicine, bioinformatics, medical informatics, primary/acute healthcare and social services. It can be applied to improve individualized healthcare and to support epidemiology study. For individualized healthcare, the HealthGrid can facilitate the access of relevant health information of a patient regardless of where the patient has been to or where he is now. The use of the computer aided tools for the specific data of the patient for the detection and diagnosis of a disease supports the physician's decision making and the definition of the most suitable therapy and treatment from the diagnosis. The HealthGrid will also facilitate the epidemiology study through the access of all relevant health knowledge of populations for both clinical, training purposes and through the assistance on the R&D of new therapies and drugs. The applications and the requirements of HealthGrid are presented more clearly in the following paragraphs.

The necessity of a medical application such as the automated diagnosis can include a check-up, a specialist examination, biosignal or genomic measurement can be provided by the utilization of the Grid Computing. Also, all the medical examinations and measurements can be linked using geographically distributed computing resources, intelligent analysis software and algorithms, databases via secure and reliable wired or wireless networks. The reason is based on the physician or the specialist who can perform analysis and diagnosis with the aid of advanced intelligent automated diagnosis machines, software and tools. Moreover, the majority of medical applications demand a lot of computational storage such as mammography for breast screening and neuroimaging. As a result, the huge medical data is difficult to manage, store, share, retrieve and may also require large scale computational resources for analyzing and processing. Projects like the EU's MammoGrid (2013), the UK's eDiaMoND (2013), and the USA's NDMA (2013) are all concerned with analysis and/or database management. The USA's BIRN (2013), Japan's MEGrid (2013). Also, Australia's NeuroGrid (Buyya, Date, Mizuno-Matsumoto, Venugopal, & Abramson, 2003), and the UK's EIT (Fritschy, Horesh, Holder, & Bayford, 2005). projects are concerned with neurological diseases and are based on Grid technology in order to improve computational speed for analysis, reconstruction and visualization.

On the one hand the necessity of Grid technology is obvious in remote medical support such as remote consultation and remote surgery. Remote consultation can provide online medical information which can be acquired by connecting to international or national medical information centers achieving to help with the diagnosis. Also, the remote consultation can be set up through the network. The remote surgery is possible via a high quality audio/video link connected to a remote surgeon specialist. Surgery, specialist and consultant units, laboratory and instrument tests are all connected to distributed databases and high performance computing resources. Comparing the results coming from clinical data and research data is a very productive process.

Both clinical and research data might be stored at different locations and have different formats and representations which can make the process of comparing it difficult. Watry and Larson (2005) have obtained an integration pass which can benefit from the ongoing efforts in the fields of metadata description and Grid Digital Repositories. Algorithms for searching and retrieving a knowledge base and for data mining can be defined properly when based on the work carried out in the Grid environment. On the other hand, in the EU GEMSS project (2013) the simulation and the visualization have a compulsory role because surgery areas of neurology, vascular and Maxillo-Facial surgery planning and/or near-real-time are critical.

The requirements of a HealthGrid can differ from other Grid applications because of the nature of Grid network. The security requirement includes the AAA frame which is the authentication process that allows us to know who is accessing Grid resources and whether this person is allowed to access the Grid network. Authorization allows applications to know what a user is allowed to do in the network or system and what kind of data he or she can access. Through auditing it is possible to record what a user did or tried to do. The privacy and confidentiality of medical data requirement can be achieved by removing sensitive patient data from files and by deidentification and encryption of data in order to guarantee the confidentiality and integrity of the data.

Also, the legal and ethical requirement can be achieved by obtaining explicit consent from patients and by gaining clearance to use data from ethics committees. Grid tools can help the enforcing of local policies and special access constraints on local data. Nevertheless the interoperability of medical data should be assured because of the heterogeneous format and nature of medical data. When considering data access and database sharing over heterogeneous networks/systems, interoperability issues between data sets at different centers/countries have to be taken into account. Current standards for medical data are incomplete. In order to achieve a pan-European HealthGrid network, there is a need for standardization of data format, data structure and data model in the future.

Finally, the Quality-of-Service (QoS) has a vital role due to the medical applications which can require response time and high audio/video/image quality such as the remote surgery. Meanwhile, the entire system requires an uninterrupted operation because it should to be available 24 hours a day and 7 days a week and thus it requires a robust and a fault tolerance design and development.

3.1 Implemented Healthcare Scenario

The practice use from the integration of WSN with Grid technologies is more obvious with the following scenario in Figure 2 which illustrates a routine process in healthcare procedure. A typical user scenario would be a nurse and/or a physician that log into the system because they intend to collect data about a patient's health status.

The authentication and authorization server (AS) will then validate the username and password just to verify that no unauthorized access is being made for confidential data. The

Figure 2. Sensor grid scenario

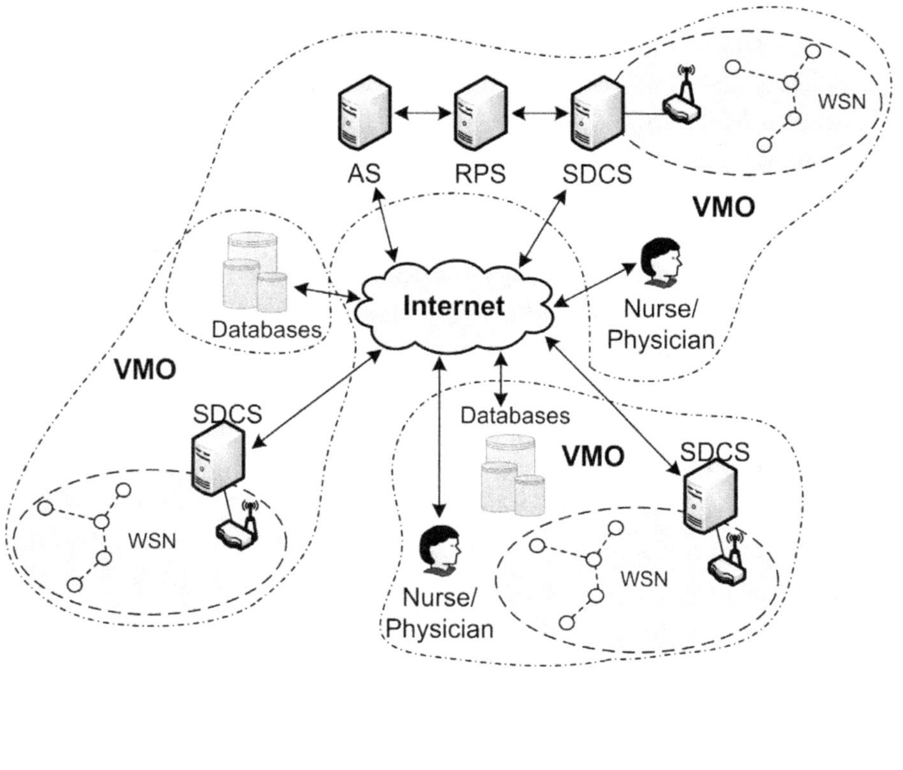

nurse/physician places the request to view i.e. the heart beat rate and the blood pressure value of a patient who has recently suffered from a cardiac arrest. After validation of the user the request is then sent to the Request Processing Server (RPS). Then, the RPS sends the request to the Sensor Data Collection Server (SDCS) which contacts the particular WSN monitoring the concerned patient to collect the data. After the data has been collected the data is sent back to SDCS and it decides whether the data needs any further processing. If it does not then it stores the data into the database and informs the RPS that the data has been collected and stored into the patients file in the Database Server (DS). Then the RPS fetches the data and sends it back to the nurse/physician who requested it.

Moreover, in the Virtual Medical Organization (VMO) scenario various medical organizations and physicians across the world can access the medical records of patients in order to refer and/or consult some critical case with some other doctor or physician who is far away from the patient site and also to come together to share resources and collaborate with each other in order to achieve a common goal.

This feature calls in for various security measures and QoS issues so that only authorized users can access the data on demand. We strongly hope that Sensor Grid will be able to greatly enhance the advantage of these two technologies for new and powerful application in the Electronic health (E-health) in order to attract the growing attention of research community. Finally, this scenario redefines the concept of VMO while focuses on the idea of integrating technologies and the storage problem while it helps us to monitor the collected by the sensors data to be stored and processed efficiently.

4. GRID STORAGE DESIGN

A Grid Infrastructure aims at storing and accessing data distributed at some storage centers when an application requires them. The responsibility of the maintenance of the reliability, scalability, manageability and the high performing network storage is provided by the Grid middleware which is responsible for ensuring these operations over a multitude of hardware and software solutions. These aspects have led to a proliferation of commercial and customized solutions.

Figure 3 illustrates the computer center on Grid Infrastructure which chooses on its own the storage system. This decision relies on the budget limitations, the experience of the vendors and their support which enhance the knowledge of system administrators. The result of this process is the high performance of the Grid through the interoperability of the devices because the variety of the interfaces and the implementation can cause a wide scale problem.

Figure 3 also shows the storage technologies used in the present time beyond the complexity of storage solution and cost. These types of systems can satisfy all users' needs for storage because they tend to use all the available resources. In these centers, the computing nodes can be equipped with a good amount of terabytes hard disks drives or with smaller but reliable storage systems. In addition, larger centers should have stronger requirements because they provide high capacity, reliability and durable storage. Some centers have to adapt proprietary backup or hierarchical storage management systems to manage in order to serve user requests and robotic libraries. In some cases, the usage of a robotic arm and an optical label reader is

Figure 3. Different types of storage solutions

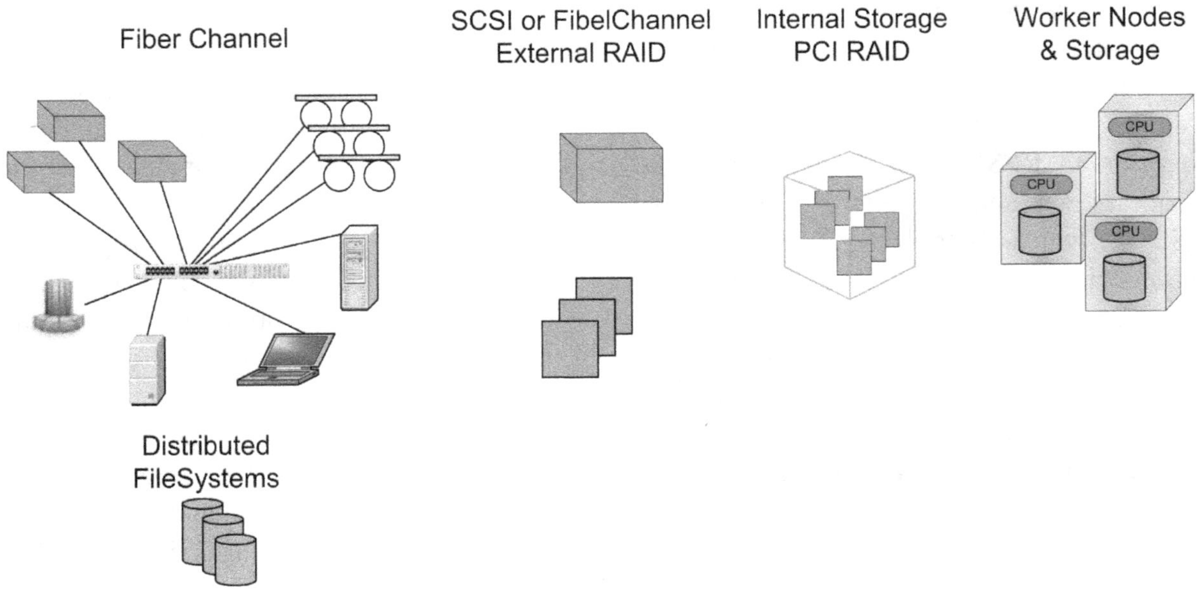

compulsory for the automatic management of the storage system.

A reduction of the system overhead may come from the adoption of commercial solutions and then the installation of Network File System (NFS) (IBM Network File System, 2013) or the Andrew File System (AFS) (AFS File System, 2013) or parallel file systems such as IBM General Parallel File System (GPFS) (IBM General Parallel File System, 2013) or Lustre (Lustre File System, 2013) is essential.

4.1 Grid Storage Element

To realize a Grid Service we have to adopt the Grid Storage Element (SE) which was obtained by Stewart, Cowan, Dunne, Elwell, and Miller (2008) and compromise a set of hardware and software solutions. Adopting this solution, the difference among specific solution can be hidden allowing users consistently and securely to store files at a Grid site. The EDG (2013) and EGEE EU (2013) projects provide a generic Grid Infrastructure to several communities of scientists which include healthcare and biology and because of the problem of storage requirements there have been created several working groups (Baseline Services Working Group, 2013). The SE is a basic storage resource which provides a uniform interface to storage in a Data Grid together with the following set of functionalities.

The migration of Grid users and applications across multiple administrative domains involves some consequences such as a transparent interface for specific applications, frequency of operations, security protocols and a set of different communication protocols to be supported at the same time. Providing efficient methods for both local and wide area access we ensure the reliability and high performance of data transfers protocols across domains. Beside the normal user who needs to store permanently his or her data, the Grid introduces a new set of users, the migratory users. These users use the local storage as intermediate storage to execute transient operations. Therefore a set of storage classes must be available and published in the information system so that applications and services can take advantage of them. A storage class is a type of storage space with specific attributes. Grid users also need to have available a set of operations for managing and reserving storage space and for filesystem-like operations as well as different QoS that need to be supported by the local storage solution. Storage services should be able to differentiate between valuable and expendable data when reservations expire. To avoid this process when a file is in use a concurrent application, called pinning is used to prevent the system from removing files.

Finally, the mechanisms of availability, capacity, content and system status may be supported. Also, the functions for management and monitoring of Grid are important for the control of services behavior. To ensure data integrity and data privacy we use a mechanism of checksum for the correctness of data even after replication or reprocessing. The mechanism of data privacy can be ensured with the support of side services that allow the storage of encryption keys on distributed servers to protect either from malicious attempts or from a specific site. A part of the solution was obtained by Shoshani et al. (2008), who presented the Storage Resource Manager (SRM) specification. An SRM is a middleware component whose function is to provide dynamic space allocation and file management on shared storage components on the Grid, but this does not solve completely the storage problem.

5. ARCHITECTURE AND IMPLEMENTATION OF THE SEGEDMA

A Sensor Grid consists of WSNs and conventional Grid resources like computers, servers, and disk arrays for the processing and storage of sensor data. The resources in the Sensor Grid are shared between several Virtual Organizations (VOs) and/or certain resources might belong to more than one VO. Users from various VOs may access the resources in the Sensor Grid, even if the resources are not owned by their VO. The architecture of our Sensor Grid and its components is illustrated in Figure 4.

We propose in the SEGEDMA framework a novel Sensor Grid architecture. This architecture is a proxy-based approach in order to achieve availability of the sensor devices on the Grid like conventional Grid services. Moreover, the proxy is a useful tool because it provides interoperability and supports a wide variety of WSN implantations.

In our implementation we use WSN proxy because it provides interoperability and acts as an interface between the wireless sensor network and the Grid network. The functions of the proxy are the exposition of the sensor resources as Grid Services that can be discovered and accessed by any Sensor Grid application and the translation of the sensor data from its native format to a suitable OGSA format. The test results show that the exposition of sensor resources becomes in a similar manner as other compute or data resources. Also, the proxy coordinates the network connectivity between the WSN and the Grid network and provides an interface between the sensor network protocols and the Internet protocols by using techniques like buffering, caching and link management.

Figure 4. Implemented of SEGEDMA architecture

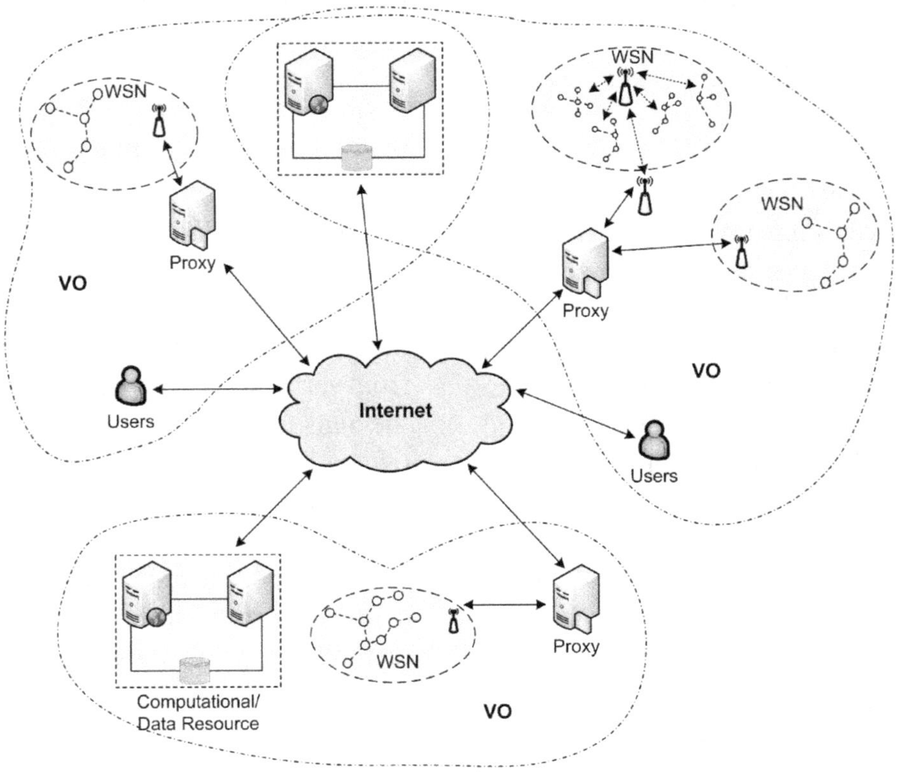

Consequently, the proxy can mitigate the effects of unexpected sensor network disconnection or long periods of disconnection. In this case, the enhancement of the Sensor Grid scalability is more obvious because new wireless sensor networks can be integrated with an existing Sensor Grid by adding proxy systems. Finally, the set of services which can be provided by using proxy includes services such as availability, power management, scheduling, security and QoS for the underlying wireless sensor network.

Figure 5 illustrates the features of the proposed SEGEDMA framework are based on a layered architecture approach where the layers represent the software components which are the basis of a Sensor Grid. Each of them defines accessible services through Application Programming Interfaces (APIs) for the application or other layers. The Grid Interface Layer supports a standard Grid middleware that enables different types of resources to communicate over the Grid network.

Regarding the user side, the access layer provides a Grid portal interface or a workflow management tool interface that both enable users to submit applications for execution on the Sensor Grid. The application consists of sensor jobs which have to be executed on the WSNs. This process takes place because the application might collect sensor data and computational jobs to process the sensor data. A Grid Meta-Scheduler, such as Community Scheduler Framework (CSF) has obtained by Smith (2003) is also used in our implementation because the involvement of CSF in routing and scheduling the jobs according to their required resources is important.

Figure 5. The sensor grid framework

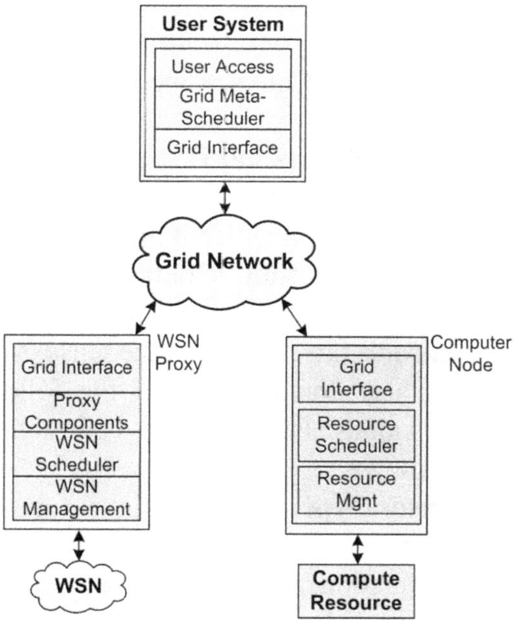

Considering the WSN Management layer, an abstraction of the specific APIs and protocols is provided in order to access and manage the underlying heterogeneous sensor resources. It manages the configuration of the sensor nodes and provides status information of the sensor nodes while it accepts sensor job requests from the Grid and invokes the specific commands to execute the jobs on the sensor nodes. The WSN Scheduler is the local resource scheduler for the sensor network and implements the low level scheduling algorithms for sensor power management and resource management. Furthermore, it controls the scheduling of sensor job requests from the users. The parameters of a sensor job include the amount of sensor resources required, desired start time, duration, priority, etc. The scheduler considers these job parameters and also checks whether the required sensor resources are available and reserves the resources for the job. It also works in conjunction with other proxy components providing services for availability and QoS.

The collaborative work of proxy components and WSN Management Layer provides important services for sensor data management, information services, network connectivity, power management, security, availability and QoS. The access and the management of computational and storage resources for the execution of Grid jobs are provided by APIs from Resource Management layer and then the Resource Scheduler performs the scheduling of the Grid jobs based on local usage policies.

5.1 OGC-Based Approach

Grid Computing is a rapidly developing web services based technology which tends to be a part of utility computing. The approach of the Service-Oriented Architecture (SOA) is the basis of our implemented system because it enables the discovery, access and sharing of the services, data, computational and communication resources in a Grid network by many different users.

On the other hand, wireless sensor networks consist of an amount of sensors which collect data about patients' health status in real-time. Until now, wireless sensors have been managed with individual specification and not by an explicit standardization of metadata. As a result the collection and communication were limited due to heterogeneous sensors. In order to solve this problem the Open Geospatial Consortium (OGC) has introduced the Sensor Web Enablement (SWE) concept that is actually a set of specifications including Sensor Model Language (SensorML), Observation & Measurement (O&M), Sensor Observation Service (SOS), Sensor Collection Service (SCS), Sensor Planning Service

(SPS) and Web Notification Service (WNS) to implement the Sensor Web. However, it is important to note that the SWE framework is not depending on the mentioned components because they can be used on their own or in conjunction with other sensor system architectures.

SensorML is an eXtensible Markup Language (XML) based language which has developed in order to overcome the difficulty to match sensor data with geographical information efficiently while combining various sensors. SensorML is a key component for enabling autonomous and intelligent sensor webs. In the SEGEDMA project we use the SensorML model and XML schema in order to define the measured features from sensors using XML-based language for that it can describe attributes of dynamic sensors such as geometric, dynamic and radiometric attributes. Moreover the sensors can be in one or several networks, can be geographically distributed, can have a variable status and can be variably grouped. For these reasons, we have designed an information structure able to contain all relevant information about sensors and the values observed by it. During the design phase, we have dealt with the following parameters:

Step 1: We chose which information is relevant to publish.
Step 2: We analyzed how the information must be represented in a relational data model.
Step 3: We designed a standard interface that allows sensors to publish its data.
Step 4: We determined how the communication can be done.

According to the SensorML standard we define a model with an objectclass named SensoGedma containing the following information:

1. **Sensor-ID:** Contains the unique ID of the sensor.
2. **Sensor-Hostname:** Describes the host name of the sensor or the host name of the resource in which it is installed.
3. **Sensor-Location:** Contains the geographic coordinate of the sensor.
4. **Sensor-State:** Describes the sensor state and also contains one of the following values: Ready, Busy, Uninstalled, Unknown.
5. **Sensor-Type:** Describes the type of the sensor and the type of supplied information.
6. **Sensor-Value:** Contains the instantaneous value (or values) of observed target.

This object is modeled by an XML schema that will be published through the network and it is written in a language supported by the sensors.

Having the SensorML in our Sensor Grid we can manage successfully the produced and stored metadata. The metadata are composed by identification, classification, limitation, features etc. Our SensorML framework is illustrated in Figure 6 and is comprised by:

1. Sensor information about data discovery.
2. Processing and analysis of the sensor measurements.
3. Support of geolocation of the measured data.
4. Characteristics about the performance.
5. Properties and assumptions regarding sensor.

Figure 6. Code generator

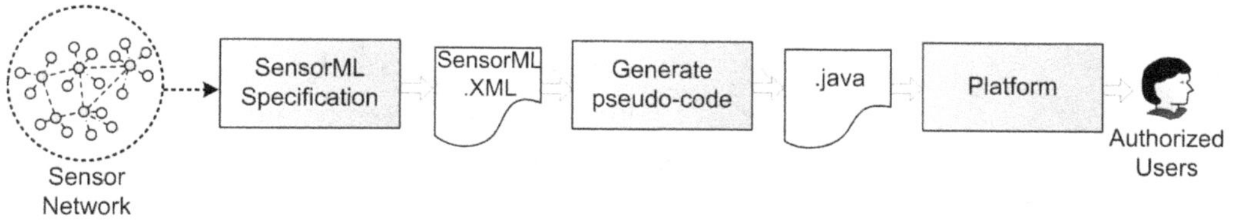

Thus, our developed prototype is based on OGC standards. The SensorML model ensures an interoperable function of the wireless sensor network eliminating the need of detailed description of hardware while supports rigorous geolocation models which can describe sensor parameters independent of platform and target as well as mathematical models which can directly map between sensor and target space. O&M defines a framework and a conceptual model, where the encoding is formalized as an application schema. Also, O&M binds a result to a feature of interest, upon which the observation was made using a procedure to determine the value of the result.

Other standards that define the services to access the sensors data are SOS and Sensor Planning Service (SPS). The SOS provides an interface to make sensors and sensor data archives accessible via an interoperable Web based interface.

The basic SOS allows the operations of GetCapabilities (request a self-description of the service), DescribeSensor (request information about the sensor itself in a SensorML document), GetObservation (request the sensor data, encoded in an O&M document). The SPS is an interface to task an asset, or an asset system. The SPS allows the operations such as GetCapabilities which retrieves the metadata about the capabilities of an SPS, DescribeTasking gets the information that is required to prepare a tasking request), GetFeasibility obtains the feasibility details about a tasking request, Submit submits a tasking request and DescribeResultAccess can retrieve the information about where observed data can be accessed from.

The compulsory usage of OGC standards in our Sensor Grid architecture ensures the support of process such as reading, controlling, processing and analyzing data from the physical world through a Grid environment achieving an uninterrupted operation of our Sensor Grid network. Figure 7 illustrates the layered architecture of our prototype in conjunction with the OGC standard.

The environment of distributed databases is fully controlled by unauthorized access. A custom java interface is developed and is presented in Section 6.2 in order to ensure access to the distributed databases of our system which are in a full controlled environment preventing access from unauthorized users. The functionalities of our java interface are spread between the service layer, the sensor access layer and the storage access layer.

The SCS specification is one of the core services in our implementation which belongs in the service layer. This component is responsible for collecting real time sensing data and then translating the resulting raw information into an XML-based O&M encoding for other services to utilize and process. The SCS is the gateway for entering into the sensor networks from outside users. The design of the SCS provides an interface to both streaming data

Figure 7. Layers in SEGEDMA framework

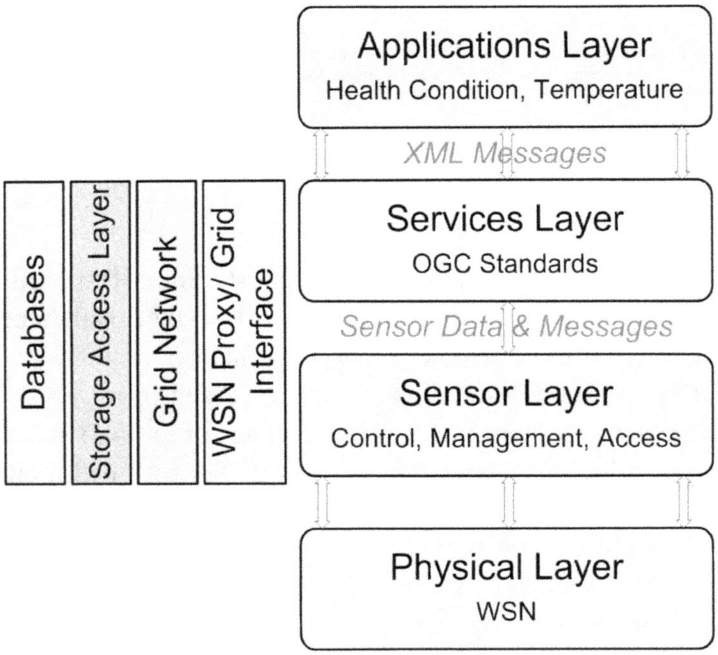

and query based sensor applications that are built on top of TinyOS.

As it is illustrated in Figure 8 the architecture of the SCS conforms to the interface definition that is described by the OGC SCS and has been designed as a Web Service which works by connecting via a proxy to either real sensors or a remote repository database. Users need to query the sensor registry service in order to retrieve an available SCS Web Services Description Language (WSDL) address. A data query request is then sent via SOAP to the SCS in order to obtain the resulting encoded observation data conforming to the O&M specification. As we mentioned the proxy acts as an agent working with various connectors that connect to the resources holding the information and which encode the raw observation into O&M compatible data. Different types of connectors have been designed to fit into different types of resources including sensor networks running on top of TinyOS and remote observation data archives.

The proxy needs to process the incoming messages from the user in order to determine what kind of connectors, either real-time based or archive based, to use. The design of the SCS is flexible and makes it simple to extend for further development if alternative sensor operating systems are adopted by the sensor networks. Besides a sensor operating system specific connector no modifications need to be made in the current system. The design of the proxy also encourages the implementation of a cache mechanism to improve the scalability and performance of the SCS. Load balancing mechanisms can be added to the system easily as well, by simply deploying the web service to different servers.

Figure 8. OGC proxy approach

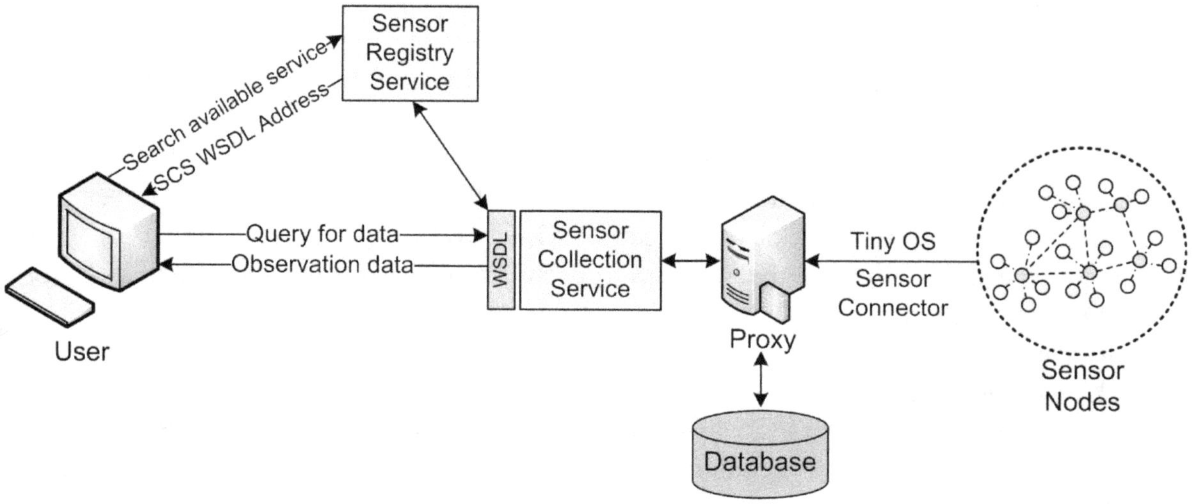

5.2 Proxy Software Architecture

In this section we discuss the provided proxy components and the important services for a Sensor Grid which are illustrated in Figure 9. First, the Data Management component handles the conversion of sensor data from its native format to a Grid friendly format like XML or other formats desired by the user. This component also performs data fusion and other optimizations to improve the quality of data collected from multiple sensors. It supports several methods for the transfer of the sensor data to the user application, such as using GridFTP or by streaming the data.

Second, the Information Services Component manages the discovery and monitoring of sensor resources. This component advertises the available sensor resources as Grid services via mechanisms such as the Indexing Service (IS) of OGSA. Users can query the availability and status of sensor resources via mechanisms such as the Monitoring and Discovery Service (MDS) of OGSA. The static and dynamic information on sensor resources is directly relevant to the WSN Scheduler. Third, the WSN Connectivity component provides services to interface the sensor network protocols with the Grid networking protocols. It buffers the transmission of sensor data, caches the routing information of sensor nodes and manages the ad hoc sensor network links.

Fourth, the Power Management Component keeps track of the power consumption of the sensor nodes. Together with the WSN

Figure 9. Proxy component

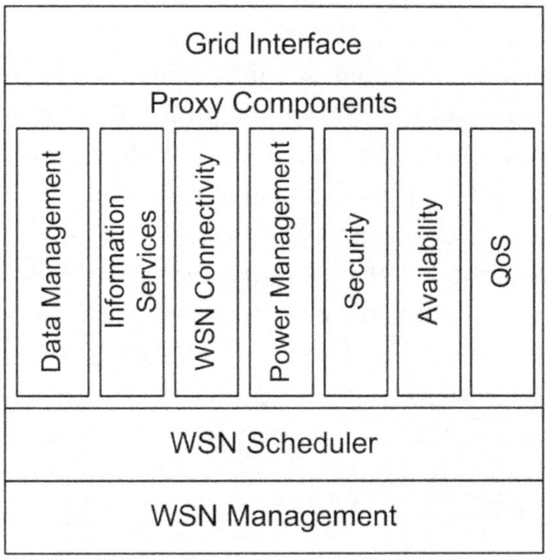

Scheduler, it performs actions to conserve power for the sensor nodes. The Security component implements OGSA compliant Grid security technologies. For example, it can use technologies such as the Generic Security Service (GSS) API to perform authentication between the proxy and the sensor nodes. Fifth, the Availability component provides services to improve the availability of the wireless sensor network. It monitors the sensor nodes to find those with possible failing hardware or weak power level and migrate the jobs in such nodes to the reliable nodes. To do so, it works closely with the WSN Scheduler. The availability component can also provide fault tolerance features such as the replication of services and the recovery of interrupted jobs.

Finally, the QoS component supports the provisioning of QoS in the Sensor Grid. In conjunction with the WSN Scheduler, the QoS component performs the reservation and allocation of sensor resources based on QoS requirements of sensor jobs. It works with the WSN connectivity of the proxy component to adapt to the varying network conditions in order to provide the desired QoS.

5.3 Distributed Databases in Healthcare Information System

This section analyses the application of Information and Communication Technologies (ICT) on the whole range of health sector activities defining the term of E-health and also simplifies the access to healthcare services while boosts their quality and effectiveness. Traditionally, the patient record was a record of care provided when a patient was ill. An Electronic Health Record (EHR) represents the electronically maintained information about a patient's lifetime health status and healthcare which are stored serving the share between multiple legitimate users of the record. Managed care encourages healthcare providers to focus on the continuum of health and healthcare from wellness to illness and recovery.

The name Health Leven 7 (HL7) came from the seventh Application Layer of the Open System Interconnection (OSI) reference model. HL7 has developed in order to succeed systems interoperability between different hospitals and other healthcare provider organizations which have different computer systems for each hospital procedure. Nevertheless, HL7 specifies a number of flexible standards, guidelines, and methodologies for various healthcare systems ensuring the interoperability. This mechanism provides an excellent ability for internetworking centrals and geographically isolated hospitals. Today most clinical data sources can deliver the clinical content as HL7 messages. Consequently, the patients' records must be integrated regarding their health and illness status which can be acquired by multiple healthcare providers across diverse Health Information Systems (HIS) settings. In addition, the patients' data should be stored in to be available at any time to any healthcare organization when needed.

Our implemented healthcare information system is based on the HL7 standard and has a patient-centric architecture achieving to prevent their possible diseases, to monitor their health status while it handles effectively both service and patient information. HL7 standard provides several functionalities for the exchange, the management, searching, sharing, retrieval and the integration of electronic health information regarding both patients and healthcare services. The implementation of this system relies on distributed databases across the interconnected hospitals through a database interface and aims at supporting medical employees to retrieve medical information. It also aims at the integration of incidental systems such as financial services and pharmaceutical prescriptions through the distributed databases in which the patients' records and his clinical data are stored.

As it is illustrated in Figure 10, two different operations have been developed. The first of them concerns the integrated data architecture from multiple sources systems while the second provides a database interface with message-handling capability and automatically codes translation from the source system to the supported code of the receiving EHR. Moreover, HL7 is strictly related with XML since it is based on coded documents in this language while it is a widely accepted standard in the marketplace (Watry, & Larson, 2005). Thus, HL7 consists the basis of the SEGEDMA architecture which ensures the interoperability between different hospital information systems. The presented architecture connects together the information systems that belong to different hospitals constituting a large-scale Grid network.

In order to access any certificated hospital the infrastructure has to register their local information service as a web service in the Grid and its users can utilize the platform finding the proper resources that they need. All the participated hospitals use one node as a Grid node which works as an information provider of the Grid and also as an agent in order to access any HIS retrieving medical information with the support of the HL7. Our system consists of following components:

Figure 10. HIS with distributed database

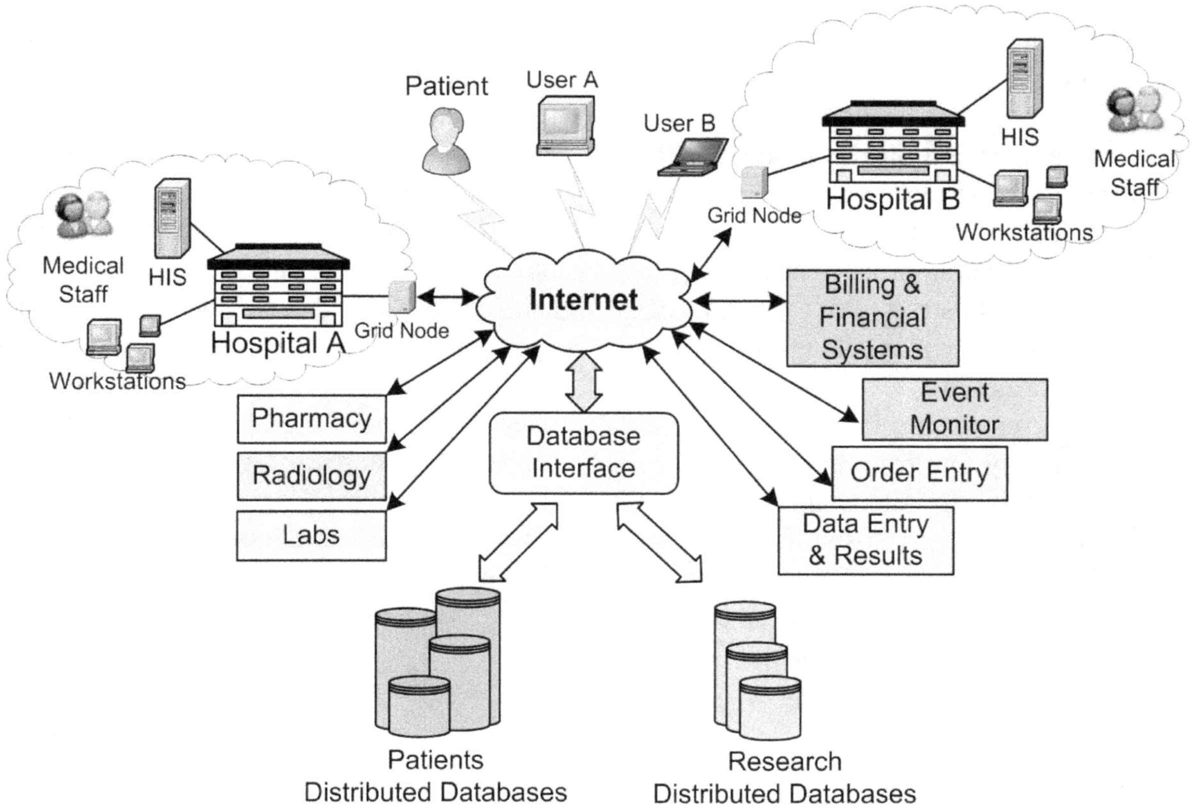

1. Patient Agent (PA), allowing a patient to submit queries for detecting services of his interest.
2. Healthcare Service Provider Agent (HCSPA), supporting a Healthcare Service Provider Manager (HCSPM) in order to maintain the corresponding service database updated.
3. Coordinator Agent (CA), cooperating with PAs and HCSPAs to detect those services appearing to be the closest to patients' queries and profiles.
4. Healthcare Service Provider Distributed Database (HCSPDD), which is associated with an HCSPM managing information about services delivered by it.
5. Patients Profile Distributed Database (PPDD), storing and handling patient profiles.

In Figure 11 is illustrated the procedure of our HL7 based healthcare system when a doctor or a patient use our infrastructure. When a patient submits a query, our system forwards it only to appropriate healthcare department through the five mentioned components. Besides this patient-centric multi-agent design a patient does not contact manually with any intermediate agent in order to advice him or monitor his health status. But the agents can interact between them exchanging patient's medical information.

In order to ensure the data security level of the presented system from unauthorized users' access each hospital installed a software configuration on each hospital Grid node. Thus different Grid users such as physicians, nurses, patients and various authorized users from the Internet or inside hospitals have different authorization level when access the infrastructure. As a result the medical staff across Sensor Grid infrastructure can exchange, request and acquire information and results with security from different local HIS and distributed databases in the desired format.

5.4 Data Management Model

Our implementation is based on the utilization of proxy systems which act as interfaces between the different networks. This architecture specifies the middleware that controls the operation of user systems, WSN proxy and computational resources connected to a Sensor Grid. As it can be seen the Figure 5 represents layers of the main middleware components that connect different types of systems to the Grid network. Those layers define accessible services via APIs for the application or other layers.

Figure 12 shows the MySQL backend is responsible for the query and retrieval services in our implementation. It provides a database extension by including a table to catalog for all sensor jobs that were executed. The contained metadata refer to sensor jobs in order to allow user's application to find out which sensor jobs were executed on the WSN. When a job is executed by sensors the information of the job is extracted in the catalog table. The query and retrieval are implemented as a Grid service. Therefore the Grid users will be able to see if a sensor job is running and then they can retrieve the desired collected data through the Grid service using the GridFTP in order to transfer data.

Figure 11. Implemented HL7-based infrastructure

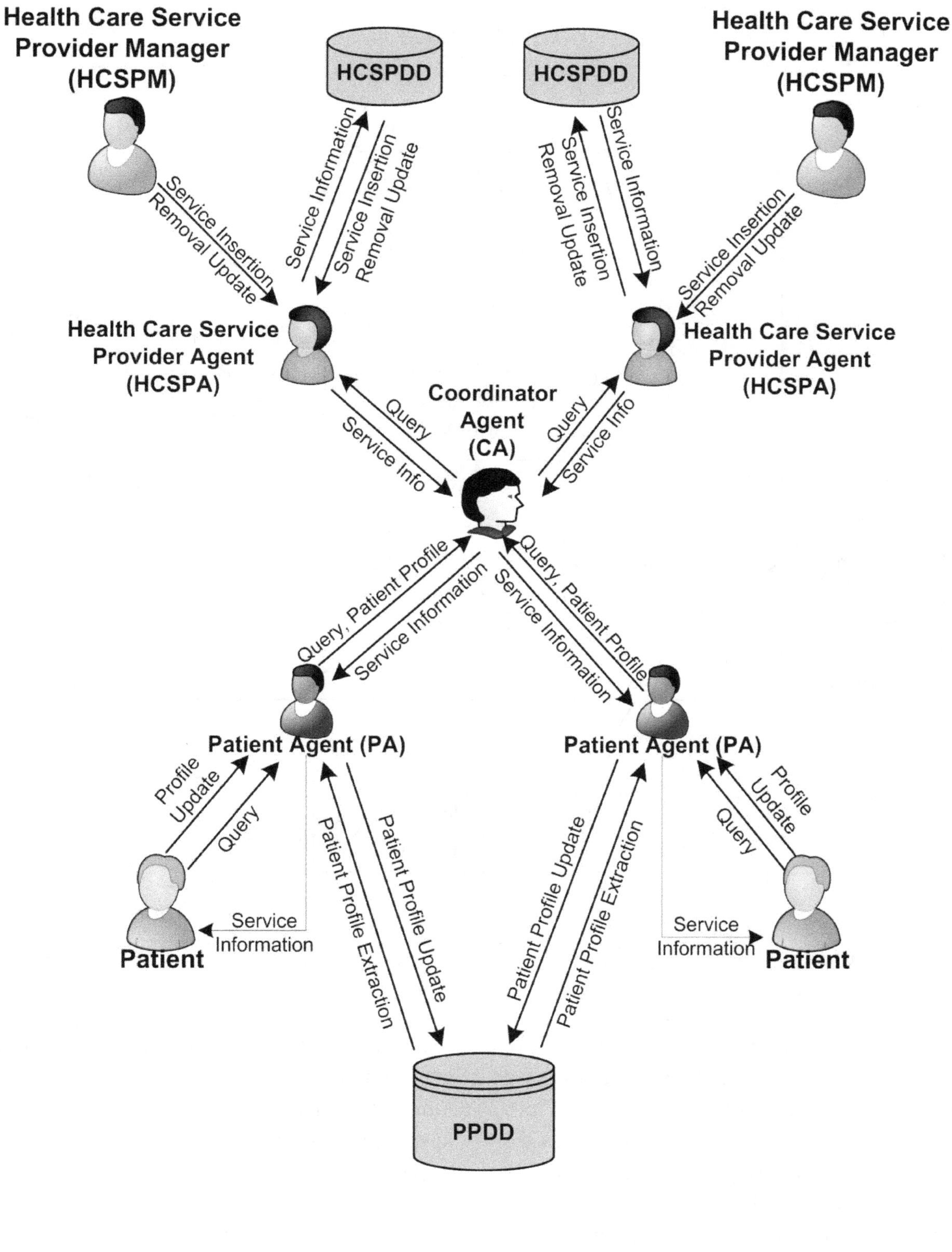

Figure 12. The data management model

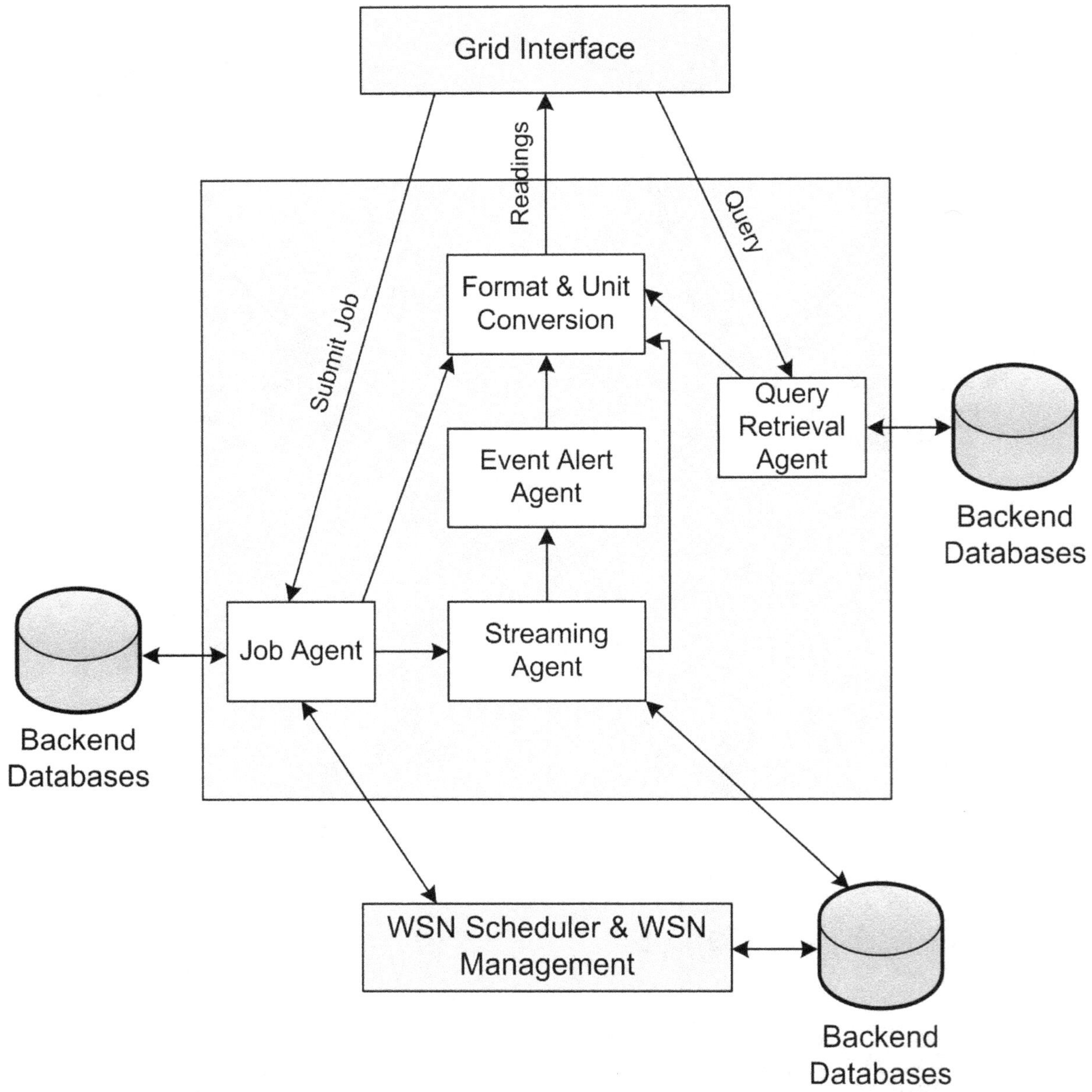

Before the implementation of the WSN management layer which is supported by Motelab we have to follow two steps. First, we have to determine how Motelab names are created for new sensor jobs and the table fields used to store the collected data. The second step is to determine how the data management component will be informed when a sensor job has finished its execution because after that the catalog update is a required process. In our Sensor Grid when an application submits a sensor job for execution, it will specify the type of data format conversion required. The service provides conversion to text or XML format. For the conversion to XML format, an eXtensible Stylesheet Language (XSL) document is also generated and transferred back to the user application along with the XML data. Over at the side of application, XSL Transformation (XSLT) is used to convert the XML data into a HTML document, allowing the user to view the collected data on a browser. Based on the application requirement for both non-streaming and streaming of sensor data, the data format will be converted on-the-fly and returned to the application. The data unit conversion is implemented using Java's polymorphism mechanism so that is easy for the developer to add or remove a data unit conversion module. When an application submits a sensor job for execution, it will specify what type of data unit conversion is required.

For our streaming service we use the Globus Toolkit mechanism which allows the notifications of users about the changes in a Grid service. In the implemented Sensor Grid a user can subscribe to the streaming service. As the sensor job is being executed in the WSN, the streaming service will detect if there are any data being collected, and stream the data back to the application in real-time. For the detection of new data, the streaming service periodically checks the backend database to see if there is new sensor data being stored by the WSN management layer. The WSN management layer is based on Motelab and uses a MySQL backend database to store information about jobs and their collected data.

Also, the streaming service can be leveraged by the Event Alert which extends this service. The extension of the streaming service is realized by filtering out those sensor data that are not of interest or importance and only sends an event notification to the user application when the data meets the interest of the application. In our Sensor Grid when a sensor job is being executed the service will detect whether any data being collected is above a threshold defined by the application and delivers the event alert to the application immediately.

6. VALIDATION TESTBED

The wireless sensor network hardware testbed deploys 16 MICA2 motes and 10 MICAz motes. The model of the MICA2 motes incorporates a 7.3MHz Atmel ATmega128L microcontroller, 128KB of program flash memory, 4KB of EEPROM, and 512 KB of flash logger memory for data. It makes use of the Chipcon CC1100 radio transceiver which operates in the 433 MHz RF frequency band.

We also use the MTS310CA sensor boards, which can be plugged into the MICA2 motes. The MICAz is an upgraded version of the MICA2 with the IEEE 802.15.4 compliant Chipcon CC2420 radio operating at 2.4 GHz and 250Kbps data rate. We use 5 MIB600 Ethernet interface boards for hosting the base station motes and to collect sensor data we use 12 MTS310CA sensor boards that are plugged onto the motes. Each sensor board contains a variety of sensors. The MICA2 and MICAz both run a small open source operating system designed for embedded wireless sensor networks, the TinyOS. The sensor applications are developed with an extension of the C programming language, the nesC.

Finally, the testbed is compromised by a Sun cluster with 4 server nodes and 25 compute nodes. The total capacity of the cluster is 15 TB of disk storage. We also use Linux-based PCs as the proxy systems and user systems. Each server node contains Intel

Xeon 2.8 GHz processors with 16 GB RAM and each compute node contains Intel Xeon 2 GHz processors with 4 GB RAM. Also, the proxy systems and the users systems are both Linux-based PCs.

6.1 Testbed Implementation

The implemented Grid Interface layer of our proposed Sensor Grid uses Globus Toolkit (GT) 4.2 which is installed on the WSN proxies, the Sun cluster and the user systems. The implemented Grid Meta-scheduler uses the CFS to route sensor and computational jobs to their destinations. The Sun Grid Engine (SGE) 6.2 plays an important role in the implementation of the WSN scheduler as well as the resource scheduler for the compute cluster. For the WSN Scheduler, we set up a SGE queue for sensor jobs. Similarly, the compute Resource Scheduler has a SGE queue for computational jobs. To pass jobs from GT 4.2 to the SGE queues, we use a toolkit for integrating GT 4.2 with SGE called EPIC (Epic-Sun Grid Engine integration with Globus Toolkit, 2013).

Another important component of our testbed is the WSN Management layer which is based on MoteLab and we have to reuse some software components of MoteLab such as database backend, the job daemon, and the data logger. Our WSN Scheduler controls the operation of these components and bypasses MoteLab's web frontend. We also implemented additional functionalities for this layer such as the status monitoring of the motes. In MoteLab, all the motes are permanently connected to the network and are programmed via MIB600 interface boards. For our testbed, five base station motes are connected to the network via MIB600 boards. The rest of the motes are programmed wirelessly over-the-air in an automated manner using XnP (Mote in Network Programming User Reference, 2003).

At present, the Sensor Grid testbed has been successfully deployed and we can execute sensor jobs to collect sensor data for process and storage. We plan to enhance the testbed in several ways. First, we will continue to work on the design and implementation of the proxy components because the majority of them have not been fully implemented yet. Second, we will develop a workflow tool to help users develop sensor applications and automate the submission of jobs. After the key enhancements to our Sensor Grid testbed are completed we intend to conduct extensive experimental studies to obtain performance measurements from the testbed and this will enable us to evaluate more the effectiveness of our implementation.

6.2 Data Management Component

The deployment of the developed data management component into existing Sensor Grid as a Grid service was a successful process. Also, Figure 13 shows the development of the Graphical User Interface (GUI) application client in order to perform validation testing of the services which are provided by the data management component.

For the query and retrieval service the application client successfully displayed past sensor jobs and their respective information from the sensor network. The application can also select which sensor job should retrieve and display the collected data in a browser.

For the testing of the streaming service, the application client submitted a streaming sensor job and successfully received the collected sensor data in real-time. For the testing of the event alert service, the application client

Figure 13. Retrieval of sensor data for display in GUI

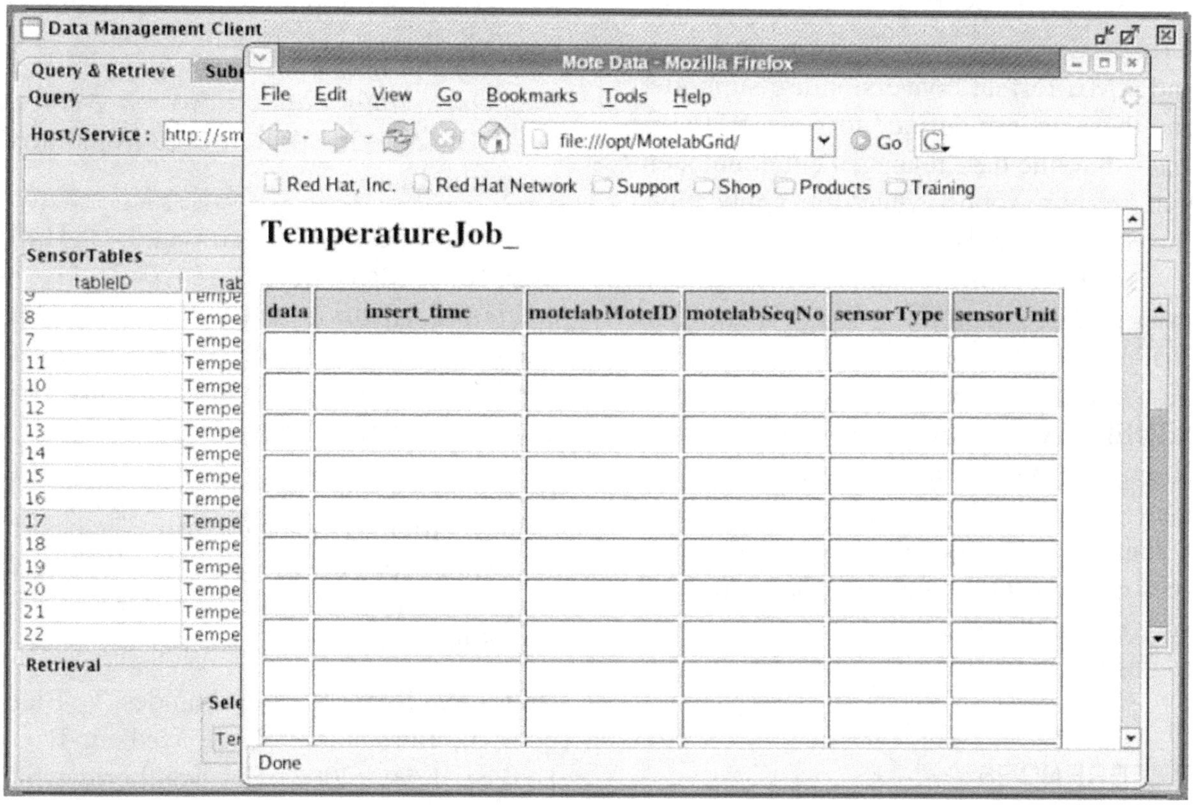

submitted an event alert sensor job and successfully received an event notification when the temperature reached above the specified threshold. Using the application client, we also successfully validated the conversion of sensor data format using the data format conversion service and the conversion of sensor data units using the data unit conversion service.

7. CONCLUSION

Wireless sensor networks and Grid computing are promising technologies that are being adopted in the industry. By the implemented integration of these technologies, Sensor Grids greatly enhance the potential of them for new and powerful applications. Thus, we believe that Sensor Grids will attract growing attention from the research community and the industry.

In this chapter, we propose SEGEDMA model which provides a novel architecture and an enhancement model for management of the stored data in Sensor Grid networks in a healthcare system. Moreover we developed a standardized Health Information System according to the OGC and HL7 directives ensuring the interoperability of the infrastructure. Nevertheless, the data management component of the proposed architecture and the important services that it should provide were discussed. The data management component was successfully developed and integrated into our implemented Sensor Grid testbed. It can be extended so that the data format conversion can provide services to convert data readings to a user specified format. Currently, only conversion to text and XML format conversion are supported and these are pre-defined formats. With this extension, the data management component will be more robust since user applications can define their own format conversion.

Finally, in this chapter we have also examined the important design issues and challenges for Sensor Grids in Healthcare. To address these design issues, we proposed SEGEDMA model for Sensor Grid networks based on proxy systems with an enhanced data management model. Also, we have developed a Sensor Grid testbed to study the design issues of our network because the testbed is a very useful research tool to study issues and to improve our architecture design.

REFERENCES

Abbas, A. (2003). *Grid computing: A practical guide to technology and applications*. Hingham, MA: Charles River Media. *AFS file system*. (2013). Retrieved from: http://lxr.linux.no/linux/Documentation/filesystems/afs.txt

Akyildiz, I. F., Weilian, Su, Sankarasubramaniam, Y., & Cayirci, E. (2002). A survey on sensor network. *IEEE Communications Magazine*, *40*, 102–114. doi:10.1109/MCOM.2002.1024422

Amendolia, S. R. (2007). Mammogrid - A prototype distributed mammographic database for Europe. *Clinical Radiology*, *62*, 1044–1051. doi:10.1016/j.crad.2006.09.032 PMID:17920862

Baseline Services Working Group. (2013). Retrieved from http://lcg.web.cern.ch/LCG/peb/BS

Biomedical Informatics Research Network (USA BIRN). (2013). Retrieved from http://www.nbirn.net

Bramley, R., Chiu, K., Huffman, J. C., Huffman, K., & McMullen, D. F. (2003). *Instruments and sensors as network services: Making instruments first class members of the grid* (Technical Report 588). Indiana University Computer Science Department.

Breton, V., Dean, K., & Solomonides, T. (2005). From grid to healthgrid: The healthgrid white paper. In *Proceedings of Healthgrid Conference* (pp. 249-321). Amsterdam, The Netherlands: IOS Press.

Breton, V., Dean, K., Solomonides, T., Blanquer, I., Hernandez, V., & Medico, E. … Herveg, J. A. (2004).The healthgrid white paper. Studies in Health Technology and Informatics, *112*, 249-321.

Buyya, R., Date, S., Mizuno-Matsumoto, Y., Venugopal, S., & Abramson, D. (2003). Composition and on-demand deployment of distributed brain activity analysis application on global grids. In *10th Proceedings of the International Conference on High Performance Computing (HiPC)* (pp.1-10). New Delhi, India: Elite Publishing House.

Charles River Media. AFS file system. (2013). Retrieved from: http://lxr.linux.no/linux/Documentation/filesystems/afs.txt</

CLEF-integrating information for the clinical E-Scientist. (2013). Retrieved from: http://www.clinical-escience.org

Crossbow Technology, Inc. (2003). Mote in network programming user reference (Technical Report). Berkeley WEbS.

Czajkowski, K., Ferguson, D., Foster, I., Frey, J., Graham, S., & Maquire, T. et al. (2004). *From open grid services infrastructure to WSResource framework: Refactoring & evolution*. IBM DeveloperWorks.

Eichelberg, M., Aden, T., Riesmeier, J., Dogac, A., & Laleci, G. B. (2005). A survey and analysis of electronic healthcare record standards. *ACM Computing Surveys*, *37*(4), 277–315. doi:10.1145/1118890.1118891

Enabling grid for E-science (EGEE). (2013). Retrieved from http://www.eu-egee.org

Epic-sun grid engine integration with globus toolkit. (2013). Retrieved from http://www.lesc.ic.ac.uk/projects/epic-gt-sge.html

EU mammogrid. (2013). Retrieved from, ftp://ftp.cordis.europa.eu/pub/ist/docs/grids/mammogrid_achievement.pdf

European data grid (EDG). (2013). Retrieved from http://www.edg.org

Foster, I., & Kesselman, C. (1997). Globus: A metacomputing infrastructure toolkit. *The International Journal of Supercomputer Applications*, *11*, 115–128. doi:10.1177/109434209701100205

Foster, I., Kesselman, C., Nick, J., & Tuecke, S. (2002). *The physiology of the grid: An open grid services architecture for distributed systems integration*. Open Grid Service Infrastructure WG, Global Grid Forum.

Foster, I., Kesselman, C., & Tuecke, S. (2001). The anatomy of the grid: Enabling scalable virtual organizations. *The International Journal of Supercomputer Applications*, *15*, 200–222. doi:10.1177/109434200101500302

Fritschy, J., Horesh, L., Holder, D., & Bayford, R. (2005). Applications of grid in clinical neurophysiology and electrical impedance tomography of brain function. In *Proceedings of Healthgrid from Grid to Healthgrid* (pp. 138–145). Amsterdam, The Netherlands: IOS Press.

IBM general parallel file system. (2013). Retrieved from: ftp://ftp.software.ibm.com/common/ssi/pm/fy/n/clf03001usen/CLF03001USEN.PDF

IBM network file system (NFS-IBM). (2013) Retrieved from: http://www03.ibm.com/servers/s390/os390/bkserv/r10pdf/nfs.html

Japan medical engineering grid (MEGrid). (2013). Retrieved from: http://www.biogrid.jp

Liu, Y., Bacon, J., & Wilson-Hinds, R. (2007). On smart-care: Services studies of visually impaired users in living context. In *1st International Conference on the Digital Society* (pp. 32-40). French Caribbean: IEEE Press.

Lustre file system. (2013). Retrieved from: http://www.sun.com/software/products/lustre

National digital mammography archive (NDMA). (2013). Retrieved from: http://rt-image.com/0825digitalmammo

Shoshani, A., Kunszt, P., Stockinger, H., Stockinger, K., Laure, E., & Baud, J. P. … Sim A. (2008). Storage resource management: Concepts, functionality and interface specification. In *International Conference on Computing in High Energy and Nuclear Physics*. Czech: IOP Publishing.

Smith, C. (2003). *Open source meta-scheduling for virtual organizations with the community scheduler framework (CSF) (Technical Report)*. Platform Computing.

Stewart, G. A., Cowan, G. A., Dunne, B., Elwell, A., & Miller, A. P. (2008). Optimising LAN access to grid enabled storage elements. In *International Conference on Computing in High Energy and Nuclear Physics*. Pennsylvania: IOP Publishing.

Syed, J., Ghanem, M., & Guo, Y. (2006). Supporting scientific discovery processes in discovery net. *Concurrency and Computation*, *19*, 167–179. doi:10.1002/cpe.1049

Tuecke, S., Czajkowski, K., Foster, I., Frey, J., Graham, S., Kesselman, C., et al. (2003). *Open grid services infrastructure (OGSI) version 1.0* (Technical report). Global Grid Forum.

UK E-Science eDiaMoND. (2013). Retrieved from: http://www.ediamond.ox.ac.uk

Warren, R., Solomonides, T., Del Frate, C., Warsi, I., Ding, J., & Odeh, M. … Estrella, F. (2013). *Grid-enabled medical simulation services (EU GEMSS)*. Retrieved from: http://www.it.neclab.eu/gemss

Watry, P., & Larson, R. (2005). Cheshire 3 framework white paper: Implementing support for digital repositories in a data grid environment. In *IEEE International Symposium on Mass Storage Systems and Technology* (pp. 60-84). Sardinia: IEEE Press.

Chapter 8
Using Agent and Workflow Technologies for the Implementation of Interoperable Healthcare Information Systems

Vassiliki Koufi
University of Piraeus, Greece

Flora Malamateniou
University of Piraeus, Greece

George Vassilacopoulos
University of Piraeus, Greece

ABSTRACT

Healthcare is an increasingly collaborative enterprise involving many individuals and organizations that coordinate their efforts toward promoting quality and efficient delivery of healthcare through the use of interoperable healthcare information systems (HIS). Service-oriented architecture (SOA) provides a cost-effective solution to implementing interoperability between heterogeneous HIS which have resulted from extensive investments that most healthcare organizations have made in system resources over the course of many years. However, issues of semantic interoperability still remain unresolved while new challenges arise regarding web service interoperability. This chapter presents a mediator-based approach for achieving data and service interoperability among disparate and geographically dispersed HIS. The proposed system architecture provides a uniform interface to the underlying HIS, thus enabling decoupling of the client applications and the server-side implementations while it ensures security in all transactions. It is a distributed system architecture based on the agent paradigm for both healthcare process management and management of interactions among the participating systems. The healthcare processes and all interactions involved in each process are described according to the workflow metaphor. Thus, robustness, high flexibility and fault tolerance are provided in an environment as dynamic and heterogeneous as healthcare.

DOI: 10.4018/978-1-4666-3000-0.ch008

INTRODUCTION

Healthcare delivery involves a broad range of in-patient, out-patient and emergency healthcare services, typically performed by a number of geographically distributed and organizationally disparate healthcare providers who often invest significant resources in the development of large and complex information systems. Technologically innovative efforts of the past have often resulted in the development of disparate, incompatible and heterogeneous systems based on the traditional transaction processing paradigm rather than on supporting business processes. However, healthcare providers' activities require increased collaboration and coordination in order to provide shared and integrated care when and where needed (Malamateniou and Vassilacopoulos, 2003). Thus, the integration of diverse and disparate information systems with emphasis on communication and collaboration is a challenge often faced by healthcare organizations (Lenz and Kuhn, 2004; Huizen and Backman, 2005). This challenge can be met by means of interoperable healthcare information systems (HIS) that support a process view of the healthcare delivery context and also facilitate communication among diverse systems on an ongoing basis, despite different purposes, structures, and underlying technologies. Such systems may assist in realizing collaboration among healthcare providers and in providing readily access to patients' longitudinal health records by authorized users at the point of care. This, in turn, will improve the quality, efficiency, and effectiveness of healthcare delivery – dimensions of healthcare in need of innovation and improvement.

When an interoperable HIS is envisaged, communication-level interoperability issues need to be solved in order to ensure that existing systems using different transport protocols and data formats can exchange information. Such interoperable HIS can be realized according to the Service-Oriented Architecture (SOA) which can solve these issues to a great extent while protecting past investments since existing information assets and applications are preserved (Wang and Wang, 2005). However, data integration issues are not fully addressed while new challenges are created regarding interoperability due to inconsistencies in web service implementations (Cohen, 2002). Thus, the movement towards such an interoperable HIS requires an architecture that implements interoperability among existing information systems in all levels, including service and data levels. The effective management of interactions in such a heterogeneous and distributed environment is a fairly complex task. The conjunction of agent and workflow technologies provides the ability to execute such complex tasks and helps managing the complexity of the distribution in terms of both administration and fault tolerance. In particular, these technologies can be used for the integration of existing systems both within and across different healthcare organizations by integrating the common data and business logic into a specific architectural layer (i.e. middleware) distinct from individual applications and accessible through the whole HIS.

This chapter presents a, compatible to the EN 12967 standard (ISO/TC 215, 2008), mediator-based system architecture that addresses HIS interoperability issues while it complies with the most stringent requirements of high performance, reliability, robustness, scalability, high flexibility and fault tolerance. The proposed system architecture utilizes both workflow and agent technologies for supporting healthcare process collaboration and coordination requirements and for resolving data integration issues. In particular, it uses a set of cooperating agents for managing healthcare processes and handling all the interactions between the client applications and the existing HIS initiated during healthcare process enactment. Moreover, java-based workflows are used for modeling both the healthcare processes and the logics of all interactions as well as the internal behavior of system participating in these interactions. The latter are workflows that may involve several tasks such as data retrieval and transformation, computations and other low level auxiliary operations needed during execution of a process handling a client request.

BACKGROUND

One of the key problems in healthcare informatics is the lack of interoperability among different HIS. Interoperability can be investigated in different categories in the eHealth domain, such as the interoperability of the messages exchanged between healthcare applications, interoperability of Electronic Healthcare Records (EHRs), interoperability of patient identifiers, coding terms, clinical guidelines and healthcare business processes. Furthermore, all these categories can be investigated in two major layers: syntactic interoperability layer and the semantic interoperability layer. Syntactic interoperability (which we term as messaging layer), involves the ability of two or more systems to exchange information. Semantic interoperability is the ability for information shared by systems to be understood at the level of formally defined domain concepts (Dogac et al., n.d.)

To address the EHR interoperability problem, there are several standards currently under development such as the Health Level 7 (HL7) Clinical Document Architecture (CDA) (Dolin et al., 2001), CEN EN 13606 EHRcom and openEHR (CEN/ISSS eHealth Focus Group, 2005; openEHR Community, n.d.). These standards aim to structure and markup the clinical content for the purpose of exchange. There is also an industry initiative called Integrating the Healthcare Enterprise (IHE) which specified the Cross-Enterprise Document Sharing (XDS) integration profile for this purpose. The IHE initiative makes a contribution to interoperability issues regarding data and services. In particular, IHE is working to refine the standards required to improve workflow and dataflow within hospitals and across a community of care. It promotes the coordinated use of established communication standards, such as DICOM and HL7 (ANSI American National Standards Institute, 2003), by clearly defining how existing standards can be implemented. However, new problems arise due to lack of flexibility for adoption to different organizational conditions and lack of security integration in its different profiles (Wozak et al., 2008).

RIDE (Dogac et al., n. d) project is a roadmap project for interoperability of eHealth systems leading to recommendations for actions and to preparatory actions at the European level. The CEN Standard Architecture for Healthcare Information Systems (ENV 12967) (ISO/TC 215, 2008), Health Informatics Service Architecture or HISA is a standard aimed at enabling the development modular open systems to support healthcare. HISA integrates the existing information assets and makes them available, facilitating the interoperability of applications. It also specifies a unified, open service architecture based on a middleware of information services independent of any specific technological environment, applicable to any type of information system of healthcare organizations and capable of integrating common data and business logic. These services are available to diverse, multi-vendor applications through many types of implementations and are able to support all aspects (i.e. clinical, organizational and managerial) of the healthcare structure, comprising all relevant information and all business workflows. HISA identifies a methodology to describe HIS through a language, notation and paradigms suitable to facilitate the planning, design and comparison of systems; and recognizes the fundamental architectural aspects enabling the openness, integration and interoperability of HIS. The architecture is intended as a basis for the description, planning and development of new systems as well as for the integration of existing information systems, both within and across different healthcare organizations. The specification, architecture and models are all open and extensible, to allow evolutions during the time according to national and local requirements and new standards.

During the last few years, research efforts regarding the realization of interoperability among existing HIS have been on the rise (Berler and Pavlopoulos, 2004; Grimson et al., 2000; Hsieh, 2007; Jin and Cordy, 2006; Jin and Winter, 2005; Li-Fan Ko, 2006; Souder and Mancoridis, 1999; Yang, 2006, Wang and Wang, 2005; Zou and Kontogiannis, 2005). Technologies used for this purpose range from low-level techniques such as RPC/RMI to provider-independent techniques based on XML/web services. These techniques have solved to a great extent the problem of interoperability of heterogeneous distributed systems but still lack the efficiency when it comes to performance issues.

Agent and Workflow Technology for Supporting Interoperability of Healthcare Information Systems

Nowadays, patients receive care from more than one healthcare organization. Furthermore, healthcare professionals often require instant access to accurate patient information which may be scattered around disparate and geographically dispersed systems. This demands an interoperable HIS which can facilitate instant access to the longitudinal medical record, when and where needed and where patients' relevant medical information can be accessed in a generally accepted standard. The conjunction of agent and workflow technologies is increasingly contributing to the development of interoperable HIS from the point of improving the quality of healthcare, facilitating the access to healthcare and reducing costs.

The Agents Paradigm

Agents are considered one of the most important paradigms that on one hand may improve methods currently used for conceptualizing, designing and implementing software systems, and on the other hand may be the solution to the legacy software integration problem.

The term *agent* or *software agent*, has found its way into a number of technologies and has been widely used, among others, in artificial intelligence, databases, operating systems and computer networks literature. Although there is no single definition of an agent, all definitions agree that an agent is essentially a special software component that has autonomy that provides an interoperable interface to an arbitrary system and/or behaves like a human agent, working for some clients in pursuit of its own agenda (Nguyen et al.,

2009). An agent system usually consists of multiple agents even though it can be based on a solitary agent working within an environment and if necessary interacting with its users (Indap and Thakre, 2007). These multi-agent systems (MAS) can model complex systems and introduce the possibility of agents having common or conflicting goals (Bergenti and Poggi, 2009). These agents may interact with each other both indirectly (by acting on the environment) or directly (via communication and negotiation). Agents may decide to cooperate for mutual benefit or may compete to serve their own interests. An agent is:

- Autonomous because it operates without the direct intervention of humans or others and has control over its actions and internal state,
- Social because it cooperates with humans or other agents in order to achieve its tasks,
- Reactive because it perceives its environment and responds in a timely fashion to changes that occur in the environment, and
- Proactive because it does not simply act in response to its environment but is able to exhibit goal-directed behaviour by taking initiative.

Moreover, if necessary, an agent can be:

- Mobile with the ability to travel between different nodes in a computer network,
- Truthful providing the certainty that it will not deliberately communicate false information,
- Benevolent always trying to perform what is asked of it,
- Rational always acting in order to achieve its goals and never to prevent its goals being achieved, and
- Adaptive adapting itself to fit its environment and to the desires of its users.

The Workflow Metaphor

Workflow technology is crucial to automating business processes and their reengineering. It is regarded as an important means of increasing the productivity of enterprises since it crosses organizational boundaries and facilitates exchange of information among units and people. A workflow describes a business process in terms of a process model that links activities (either manual that necessitates user intervention or automatic) with participant users within the overall organizational framework. In BPM (Business Process Management) environments, the workflow metaphor is used for representing business processes and orchestrating a number of existing systems typically (but not necessarily) accessible by means of Web Service interfaces (Buhler and Vidal, 2005). However, the workflow approach can be brought from the business process level to the level of system internal logics. That is, it can be used not only for the high level orchestration of services provided by different systems, but for the implementation of the internal behaviour of each single system as well. Thus, the execution of possibly long and fairly complex tasks is facilitated while ensuring that the most stringent requirements of high performance, reliability, security, robustness, scalability, high flexibility and fault tolerance are met.

The key aspect of the workflow metaphor is the fact that the execution steps as well as their sequencing are made explicit. This makes it possible to give a graphical representation of a process defined as a workflow. Such representation is clearly extremely more intuitive with respect to a piece of software code and in general is understandable by domain experts as well as by programmers. Domain experts can therefore validate system logics directly and not only on documents that most of the time are not perfectly up to date. In some cases they could even contribute to the actual development of the system without the need for any programming skill. Another important characteristic is that, being the execution steps explicitly identified, the workflow engine (i.e. a system able to automatically execute a process defined as a workflow) can trace them. This makes it possible to create automatic mechanisms to facilitate system monitoring and problem investigation. Additionally, when processes have to be executed within the scope of a transaction, semi-automatic rollback procedures can be activated in case of unexpected fault. Finally, since workflows are fully self-documented, workflow-based development releases the development team of the burden of keeping documentation aligned each time design choices must be revisited to face implementation details or evolving requirements.

Workflows and Agents Development Environment

Workflows and Agents Development Environment (WADE), which is the main evolution of Java Agent Development Environment (JADE) (Java Agent Development Framework, 2010), is a software platform suitable for the development of mission critical applications by exploiting agent and workflow technologies (Caire, 2008). In particular, it facilitates the development of interoperable multi-agent systems where agent tasks can be defined according to the workflow metaphor. In WADE each workflow is expressed as a Java class with a well defined structure, thus combining the advantages of workflow technology with the power and flexibility of an actual programming language like Java. Unlike the majority of existing workflow systems that provide a powerful centralized engine, in WADE each agent can embed a "micro workflow engine" and a complex process can be carried out by a set of cooperating agents each one executing a piece of the process (Caire, 2008). This improves significantly performance which is a matter of prominent importance in the healthcare field.

MOTIVATING SCENARIO

The basic motivation for this research stems from our involvement in a recent project concerned with defining and automating cross-organizational healthcare processes spanning a health district in order to implement a district-wide, process-oriented HIS. The interoperability requirements and the stringent needs for a secure, reliable and high performance system that provides real-time access to sensitive patient information motivated this work and provided some of the background supportive information for developing the prototype presented in this chapter.

Typically, a health district consists of one district general hospital (DGH) and a number of peripheral hospitals and health centers. As patient information is scattered around disparate and geographically dispersed systems and patient referrals are usually made among various healthcare providers within a district (e.g. for hospitalization, for outpatient consultation or for performing specialized medical procedures), there is a need to ensure that a high performance interoperable environment is created and that authorized access to healthcare services and data is provided.

Suppose a healthcare delivery situation where a physician situated within a health district issues a radiological request for one of his/her patients. The request is submitted to a radiology department of a hospital which schedules the radiological procedure requested and notifies the requesting physician on the date and time scheduled. After performing the radiological procedure requested, the radiologist consults the relevant portion of the patient's medical record and writes a radiological report, incorporating both the radiological images and the associated text, which is sent to the requesting physician. Figure 1 shows a high-level view of the radiological request process model using Workflow Life Cycle Management Environment (WOLF), a graphical development environment for WADE based applications (Caire, 2008). This process consists of four tasks: *IssueRadRequest*, *ScheduleRadProc*, *IssueRadReport* and *ReceiveRadReport*.

SYSTEM ARCHITECTURE

Figure 2 illustrates a high-level view of the system architecture in terms of a three-tier model which comprises the client application (i.e. web portal), the mediator and the health district information systems. The latter are, in general, heterogeneous and reside in geographically distributed and organizationally disparate healthcare providers within the health district. Moreover, their functionality is exposed by means of web services. The mediator lies between the client and the health district's information systems.

In essence, the mediator is a distributed, multi-agent system that enables client interactions with the existing information systems. Mediator agents are built using the WADE platform and are held in containers which run on various servers that reside at the DGH and other healthcare organizations within the boundaries of the health district. In each server, containers are activated by a BootDaemon process and container agents are, then, employed to process access requests to existing information systems and to decide whether each request should be permitted or denied. This access control process, that involves the execution of a number of agent tasks, has been defined according to the workflow metaphor.

One of the containers is hosted at the DGH site and is called the main container while the rest of the containers, hosted at the DGH site and elsewhere, are called peripheral. The main container holds the WADE-specific agents, namely the Agent Management System (AMS), the Directory Facilitator (DF) and the Configuration Agent (CFA) (Java Agent Development Framework, 2010). The AMS represents the authority in the platform, namely it is the only agent that can activate platform

Figure 1. A high-level view of the radiological request process

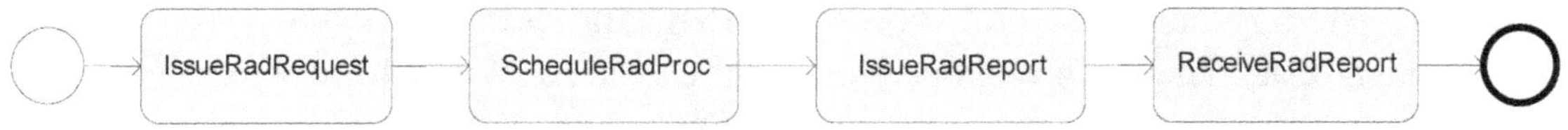

Figure 2. System architecture

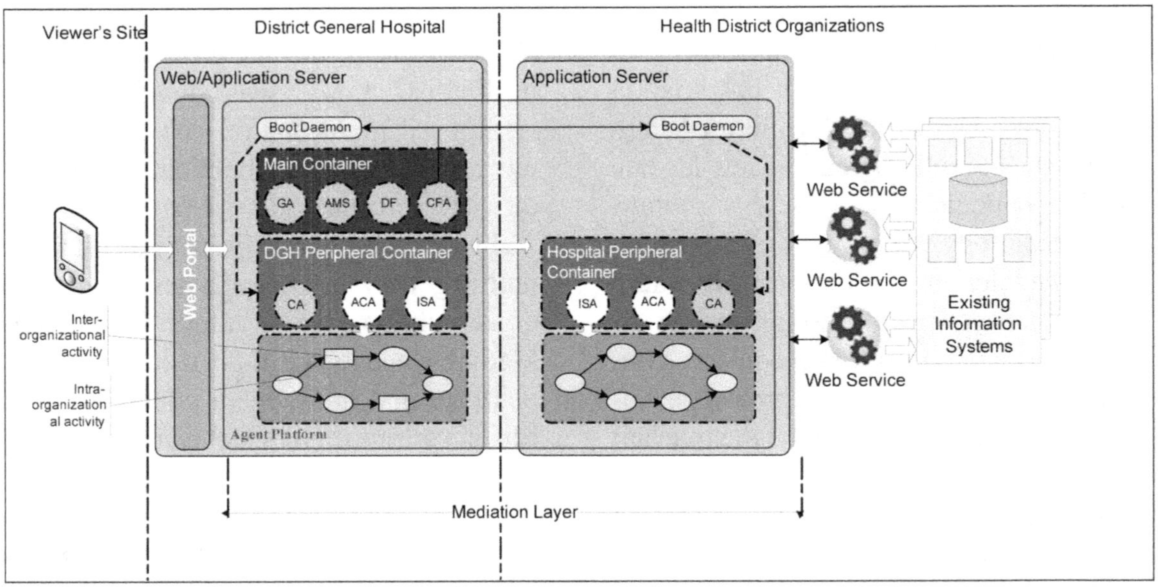

management actions such as creating/killing other agents, killing containers and shutting down the platform (Java Agent Development Framework, 2010). The DF implements the yellow pages service by means of which the other agents advertise their services and find other agents offering services they need (Java Agent Development Framework, 2010). The CFA is responsible for interacting with the boot daemons and controlling the application lifecycle. Moreover, the main container holds one application-specific agent, namely the Gateway Agent (GA), which enables the communication between the client portal and the mediator.

Each peripheral container holds a WADE-specific agent, namely Controller Agent (CA) (Java Agent Development Framework, 2010), and two application-specific agents, namely Information System Agent (ISA) and Access Control Agent (ACA). The CA is responsible for supervising activities in the peripheral container and for all the fault tolerance mechanisms provided by WADE.

The ISA hosted at the DGH peripheral container (i.e. DGH ISA) is responsible for the management of the workflows pertaining to a number of healthcare processes. Moreover, each time a workflow task is picked for execution, the DGH ISA performs all actions required for the successful execution of the task. In particular, if the task execution requires interaction with existing information systems operating within the health district, the DGH ISA cooperates with the relevant local ISAs (i.e. hospital peripheral container ISAs), which wrap the functionality of each HIS, in order to handle these interactions. That is, DGH ISA contacts the relevant local ISAs in order to assign them the tasks that need to be executed in order for the request to be fulfilled. On arrival of an access request to an existing information system of a healthcare organization, the local ISA handles the request in collaboration with the local ACA which enforces access control. Essentially, ISA provides a standard interface to the underlying database(s) and applications, facilitating interoperability in terms of service accessibility and data semantics. For example, upon request concerning the retrieval of a portion of a patient's medical record, the DGH ISA uses a district-wide directory in order to locate the various HIS where pieces of the requested information are stored and then commands the relevant ISAs to retrieve and deliver the requested pieces of information to the DGH ISA.

Each application agent announces to the DF a number of services through which he carries out the tasks he is responsible for. In particular,

- DGH ISA, in addition to the services pertaining to the execution of healthcare processes, announces to the DF the following two services:
  - "LocateLocalISA": it locates the local ISAs that wrap the functionality of the various HISs where pieces of the requested information are stored.
  - "ProcessTransaction": it contacts the local ISAs located by the "locateLocalISA" service in order to assign them the task they are required to perform and receives the relevant output.
- Local ISA announces to the DF one service, namely "performAction", which executes the tasks assigned to him by the DGH ISA (e.g. a query to the database of an existing HIS).
- ACA is responsible for making access control decisions regarding the execution of process tasks and the invocation of the associated web services. To this end, the acquisition and interpretation of context information that influence decision making may be required. To this end, the following services are used, which are announced to the DF:
  - "AcquireContext": it collects the required context information.
  - "InterpretContext": it interprets the collected context information.

More details regarding the context information model are provided in the following section.

Besides autonomy, which constitutes the fundamental agent attribute, ACA incorporates an important attribute, namely cognition as it performs context information processing and reasoning, based on its internal knowledge base which comprises a number of rules that have been defined during system configuration. For example, upon request for access to a patient's medical record through a wireless device, ACA obtains the IP of the wireless access point providing network connection to the device and compares it to a predefined set of IPs that correspond to the wireless access points set up within the hospital premises. If this IP is contained in this set, the terminal is characterized as "InPremises" and the user is provided with the requested information.

The low level internal structures of all application-specific agents and the high level interactions between these agents and the DGH ISA are modeled as workflows. Hence, all agents are designed to include a light workflow engine that executes these workflows. The workflows modeling the low level internal structures of each ISA are executed by the workflow engine embedded in it and involve, among others, tasks such as data retrieval and transformation (including computations and other low level auxiliary operations) in accordance to the reference information model defined by the EN 12967 standard. Thus, semantic interoperability can be realized. Each time a modification occurs in the database(s) and/or applications of a HIS, a new or modified workflow reflecting this modification can be deployed at runtime, thus immediately enabling the local ISA to access it. The workflows modeling the healthcare processes and the high level interactions between agents and the DGH ISA are executed by the workflow engine embedded in the DGH ISA. The interactions between agents and the DGH ISA involve, among others, tasks such as the integration of the portions of a patient's medical record delivered to it by ISAs.

Security Issues

As mentioned above, in the proposed architecture, authorization decisions are taken by ACA which, during a user interaction with the system, determines whether access of a given subject (healthcare professional) to a given object (web service or data) should be permitted or denied by taking into account the acquired by the subject and current context. The contextual information influencing authorization decisions is determined by a pre-defined set of attributes that may relate to the user (e.g. user roles, user/patient relationship), to the environment (e.g. client location and time of attempted access) and to the data resource provider (e.g. the healthcare organization's security policy). For example, the permissions of a physician accessing the system via his/her PDA, are adapted depending on his/her identity, location and time of access as well as the security policy of each healthcare organization where a portion of the requested information is stored. The whole access control process performed by ACA in order to ensure authorized access to the target objects is also modeled as a workflow process.

Due to the stringent security requirements on medical data, the specification of access control policies not for the entire record but for its components (i.e. data objects) is of outmost importance. Since medical data is accessed during workflow execution by means of web services, there is a need to specify access control policies on web service invocations and associated method executions. In the proposed architecture, access control policies are specified by means of XACML profile (OASIS, 2005). XACML is an access-control policy language that allows standard specification of rules about who can do what, and when. XACML provides for fine-grained control of activities based on common types of criteria, such as entity attributes, authentication mechanisms, and the protocol employed(OASIS, 2005). Moreover, it defines a vocabulary for expressing these policies as XML constructs. Each policy defines individual rules as the basic unit of management. Each rule evaluates some combination of characteristics of the requester, the requested resource, the desired action and the current environment. In the proposed access control mechanism, access control decisions concerning a certain user holding a certain role result from the evaluation of the aforementioned context information against XACML policies.

Suppose that the medication prescribed to the patient is accessible through a web service with URI https://localhost:8443/services/Medication and the web service method for retrieving medication is getPatientMedication. An excerpt of the access control policy on this method for a user holding the role "physician" is illustrated in Figure 3. This policy states that a physician is authorized to access the medication web service (specified within the tag <Resource>) for a specific patient provided that the physician (a) is on duty, and

(b) initiates the relevant transaction while in the hospital premises. These contextual constraints for the role "physician" are declared within the tag <Condition>.

Data Interoperability

One major problem regarding information retrieval from several distributed databases is the diversity of data formats and semantics used by each database. Hence, a need arises for ensuring data interoperability, namely for enabling automatic interpretation of the retrieved information in a meaningful and accurate manner. Thus, it is ensured that the produced results are as defined by the system from which they were originally retrieved. To achieve data interoperability, all health district organizations must use common terminology for data manipulation. To this end, they must refer to a common reference information model. In the proposed architecture the reference information model used is compatible to the EN 12967 standard and contains a number of data elements (virtual data elements), the mappings of which to the actual data elements (used in the databases of each HIS) is declared by means of an XML file. In the XML file a virtual name is assigned to each data element and mappings are defined between the data types of the actual data elements and the data types of the virtual data elements (where applicable). Figure 4 illustrates an excerpt of the XML file which resides at a server hosted at each health district organization.

Figure 3. Sample access control policy for medication web service

```
<Resource>
  <ResourceMatch MatchId="&function;string-equal">
   <AttributeValue DataType="anyURI "> https://localhost:8443/services/Medication/getPatientMedication
    </AttributeValue>
...
  </ResourceMatch>
 </Resource>
  ...
 <Action>
   <ActionMatch MatchId="&function;string-equal">
    <AttributeValue DataType="&xml;string">execute</AttributeValue>
   ...
   </ActionMatch>
 </Action>
 <Condition>
   <Apply FunctionId="&function;and ">
     <Apply FunctionId="&function;string-equal">
      <EnvironmentAttributeDesignator AttributeId="urn:oasis:names:tc:xacml:2.0:environment:staffStatus"
        DataType="&xml;string"/>
       <AttributeValue DataType="&xml;string">onDuty</AttributeValue>
     </Apply>
     <Apply FunctionId="&function;string-equal">
      <EnvironmentAttributeDesignator AttributeId="urn:oasis:names:tc:xacml:2.0:environment:terminal"
        DataType="&xml;string"/>
    <AttributeValue DataType="&xml;string">inPremises</AttributeValue>
    </Apply>
  </Apply>
 </Condition>
```

The adoption of a, compatible to the EN 12967, information model provides the ability to describe important information deemed necessary for all healthcare organizations, hence making a substantial contribution to data interoperability. An alternative approach to data interoperability could be provided by means of structures called archetypes. These structures are computable expressions of a domain content model of medical records and constitute a fundamental component of the EN 13606 standard (Karla, 2009). Essentially, EN 13606 is a five part standard that defines the logical models and interfaces required to support the generic communication of EHR data and archetypes between heterogeneous EHR systems (Karla, 2009). However, since the purpose of our research is the implementation of interoperable health information systems, the EN 12967 standard has been considered more suitable as it constitutes a multi-part standard that provides guidance for the description, planning and development of new systems as well as for the integration of existing information systems, both within one enterprise and across different healthcare organizations (CEN/TC 251, 2007). This is achieved through an architecture integrating the common data and business logic into a specific architectural layer (i.e. the middleware), distinct from individual applications and accessible throughout the whole information system through services (CEN/TC 251, 2007).

Figure 4. Excerpt of XML file storing the mapping of virtual data elements to actual ones

```
xml version="1.0" encoding="ISO-8859-1"?>
  <terms>
    <table>
      <virtual_name>patient</virtual_name>
      <local_name>pat</local_name>
      <columns>
        <column1>
          <patient_id>pat_id/<patient_id>
          <virtual_data_type>int</virtual_data_type>
          <local_data_type></local_data_type>
        </column1>
        <column2>
          <patient_name>pat_name</patient_name>
          <virtual_data_type>varchar(20)</virtual_data_type>
          <local_data_type>varchar(15)</local_data_type>
        </column2>
        ...
      </columns>
    </table>
  </terms>
```

Service Interoperability

The diversity among the web service implementations used for exposing each HIS's functionality introduces new interoperability challenges. A solution to this problem is the virtualization of provided web services in order to hide technical details from users and applications and to support application-level interoperability among different healthcare resources. The proposed mediator realizes this virtualization by providing a uniform interface to each one of the remote web services. When a request for a web service invocation is issued, it is captured by the local ISA which performs a number of activities in order to determine the way this service should be invoked considering information such as the WSDL file). These activities are defined according to the workflow metaphor as illustrated in Figure 5. This workflow is java-based and constructed using WOLF.

According to this workflow, each time a request is issued for a task execution, the following activities are being executed:

1. **GET_WEB_SERVICE_INVOCATION_DETAILS**: Each request for a web service invocation has a standard format irrespective of the underlying web service implementations. The local ISA intercepts such requests in

Figure 5. Workflow of actions taken by the ISA

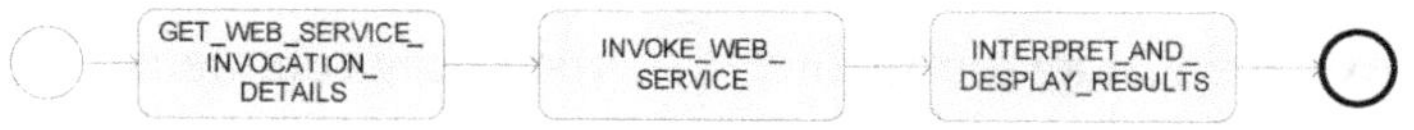

order to determine their actual format (i.e. Uniform Resource Identifiers - URIs). To this end, it queries the server where the web service is deployed in order to acquire the file containing all the relevant information (i.e. WSDL file).

2. **INVOKE_WEB_SERVICE**: The local ISA forms the request to be issued for the web service invocation by taking into account the WSDL file acquired in the previous activity. If the execution of the web service involves data access (insertion, update or deletion), the SQL query to be executed is passed as a parameter to the web service. Initially, this query is formed in accordance with the reference information model. That is, it uses the virtual data elements for determining the pieces of data to be accessed. Hence, prior to invoking the web service, ISA needs to reform the SQL query by replacing the virtual data elements with the actual data elements used in the local HIS. To this end, ISA uses the XML file containing the mappings of the virtual data elements to the actual ones.. After all the required transformations have been performed, the request for the web service invocation is issued and the ACA is contacted in order to enforce access control. Depending on the access control decision retuned by ACA, ISA caries on with the web service invocation.
3. **INTERPRET_DATA**: In case of data retrieval, the data retrieved from a health district organization's information system by means of a web service, need to be interpreted according to the reference information model. This is performed by the local ISA at the remote host, prior to delivering the data to the DGH ISA. To this end, the XML file containing the mappings of the virtual data elements to the actual data elements is used. The data delivered to the DGH ISA are being consolidated with the data retrieved by the other local ISAs and are being returned to the requesting client.

IMPLEMENTATION ISSUES

A prototype based on the architecture presented in this chapter has been developed in a laboratory environment using WADE 2.0. The latter is built on top of JADE (Java Agent Development Framework, 2010) and uses Java Runtime Environment 1.5.0 for executing the workflows that define agent tasks. Moreover, Apache/Tomcat was used as Web/Application Server and both PostGres SQL and MySQL were used for the development of a number of sample databases considered as the databases used by the existing information systems.

In order to achieve security in the agent-based mediation framework envisaged, certain security features have been incorporated. In particular, authentication is performed by means of X.509 certificates and all subsequent web transactions are executed under the Secure Socket Layer (SSL) via HTTPS. In addition, security in the communication among the agents of the agent platform is ensured by setting up a secure, confidential and mutually authenticated, connection amongst containers of the agent platform by leveraging TLS/SSL support provided by Java (Java Agent Development Framework, 2010).

System Functionality

Suppose that a physician working at a hospital within a health district needs a number of radiological procedures to be performed on one of his/her patients. To this end, the physician uses his/her PDA client in order to instantiate the healthcare process illustrated in Figure 1. To this end, the DGH ISA creates an instance of the relevant workflow and initiates the "IssueRadRequest" task. As soon as the required information regarding the radiological request are provided by the physician (e.g. radiological procedures, radiological department), the DGH ISA contacts the local ISA hosted in the peripheral container of the hospital where the radiological department belongs. In turn, the local ISA queries the hospital server in order to acquire the WSDL file of the web service responsible for handling the radiological requests. Thus, the URI for the web service invocation is determined. The web service takes as a parameter the SQL query for the insertion of the radiological request data in the local HIS database. Initially, this query is formed by the DGH ISA, in accordance with, the reference information model and then it is passed to the local ISA. In turn, the local ISA reforms the SQL query by replacing the virtual data elements of the reference information model with the actual data elements used in the local HIS database. Upon successful completion of all the aforementioned actions, the local ISA invokes the web service.

After the radiological request has been issued the "ScheduleRadProc" task is initiated by the DGH ISA. The requested procedures are being scheduled and the DGH ISA issues a request for the web service invocation regarding the appointment's details (e.g. date and time). To this end, the DGH ISA contacts the relevant local ISA which will acquire the relevant WSDL file and will reform the relevant SQL query concerning data insertion. This will be performed in a similar way as in "IssuesRadRequest" task. Finally, the web service is invoked having as a parameter this SQL query.

After scheduling the radiological request, the "IssueRadReport" task is initiated. The radiological procedures requested are performed by a radiologist who consults the relevant portion of the patient's medical record in order to compose the corresponding radiological report. In order for the requested portion of the patient's medical record to be retrieved, the DGH ISA locates the various pieces of the requested information using a district-wide directory and commands the relevant local ISAs to retrieve (by means of web services) and deliver the requested pieces of information to the DGH ISA. Upon request for a web service invocation, each local ISA queries the server hosting the service in order to acquire the relevant WSDL file. Thus, the specific URI to be used for the web service invocation is determined. Then, the SQL query used for the data retrieval is formed in the way described above and the web service is invoked having as a parameter this SQL query. During this transaction, the ISA collaborates with ACA in order to enforce access control. In particular, ACA determines whether access to portions of patient's medical record should be permitted or denied by taking under consideration the current context. Depending on the access control decision retuned by ACA, ISA caries on with the web service invocation. If access to the web service is permitted, data retrieved are transformed by the local ISA according to the reference information model and then they are delivered to the DGH ISA. The DGH

Figure 6. Sequence diagram for actions involved in patient medical record retrieval taking place during the execution of "IssueRadReport" task

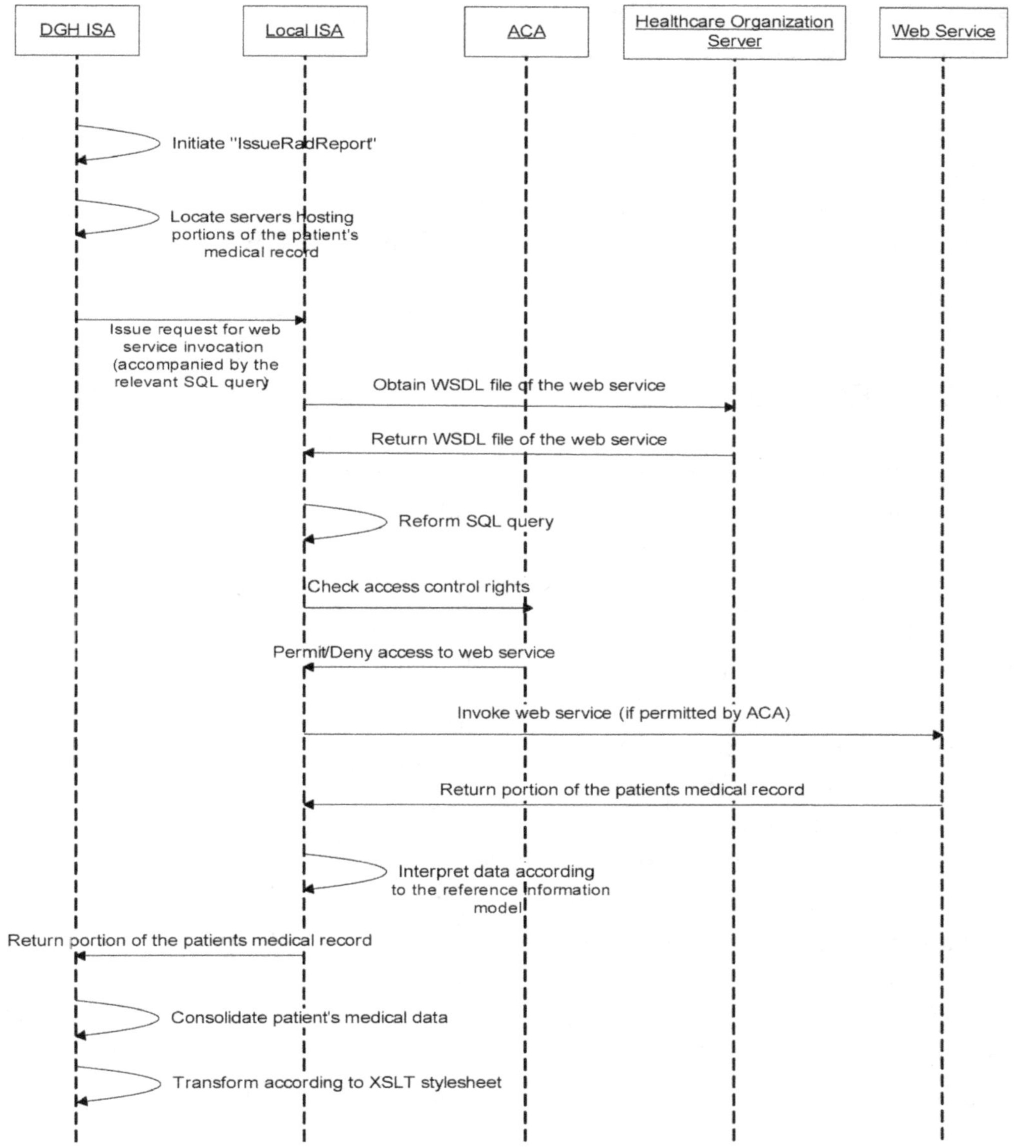

ISA consolidates the portions of the patient's medical record obtained by all the local ISAs, transforms them according to the XSLT stylesheet corresponding to the radiologist's device type and displays them on the screen.

The radiologist writes a radiological report, incorporating both the radiological images and the associated text, and sends a message to the requesting physician. After completing this task, the "ReceiveRadReport" task is initiated by the DGH ISA which, depending on the physician's device type, transforms the data in accordance with the relevant XSLT stylesheet. Thus, both the radiological images and the report are displayed on the physician's display.

The sequence of actions taking place during the execution of "IssueRadReport" task and involve the retrieval of the patient's medical record is illustrated in Figure 6, by means of a sequence diagram.

CONCLUDING REMARKS

In healthcare, the ability to share relevant information among diverse healthcare systems and provide consistent data across applications will improve the quality of care, the patient safety and reduce cost. Thus, building an interoperable health information system is of paramount importance since it can facilitate instant access to patients' longitudinal medical records, when and where needed. To this end, many healthcare organizations are looking to leverage their existing investments and incrementally adopt SOA in heterogeneous environments without needing to remove or replace existing systems. Thus, the current level of expenditure for health can be controlled and optimized whilst the quality of service provided to patients will be improved. Although, SOA and web services can resolve many of the long-standing issues facing healthcare organizations today, they raise new challenges with regard to interoperability in terms of service accessibility and data semantics. To this end, the proposed system architecture implements a workflow-based mediation framework in an attempt to resolve these interoperability issues. The proposed system utilizes agent and workflow technologies, in order to provide an interoperable healthcare information system environment that enables integrated and secure access to medical information irrespective of the location it resides and that meets the requirements of high performance, reliability, security, robustness, scalability, high flexibility and fault tolerance.

REFERENCES

ANSI American National Standards Institute. (2003). *HL7 messaging standard version 2.5*. Retrieved June, 2010, from http://webstore.ansi.org/FindStandards.aspx?Action=displaydept&DeptID=3104&Acro=HL7&DpName=HL7:%20Health%20Level%20Seven&source=google&adgroup=hl7&keyword=hl7%20standard&gclid=CJ6Vm8Gv_aICFZUA4wode3pXnA

Bergenti, F., & Poggi, A. (2009). *Multi-agent systems for e-Health: Recent projects and initiatives*. Paper presented at the Tenth National Workshop From Objects to Agents (WOA 2009), Parma Italy.

Berler, D. K. A., & Pavlopoulos, S. (2004). *Design of an interoperability framework in a regional healthcare system*. Paper presented at the 26th Annual International Conference of the IEEE Engineering in Medicine and Biology Society (IEMBS '04), San Francisco, CA.

Buhler, P. A., & Vidal, J. M. (2005). Towards adaptive workflow enactment using multiagent systems. *Information Technology Management*, *6*(1), 61–87. doi:10.1007/s10799-004-7775-2

Caire, G., Gotta, D., & Banzi, M. (2008). *WADE: A software platform to develop mission critical applications exploiting agents and workflows*. Paper presented at the 7th International Conference on Autonomous Agents and Multiagent Systems - Industry and Applications Track (AAMAS 2008), Estoril, Portugal.

CEN/ISSS eHealth Focus Group. (2005). *Report from the CEN/ISSS eHealth Standardization Focus Group: Current and Future Standardization Issues in the eHealth Domain: Achieving Interoperability*. Retrieved June, 2010, from ftp://ftp.cen.eu/CEN/Sectors/List/ICT/FocusGroups/eHealthStandardization-ExsummaryFinal.pdf.

CEN/TC251, (2007). *ISO/CD12967-2 - prEN 12967-2 HISA information view*. Retrieved February, 2009, from http://www.google.gr/url?sa=t&source=web&cd=1&ved=0CBYQFjAA&url=http%3A%2F%2Fwww.kith.no%2Fupload%2F4120%2FISOTC215_pCD_12967-2_HISA-20070208.doc&ei=XpIzTe2hDYfMswb3_KyTCg&usg=AFQjCNE3O TP0sJou-6b04AB3dD5GGg0zs7g.

Cohen, F. (2002). *Understanding Web service interoperability*. IBM Technical Library.

Dogac, A., Namli, T., Okcan, A., Laleci, G., Kabak, Y., & Eichelberg, M. (n.d.). *Key issues of technical interoperability solutions in eHealth and the RIDE project*. Retrieved July, 2010, from http://ec.europa.eu/idabc/servlets/Doc?id=27836.

Dolin, R. H., Alschuler, L., Beebe, C., Biron, P. V., Boyer, S. L., & Essin, D. et al. (2001). The HL7 clinical document architecture. *Journal of the American Medical Informatics Association*, *8*(6), 552–569. doi:10.1136/jamia.2001.0080552 PMID:11687563

Grimson, J., Grimson, W., & Hasselbring, W. (2000). The SI challenge in health care. *Communications of the ACM*, *43*(6), 49–55. doi:10.1145/336460.336474

Hsieh, S. H., Hsieh, S. L., Weng, Y. C., Yang, T. H., Feipei, L., Cheng, P. H., et al. (2007). *Middleware based inpatient healthcare information system*. Paper presented at the 7th IEEE International Conference in Bioinformatics and Bioengineering (BIBE 2007), Boston, MA.

Huizen, V. G., & Backman, A. J. (2005). *SOA: First principles. SONIC software*. Paper presented at the Conference of Oracle Global Business and Technology, Mumbai, India.

Indap, S. M., & Thakre, V. S. (2007). Weather monitoring system using JADE (Java Agent Development Environment), *Project Report*.

ISO/TC 215. (2008). *CEN 12967 Health Informatics - Service Architecture*.

Java Agent DEvelopment Framework. (n.d.). Retrieved June, 2010, from http://jade.tilab.com.

Jin, D., & Cordy, J. R. (2006). *Integrating reverse engineering tools using a service-sharing methodology*. Paper presented at 14th International Conference on Program Comprehension (ICPC 2006), Athens, Greece.

Jin, D., & Winter, A. (2005). *Working session on interoperable reengineering services*. Paper presented at the 13th International Workshop on Program Comprehension (IWPC 2005), St. Louis, USA.

Karla, D. (2009). *ISO EN 13606 electronic health communication (EHRCOM): The contribution of archetypes towards eHealth semantic interoperability*. Retrieved February, 2009, from http://www.kith.no/upload/5414/EHRCOM-Archetypes-Dipak-Kalra-20091126.pdf

Lenz, R., & Kuhn, K. A. (2004). Towards a continuous evolution and adaptation of information systems in healthcare. *International Journal of Medical Informatics*, *73*, 75–89. doi:10.1016/j.ijmedinf.2003.09.003 PMID:15036081

Li-Fan Ko, E. A. (2006). *HL7 middleware framework for healthcare information system*. Paper presented at the 8th International Conference on e-Health Networking, Applications and Services (HEALTHCOM 2006), New Delhi, India.

Malamateniou, F., & Vassilacopoulos, G. (2003). Developing a virtual patient record using XML and Web-based workflow technologies. *International Journal of Medical Informatics*, *70*(2), 131–139. doi:10.1016/S1386-5056(03)00039-X PMID:12909164

Nguyen, M. T., Fuhrer, P., & Pasquier-Rocha, J. (2009). Enhancing E-health information systems with agent technology. *International Journal of Telemedicine and Applications*, 2009. PMID:19096509

OASIS. (2005). *eXtensible Access Control Markup Language (XACML) version 2.0*. Retrieved July, 2009, from http://docs.oasis-open.org/xacml/2.0/access_control-xacml-2.0-core-spec-os.pdf.

openEHR Community, (n.d.). *OpenEHR. Future proof and flexible EHR*. Retrieved June, 2010, from http://www.openehr. org.

Souder, T., & Mancoridis, S. (1999). *A tool for securely integrating legacy systems into a distributed environment*. Paper presented at the Sixth Working Conference on Reverse Engineering, Atlanta (WCRE '99), Georgia.

Wang, W., & Wang, M. (2005). *Healthcare information system integration: A service oriented approach*. Paper presented at the International Conference on Services Systems and Services Management, ICSSSM '05, 1475–1480.

Wozak, F., Ammenwerth, E., Hoerbst, A., Soegner, P., Mair, R., & Schabetsberger, T. (2008). *IHE based interoperability – Benefits and challenges*. Paper presented at the 1st International Workshop on Describing Medical Web Resources (MIE 2008), Gotenburg, Sweden.

Yang, E. A. T. H. (2006). *A scalable multi-tier architecture for the National Taiwan University Hospital Information System based on HL7 standard*. Paper presented at the 19th IEEE Symposium on Computer-Based Medical Systems (CBMS'06), Utah, USA.

Zou, Y., & Kontogiannis, K. (2001). *Towards a Web-centric legacy system migration framework*. Paper presented at the 3rd International Workshop on Net-Centric Computing(NCC 2001), Toronto, Canada.

ADDITIONAL READING

Australia National E-Health Transition Authority. Retrieved June, 2010, from http://www.nehta.gov.au/.

Bellifemine, F., Poggi, A., & Rimassa, G. (2001). Developing multiagent systems with a FIPA-compliant agent framework. *Software, Practice & Experience*, *31*(2), 103–128. doi:10.1002/1097-024X(200102)31:2<103::AID-SPE358>3.0.CO;2-O

Canada Health Infoway. Retrieved June, 2010, from http://www.infoway-inforoute.ca/lang-en/.

Cao, F., Archer, N. A., & Poehlman, W. F. S. (2009, November). An Agent-based Knowledge Management Framework for Electronic Health Record Interoperability. *Journal of Emerging Technologies in Web Intelligence*, *1*(2), 119–128. doi:10.4304/jetwi.1.2.119-128

Davis, E. (2003). Avoiding the 'dataset mentality'. *Informatics in Primary Care*, *11*(4), 49–52. PMID:14567870

Follen, M., Castaneda, R., Mikelson, M., Johnson, D., Wilson, A., & Higuchi, K. (2007). Implementing health information technology to improve the process of health care delivery: a case study. *Disease Management*, *10*(4), 208–215. doi:10.1089/dis.2007.104706 PMID:17718659

Healthcare Information Technology Standards Panel, Retrieved June, 2010, from ards_boards_panels/overview.aspx?menuid=3

Interoperability Definition and Background. (2005). Retrieved June, 2009, from http://www.himss.org/content/files/interoperability_definition_background_060905.pdf.

Kass-Hout, T. A., Gray, S. K., Massoudi, B. L., Immanuel, G. Y., Dollacke, M., & Cothren, R. (2007). NHIN, RHIOs, and public health. *Journal of Public Health Management and Practice*, *13*(1), 31–34. doi:10.1097/00124784-200701000-00006 PMID:17149097

Kuziemsky, C. E., & Weber, J. H. (2009, November). An eBusiness-based Framework for eHealth Interoperability. *Journal of Emerging Technologies in Web Intelligence*, *1*(2), 129–136. doi:10.4304/jetwi.1.2.129-136

Lopez, D. M., & Blobel, B. (2009). A development framework for semantically interoperable health information systems. *International Journal of Medical Informatics*, *7*(8), 83–103. doi:10.1016/j.ijmedinf.2008.05.009 PMID:18621574

Maass, M., Asikainen, P., Mäenpää, T., Wanne, O., & Suominen, T. (2008). Usefulness of a regional health care information system in primary care: a case study. *Computer Methods and Programs in Biomedicine*, *91*(2), 175–181. doi:10.1016/j.cmpb.2008.04.005 PMID:18514363

Mäenpääa, T., Suominena, T., Asikainenb, P., Maassb, M., & Rostilac, I. (2009). The outcomes of regional healthcare information systems in health care: A review of the research literature. *International Journal of Medical Informatics*, *7*(8), 757–771. doi:10.1016/j.ijmedinf.2009.07.001

Marchibroda, J. M. (2007). Health information exchange policy and evaluation. *Journal of Biomedical Informatics*, *40*(6), 11–16. doi:10.1016/j.jbi.2007.08.008 PMID:17981099

National Alliance for Health Information Technology. (2005). What is Interoperability?
Noblin, A.M. (2007). Privacy policy analysis for health information networks and regional health information organizations, *Health Care Manager,* 26 (4) (2007) 331–340.

Overhage, J. M., Evans, L., & Marchibroda, J. (2005). Communities' readiness for health information exchange: the National Landscape in 2004. *Journal of the American Medical Informatics Association, 12*(2), 107–112. doi:10.1197/jamia.M1680 PMID:15561785

Pallapa, G., Roy, N., & Das, S. (2007, May). *Precision Privacy Enhanced Context-Aware Information Fusion in Ubiquitous Healthcare*, Paper presented at the First International Workshop on Software Engineering for Pervasive computing Applications, Systems, and Environments (SEPCASE'07), Minneapolis, USA.

Shapiro, J. S., Kannry, J., Lipton, M., Goldberg, E., Conocenti, P., & Stuard, S. et al. (2006). Approaches to patient health information exchange and their impact on emergency medicine. *Annals of Emergency Medicine, 48*(4), 426–432. doi:10.1016/j.annemergmed.2006.03.032 PMID:16997679

Solomon, M. R. (2007). Regional health information organizations: a vehicle for transforming health care delivery. *Journal of Medical Systems, 31*(1), 35–47. doi:10.1007/s10916-006-9041-0 PMID:17283921

Spyrou, S., Bamidis, P., Chouvarda, I., Ogou, G. G., Tryfon, S. M., & Maglaveras, N. (2002). Health care informatics standards: comparison of the approaches. *Health Informatics Journal, 8*(1), 14–19. doi:10.1177/146045820200800103

Wang, W., Wang, M., & Zhu, S. (2005, June). *Healthcare Information System Integration A Service Oriented Approach*, Paper presented at the 2005 International Conference on Services Systems and Services Management (ICSSSM '05), Chongqing, China.

Yang, T. H., Sun, Y. S., & Lai, F. A. (2009). Scalable Healthcare Information System Based on a Service-oriented Architecture. *Journal of Medical Systems*. PMID:20703551

Yasnoff, W. A., Humphreys, B. L., Overhage, J. M., Detmer, D. E., Brennan, P. F., & Morris, R. W. et al. (2004). A consensus action agenda for achieving the national health information infrastructure. *Journal of the American Medical Informatics Association, 11*(4), 332–338. doi:10.1197/jamia.M1616 PMID:15187075

KEY TERMS AND DEFINITIONS

Access Control: Any mechanism by which a system grants or revokes the right to access data, or perform an action.

Agent: A complex software entity that is capable of acting with a certain degree of autonomy in order to accomplish tasks on behalf of its user.

Context: The surroundings, circumstances, environment, background, or settings which determine, specify, or clarify the meaning of an event.

Data Virtualization: The presentation of data as an abstract layer, independent of underlying database systems, structures and storage.

Health Information System (HIS): The intersection of information science, computer science, and health care. It deals with the resources, devices, and methods required to optimize the acquisition, storage, retrieval, and use of information in health and biomedicine. Health informatics tools include not only computers but also clinical guidelines, formal medical terminologies, and information and communication systems. It is applied to the areas of nursing, clinical care, dentistry, pharmacy, public health and (bio)medical research.

Interoperability: The ability of two or more systems or components to exchange information and to use the information that has been exchanged.

Java Agent Development Environment (JADE): An open-source software framework, aiming at assisting the development and execution of agent-based applications in compliance with the Foundation for Intelligent Physical Agents (FIPA) specifications for interoperable multi-agent systems.

Process: A collection of related, structured activities or tasks that produce a specific service or product (serve a particular goal) for a particular customer or customers.

Standard: An established norm or requirement. It is usually a formal document that establishes uniform engineering or technical criteria, methods, processes and practices.

Workflow: A depiction of a sequence of operations, declared as work of a person, a group of persons, an organization of staff, or one or more simple or complex mechanisms. Workflow may be seen as any abstraction of real work, segregated in work share, work split or other types of ordering.

Workflows and Agents Development Environment (WADE): A software platform based on Java Agent Development Framework (JADE) that provides support for the execution of tasks defined according to the workflow metaphor.

Chapter 9
Enabling Interoperability of Patient Summaries across Europe with Triplespaces

Alessio Carenini
CEFRIEL, Italy

Davide Cerri
STI Innsbruck, University of Innsbruck, Austria

Reto Krummenacher
STI Innsbruck, University of Innsbruck, Austria

Elena Simperl
STI Innsbruck, University of Innsbruck, Austria

ABSTRACT

Healthcare services are naturally distributed, both from a geographical and an organisational point of view; they include various national and local authorities, as well as different actors ranging from general hospitals to individual physicians. One of the main items on the eHealth agenda of the European Union is the establishment of electronic patient summaries as an instrument to facilitate the pervasive delivery of healthcare and to guarantee its continuity across national boundaries. This chapter analyses several existing large-scale eHealth systems, chosen among the most prominent and established ones in Europe, and analyses their ability to cope with the high heterogeneity challenges of a Europe-wide solution. It then introduces triplespaces, a new-generation middleware based on the concept of semantic spaces, and presents a possible realisation of a European Patient Summary based on a triplespace infrastructure. The chapter shows that this solution can cope with the decentralisation, asynchronicity, subsidiarity, and security requirements arising in the European Patient Summary setting.

DOI: 10.4018/978-1-4666-3000-0.ch009

INTRODUCTION

Healthcare infrastructures are commonly decentralised and heterogeneous in terms of information management, document structures, protocols and language bindings. Interoperability of medical information systems has been recognised as a key challenge and a fundamental need for citizens, healthcare professionals, and governmental authorities.

This is also reflected in the agenda of the European Union in the field of eHealth (Commission of the European Communities, 2004), which includes the design and promotion of *electronic patient summaries*. This is a first step towards the realisation of a European eHealth infrastructure that is capable of integrating information and applications across different countries, in order to facilitate the pervasive delivery of healthcare services and to ensure patient mobility within the European Union. Current efforts in this area (such as project epSOS [n. d.]) aim at providing recommendations for such an infrastructure.

The technical realisation of a European Patient Summary (EPS) infrastructure needs to build on a middleware layer which can provide the needed integration features, and which is able to deal with the key design principles specified in the European Interoperability Framework (2004): multi-laterality, subsidiarity, multilingualism and security. Based on these principles, we identify the following requirements for an efficient EPS infrastructure:

- A decentralised and distributed infrastructure is a prerequisite for respecting the multi-laterality principle, allowing all healthcare authorities to become parties to the same common network and efficiently publish and retrieve patient information independently of their location.
- Asynchronous interaction among institutions is equally important to enable the access and exchange of patient information at any time, and independently of the momentary availability of the communication partners.
- In order to keep the EPS infrastructure as minimally invasive as possible, and to guarantee the subsidiarity principle, the middleware should be able to provide flexible data and service integration to cope with the inherent heterogeneity problems that occur both at the data level (e.g., different encoding schemes and terminologies) and at the service level (e.g., different protocols).
- Support for appropriate security mechanisms is important with respect to regional, national and European regulations for the treatment of citizen data.

National healthcare information systems, which exist or are currently under development in various member states of the European Union, need, to some extent, to address the same challenges when integrating different information systems from different organisations (such as hospitals and local health authorities). A Europe-wide infrastructure to share patient summaries takes such issues to a new level, compared to its nationals counterparts; requiring all the European countries to redesign their national systems, or even just to adopt a unique standard for messaging and medical vocabularies, would be very inefficient, and probably unrealistic. In addition, in a Europe-wide context, security constraints become more complex, as they have to reflect different national regulations concerning access to medical data of the citizens.

The goal of this chapter is to present a possible European Patient Summary realisation based on a triplespace middleware, as a solution to cope with the requirements we identified. For this purpose, we also analyse some existing national healthcare systems in the light of the requirements we identified, and compare them with our approach.

BACKGROUND

Healthcare services are naturally distributed, both from a geographical and an organisational point of view; they include various national, regional, and local authorities, and actors ranging from complex centres such as general hospitals to individual physicians. The ultimate objective of a healthcare system is to support a network of complementary parties spread over the specific territory, in order to effectively meet the medical needs of its inhabitants. Historically, the distributed nature of healthcare services led to a lack of homogeneity in healthcare information systems, because different authorities implemented isolated technical and organisational solutions. This lack of homogeneity, in turn, leads to interoperability problems when having to cross the boundaries of a single system or organisation.

In this section we discuss how these problems are addressed in three different large-scale eHealth systems, chosen among the most significant and established, which are currently in use in different European countries: NHS Spine (United Kingdom), NICTIZ AORTA (Netherlands), and CRS-SISS (Lombardy Region, Italy).

NHS (United Kingdom)

NHS Connecting for Health (NHS, n. d.) which came into operation on April 1, 2005, is an agency of the Department of Health in the UK. Its primary role is to deliver integrated IT systems and services to the UK National Health Service. One of the key software components of Connecting for Health is the NHS Care Record (NCR) (Booth, 2003), which ensures that the most relevant information about the care and treatment of each citizen is held in a single electronic record. The core elements of the Care Records Service are:

- The Detailed Care Record, which contains the person's electronic records for that organisation, and elements of all electronic records relating to that person from other organisations;
- The Summary Care Record, which contains the essential elements of a person's electronic record, extracted from general practitioners' notes, and from the other organisations where the person receives care;
- The Healthspace, which is a health organiser and protected link to the patient's Summary Care Record, for every person who chooses to have one.

Detailed Care Records are aimed to be built automatically from information held by disparate sources. On top of Detailed Care Records, Summary Care Records are also provided, in order to support first contact care, and less complex care operations where a complete health record of a patient is not necessarily required. A summary of care and clinical history is kept in a national database known as the Spine, to ensure that vital patient information is always accessible, while the Summary Record provides links to local information. Additional in-depth details are held locally where most care is delivered. Whenever any significant data is changed on the general practitioner's clinical system, a new summary is generated and is uploaded to the Spine.

Personal Demographics Services (PDS) are another component of NHS, providing the prime source of NHS patient demographics. This service provides all personal and demographic information for each patient and is managed centrally at the national level. Health practitioners and institutes are identified via the Spine Directory Services (SDS), which holds a unique ID for NHS resources (such as staff members and organisations). Access control and authorisation on the clinical data of a patient are managed by the Legitimate Relationship Service (LRS) of Spine, which is also centrally managed. This component provides a single log-in and a record of each healthcare professional accessing a patient's NHS Care Record. All the information is provided per request, based on a "legitimate relationship" of the user with the patient. In order to do so, LRS stores the details of the relationships between healthcare professionals and patients, as well as the patients' preferences on information sharing.

The Transaction and Messaging Spine (TMS) component of Spine routes all the clinical messages delivered through the Spine; message flows from the local services to NCR and from NCR to local systems (if applicable) are routed via the TMS. Clinical messages are based on the HL7 v3 messaging standard. Regarding the medical vocabulary, all coded entries of the Summary Care Record are recorded as SNOMED-CT codes.

AORTA (Netherlands)

The core of AORTA, the Dutch Healthcare information system (NICTIZ, n. d.) is the National Healthcare Information Hub. One of the basic assumptions made when creating the Hub is the fact that care-related data are created under the responsibility of healthcare providers, and should be stored in the providers' system. Data should reside where they were created, and preferably not be duplicated. Dutch privacy laws do not allow for centralised collections of healthcare data, therefore data have to be stored in the system of the responsible author, and not in a centralised database. If a healthcare provider requires access to all information related to a specific patient, he directly issues the request to the Hub. The Hub responds by sending any available document to the requester, behaving as a virtual gateway to all available data within systems other than that of the requester.

AORTA is designed to have a single, role-based, access control decision point, which is centrally managed at the level of the Hub. The Hub fetches data from local systems on behalf of the users, and local systems have to comply with the requirements from NICTIZ (the Dutch National ICT Institute for Healthcare) in order to join AORTA. This means that a trust relationship exists between the local systems and the central authority, which is exploited when accessing the data. Access control decisions taken in the Hub are indeed valid also for the local systems. This design decision implies that the central authority must be at all times aware of both the users and their roles in the local organisations.

Data exchange between the components of the AORTA architecture is based on HL7 v3; specifications are constantly revised and published with a bi-annual release schedule. Regarding the medical vocabularies used to represent the terms within the messages, AORTA uses the SNOMED-CT and LOINC standards.

CRS-SISS (Italy)

The Italian healthcare system is largely organised on a regional basis, with a central coordination at the national level. With almost ten million inhabitants, Lombardy is the most populated region of Italy. The Lombard regional government is in charge of the administrative management of the regional healthcare system, including the planning and provisioning of healthcare services, and the monitoring of the quality of the delivered services. The healthcare information system used in Lombardy is called CRS-SISS (CRS-SISS, n. d.).

In CRS-SISS, the regional healthcare authority acts as a coordinator for the local systems, as it maintains all citizens' and healthcare professionals' identification information, and a centralised index for clinical data stored in local systems. When a user wants to access a clinical document, a search is performed based on the centralised index in order to discover its actual location. After obtaining the location, the request is routed to the local system where the document is stored. This allows the local systems to actually store the data, as required by Italian data retention and privacy laws. Data used for tracking reimbursement claims and for statistical purposes are managed by the central regional authority.

Citizens and healthcare professionals access the network by means of the regional service card (CRS), a smart-card issued by the regional government. The access control model of CRS-SISS is role-based and leverages the cooperation between the central authority and the local systems. When accessing data, requests are routed to the authentication and authorisation module of the central system. There is a centralised database containing all the identities and the corresponding roles of the users, which can thus enforce a global access control policy, valid throughout the region. If the request is authorised, the access control module of the central system forwards the request to the access control module of the local system. If this second step is also authorised, the client system receives a set of credentials that can be used on the local system to access the requested information.

In CRS-SISS there are two main information flows: the one between users and local systems and the one between local systems and the regional health authority. In the first one, exchanged messages must conform to HL7 v2.5 standard, while the terms use a custom vocabulary defined by the national health authority. Regarding the second information flow, applications are currently being ported to HL7 CDA v2.0, a standard derived from the Reference Information Model of HL7 v3. The terms used in reporting messages, regarding the classification of diseases, traumas and medical interventions, conform to ICD-9-CM.

Summary and Comparison

Three aspects related to interoperability are particularly important for our analysis of the previously surveyed systems:

- Data distribution (e.g., centralised vs. distributed architecture);
- Security policies (e.g., single policy decision point vs. multiple decision points); and
- Communication standards (e.g., support for a single standard vs. for multiple standards).

Data distribution is handled differently in the three systems. The data distribution strategy is heavily affected by national regulations about privacy and medical data retention. Italian laws state that the data originator is the responsible entity for the retention of data of any kind (thus including medical data), therefore medical data in CRS-SISS are kept only in local systems. The only data available in a centralised repository, belonging to the regional healthcare authority, are those related to reimbursement claims of the local healthcare organisations to the regional healthcare authority. In the Netherlands, the law forbids a central database of medical data, which results in the decentralised design of the AORTA system, where data is always kept in local systems. This fact did not however prevent to design the overall system to behave like a central repository, since there is a central access point that is in charge of collecting data from the local systems. The design of NHS Spine leveraged on English laws, which do not impose strict requirements on data retention. The system is therefore able to operate both in a centralised fashion (as demonstrated by the centralised implementation of the patient summary) and in a decentralised one. In order to ease the migration to the new system, indeed, local healthcare authorities can use the Spine as a central repository while adapting their own infrastructures. When dealing just with the patient summary, it is clear that none of these systems could be used as-is for a European infrastructure, as the requirements on data distribution are not meant to be automatically compatible.

Regarding security, all the analysed systems use smart-cards for user authentication, relying on a public key infrastructure. The information contained in these cards is used to assign certain roles to their owners, which are in turn used by the access control systems when an actor tries to perform an operation on a resource. The identities are centrally controlled by the national healthcare authorities, which also define the roles that are valid throughout the country, and the local systems have to be adapted to integrate with the national eHealth platforms. All the analysed systems rely on the assumption that the identification means of a patient must be provided by a single identity provider. Furthermore, each of these systems assumes that the relationship between the identity provided by an actor and his corresponding roles is centrally known. As the roles are defined on a national basis, the central authority decides whether an actor has the right to access some given information or not. In a multi-national scenario, characterised by multiple identity providers, roles and users cannot be managed at a central level, and thus there cannot exists a central decision point when dealing with authorisation.

With respect to communication standards, all the examined systems adopt HL7 for message exchange, even though with different versions:

- Version 2.5 is used by CRS-SISS for exchanging data between users and local systems;
- Version 3 is used by NHS Spine and AORTA; in CRS-SISS it is used only for the message exchange, related to accounting information, between local systems and the regional authority.

Although the standardisation body is the same, these two versions of HL7 are incompatible. The main feature of HL7 version 2.5 is the possibility to use XML for representing the information contained in the messages. However, it lacks a common reference model to bind the content of the messages to a set of common concepts. Starting with version 3 of HL7, a methodology has been defined in order to formally derive all the possible message structures from a normative Reference Information Model (RIM). The methodology also describes how the messages already defined by the standard can be further customised, in order to meet the users' requirements. Once a system adopts customised messages, it cannot interoperate easily with one adopting the plain standard (or worse, a differently customised version). The methodology just guarantees that, given a certain element in a document, it is always possible to link it to an object in the RIM, but the interpretations of the customisation are obviously left to the systems adopting them. Therefore, as AORTA and NHS use customised versions of the same standard, their messages are not necessarily compatible. The process of refining and customising the RIM is time-consuming and requires a significant effort also in the implementation phase. Therefore, countries that are developing large eHealth infrastructures are not willing to heavily revise their standards, as that would mean undermining years of investments in the implementation of their solutions.

A TRIPLESPACE INFRASTRUCTURE FOR THE EUROPEAN PATIENT SUMMARY

In this section we introduce the triplespace platform, and show how it can be used to concretely realise a European Patient Summary infrastructure, addressing the requirements we identified. Triplespaces enable a semantics-enriched communication and coordination paradigm, and provide a platform of virtual spaces in which autonomous actors can share information via the publication and retrieval of persistent information artefacts.

The Triplespace Paradigm

Information systems often depend largely on synchronous message exchange between information producers and consumers. The World Wide Web is instead based on a "persistently publish and read" paradigm, which allows a much greater degree of decoupling between different actors. Traditional Web services, despite referring to the Web in their name, typically rely on message exchange, establishing tightly coupled communication cycles and sending directed messages back and forth. Such message-based interaction pattern requires point-to-point communication, and breaks if one of the parties becomes unavailable. Furthermore, once a message is delivered, there is not necessarily any retrievable representation of that message available to the communicating partners. Therefore, if an exchange fails, it is not guaranteed that the related messages can be traced back and interpreted. For any situation that is more complex than a single client executing a single operation on a single Web service, coordination becomes necessary. Thus, coordination is typically implemented in a middleware stack which takes over responsibility for mediating between the interacting services. Web services could benefit from the possibility of communicating through the publication-based paradigm of the Web, which allows interactions between services to be decoupled in time and reference (Fensel, 2004). This considerations motivated a new communication paradigm, the *triplespace*, which brings together *space-based computing* and *Semantic Web technologies* into a new-generation middleware based on the concept of semantic spaces.

Space-based computing has its origin in the field of parallel computing with the Linda tuplespace model (Gelernter, 1985), as a means to enhance sequential programming languages in order to handle concurrency. Linda consists of coordination primitives and a shared data space (*tuplespace*) which contains data (*tuples*). A tuple is an ordered list of typed fields. The coordination primitives are a small set of operations that permit agents to emit a tuple into the space (*out* operation) or retrieve tuples, either removing them from the space (*in* operation) or not (*rd* operation). Retrieval is governed by an associative matching technique: tuples are matched against a tuple template that specifies the values or the types of a subset of the tuple fields. A match occurs when the template and the tuple have the same number of fields, the field types are the same, and the values of constant fields are identical. For example, the tuple <"temperature", "Innsbruck", "20"> matches the template <"temperature", "Innsbruck", ?t> (Figure 1). Retrieval operations are blocking, i.e., they return a result only when a matching tuple is found. In this way, Linda combines synchronisation and communication in an extremely simple model with a high level of abstraction.

A tuplespace thus supports asynchrony and concurrency (the producers and consumers of a tuple do not need to know one another's address, nor exist concurrently), and permits associative addressing (data are retrieved on the basis of the type of data requested, rather than on which specific data are referenced). Hence, tuplespace systems are a viable candidate to meet the decentralisation and distribution needs of the EPS scenario. However, while a number of implemented tuplespace systems – e.g., JavaSpaces (Freeman, Hupfer, & Arnold, 1999), TSpaces (Wyckoff, McLaughry, Lehman, & Ford, 1998), or GigaSpaces (Cohen, n. d.) – clearly address the communication and coordination requirements we stated, none of them explicitly copes with the possible het-

Figure 1. Tuplespace example

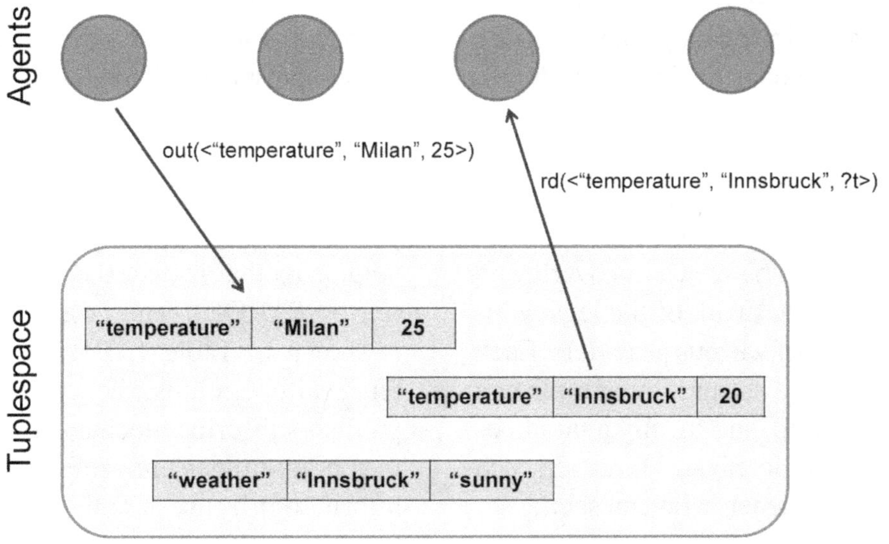

erogeneity of encoding systems and message types, which is an intrinsic challenge of the eHealth domain. Semantic technologies can provide solutions and techniques to address these challenges. In particular, semantics can help in unambiguously defining the meaning of medical concepts, in structuring the patient records, and in mediating between heterogeneous resources.

Summing up, while tuplespaces allow distributed sharing of information without requiring synchronous connections, Semantic Web technologies extend the Web with machine-processable semantic data, allowing data exchange in heterogeneous application fields. The combination of the two results in a communication paradigm with persistent and asynchronous dissemination of machine-understandable data at its core: triplespaces (Fensel, 2004). The communication and coordination space provided by triplespaces is tailored to the needs of machines, and integrates optimised storage facilities for semantic data, mediation, and reasoning engines. Information shared in triplespaces is represented as RDF (Resource Description Framework) triples, which reference ontologies that capture the meaning (i.e., the semantics) of the published information. The use of ontologies and RDF enables the application of additional semantic technologies such as data mediation, inference, or consistency checking.

A triplespace system is conceptually organised as a hierarchy of spaces that, as a whole, establish a network of virtual information resources, which can be seen as an overlay on top of the physical network of the legacy information systems of various providers. Each space can be targeted at a particular topic or a particular user group, and locally guarantees scalability and completeness. Moreover, each space can have its owner, who can set the security policy of the space in order to control access to that space. This allows particular groups of users or organisations to create their own spaces and to collaborate via their chosen spaces under their chosen security policies. Moreover, the triplespace security model allows the definition of mapping rules between attributes provided by users accessing the system (e.g., to assert the organisation to which they belong) and roles used to define the access control policy of the space. The access control policy is thus decoupled from the user attributes, and there is no need for a central authority that manages identities and access rights (Cerri & Corcoglioniti, 2009).

Data in the triplespace are represented using three-fielded tuples that model the <subject, predicate, object> triples of RDF. Moreover, in RDF triples are grouped into graphs, and this structure is taken over to triplespaces. Hence, an agent has no longer to read and write single tuples, but can rather read and write whole constructs of semantic data. The usage of RDF also implies a more expressive retrieval scheme than the traditional tuplespace template matching, because triples cannot be distinguished from one another in terms of the number or the type of their fields. Indeed, the application of Semantic Web technology allows the space to perform more sophisticated, knowledge-driven, matching: not only the structure, but the meaning of data can be taken into account. We therefore extend the traditional tuplespace retrieval primitives to support RDF-specific query languages that reflect the semantics of data (e.g., SPARQL). The core triplespace API is shown in Table 1. Besides the blocking retrieval operations, the triplespace offers a publish-subscribe mechanism with semantic matching: an agent may subscribe to particular information by use of semantic templates, and

Table 1. Core triplespace API

out(Set<Triple>triples, URI space):void	Inserts the given *triples* into the given *space*.
rd(Template t, [URI space,] int timeout):Graph	Returns a single match to the *template* provided. A template is a query that follows some implementation-specific syntax, e.g. a single triple pattern or a SPARQL (graph pattern) query. The scope of the query is restricted to the given *space*, if indicated. Otherwise the request is resolved in best effort over all known spaces. The *timeout* is used as a means to restrain the blocking characteristics of the operation to a finite time period.
rdmultiple(Template t, URI space, int timeout):Graph	Operates as rd but it is not restricted to returning a single match. Rather, it attempts to return as many matches as can be found within the scope of the query and the given timeout.

then be informed whenever relevant data is published in the space.

The actual realisation of a triplespace infrastructure is delivered by triplespace *kernels*, which are responsible for (i) exposing the coordination primitives defined by the triplespace API to clients, (ii) providing access to security policies and configuration functions via a separate Management API, (iii) coordinating connected clients, (iv) guaranteeing secure and persistent data exchange, (v) mediating between different data formats, and (vi) retrieving required data from kernels that collaboratively manage the published data. The latest carries along the advantage that a client does not have to know the particular kernel that manages the requested data, but that any kernel is able to respond to any client request. Triplespace kernels constitute therefore an overlay network, as shown in Figure 2.

Figure 2. Network of triplespace kernels

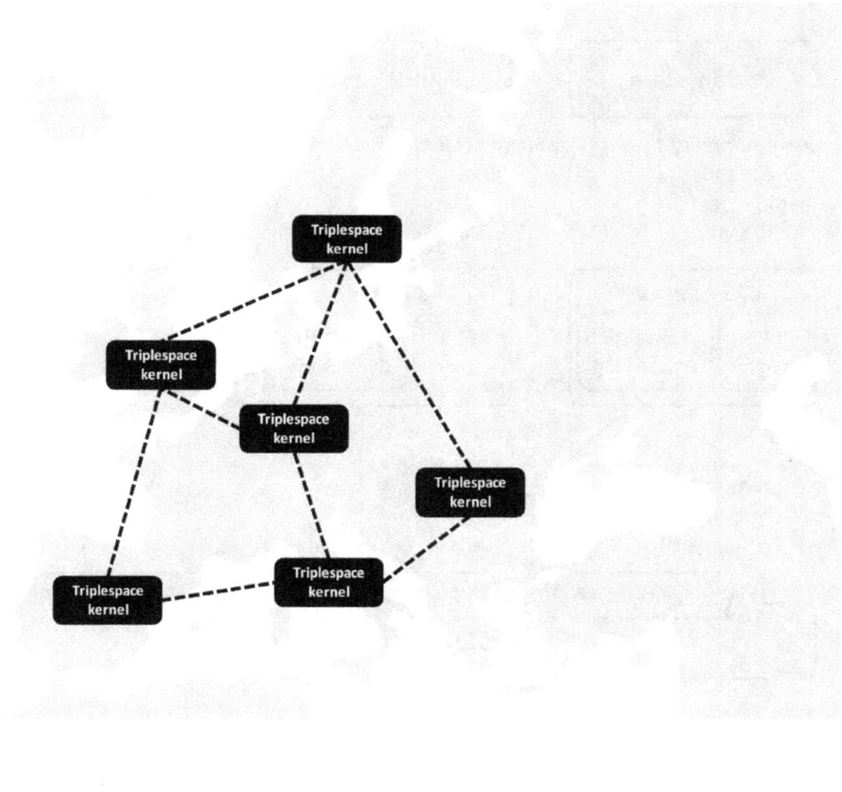

A European Patient Summary Architecture Using Triplespaces

In this section we propose a realisation of the European Patient Summary scenario using triplespaces. The triplespace infrastructure briefly presented in the previous section provides the middleware layer for a large-scale information space that enables pervasive access to patient information across regional and national borders. The EPS system is realised on top of the triplespace middleware as an integrated collection of various medical information systems and electronic health record software, which can communicate with the triplespace infrastructure by means of EPS Adapters (Figure 3). Patient data, as well as associated coding systems and message types, are represented using machine-understandable representation languages (such as RDF(S), OWL) and ontologies. This enables support for semantic mediation between heterogeneous data formats and reasoning over the information in the system to infer new knowledge.

Our EPS system architecture is based on a three-tier realisation (Figure 3). The top tier, i.e. the user front-end, is realised by *existing medical applications and services*: eHR, Hospital and Laboratory Information Systems (HIS and LIS), and similar legacy applications. These systems exchange patient data with the EPS infrastructure through existing eHealth standards for the communication of clinical patient information, including HL7 Clinical Document Architecture, OpenEHR, and ASTM CCR. Each of these standards focuses on a specific part of the healthcare domain, ranging from exchanging general-purpose clinical documents to patient summary information.

The middle tier of the EPS architecture is constituted by *EPS Adapters*, which mediate between existing eHealth information systems and the underlying triplespace infrastructure.

Figure 3. EPS system architecture

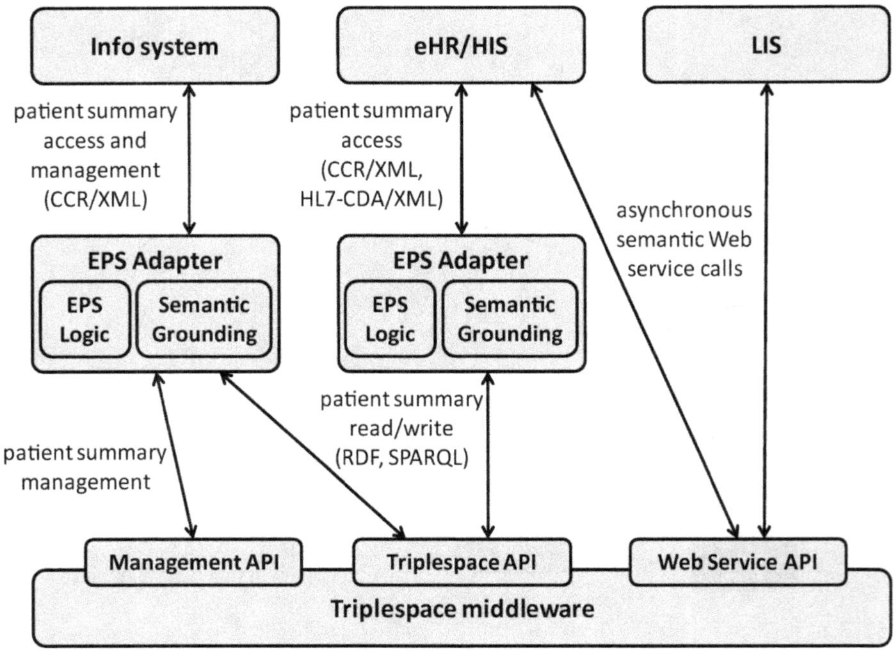

The triplespace middleware requires the published data to be represented in RDF, while the mentioned eHealth standards are based on XML syntax. Therefore, the EPS Adapter includes a *Semantic Grounding* component that is able to translate HL7 CDA, CCR and OpenEHR messages into their corresponding RDF versions. In order to perform this step, we developed formal models (in the form of ontologies) and mappings that capture both the structure of the messages and their meaning. As for the content of the messages based on ontologies, we use an ontologised version of the Unified Medical Language System (UMLS) as a reference vocabulary in the prototype, since it already includes well-defined mappings to other vocabularies, such as ICD (International Classification of Diseases) 9 and 10. The EPS Adapter also contains an *EPS Logic* component that is in charge of delivering the logic bindings between the native information systems and the shared information space. Whenever an information system needs to access or update a patient summary, the EPS Logic component takes over the communication with the triplespace and uses the Semantic Grounding component to resolve the necessary translations. An extension beyond the pure integration of legacy information systems via EPS Adapters is the use of the triplespace Web Service API. The Web Service API provides a means of binding asynchronous Semantic Web service calls to EPS interaction patterns in order to integrate data delivered by external knowledge and service providers, e.g. the exchange of laboratory examination data from different health authorities.

The triplespace middleware constitutes the bottom tier of the architecture. The hierarchical organisation of the spaces is shown in Figure 4. The global EPS space is virtually one big space, divided into many subspaces following the natural structure of health authorities in Europe. There are several nations with national authorities, which in turn are subdivided into regions and cities. Although the number of levels may vary from country to country, the overall structure remains the same. Thus, the EPS triplespace structure consists of a tree of spaces with the root representing all of Europe, and the leaves delivering the individual citizens' patient summaries. Every summary is further divided into three subspaces: two for the parts of the patient summary related to administrative data and clinical data, protected according to public regulations, and a third subspace protected by patient's specific access policies. Indeed, the hierarchy of spaces, which represents a hierarchy of authorities, is also significant from a security perspective: according to the triplespace security model, each authority can associate to its space its own policy for what is allowed by the higher level policies, and can also inherit role definitions from higher level policies, and add its own ones.

Reconsidering Figure 2 leads to a view of the EPS realisation in which every patient summary is stored on a triplespace kernel that manages the space of the local health authority with which a citizen is associated. Consequently, the kernels that collaboratively manage the EPS system would be distributed all over Europe. While this is clear from the details of the EPS infrastructure, it is absolutely transparent to client applications. Hidden behind the triplespace API, the kernels take over the request propagation, kernel discovery, and query resolution tasks. This distributed nature of the triplespace-based EPS has clear advantages with respect to scalability and dynamism, while the advantage with respect to heterogeneity comes from the embedded

Figure 4. EPS space hierarchy

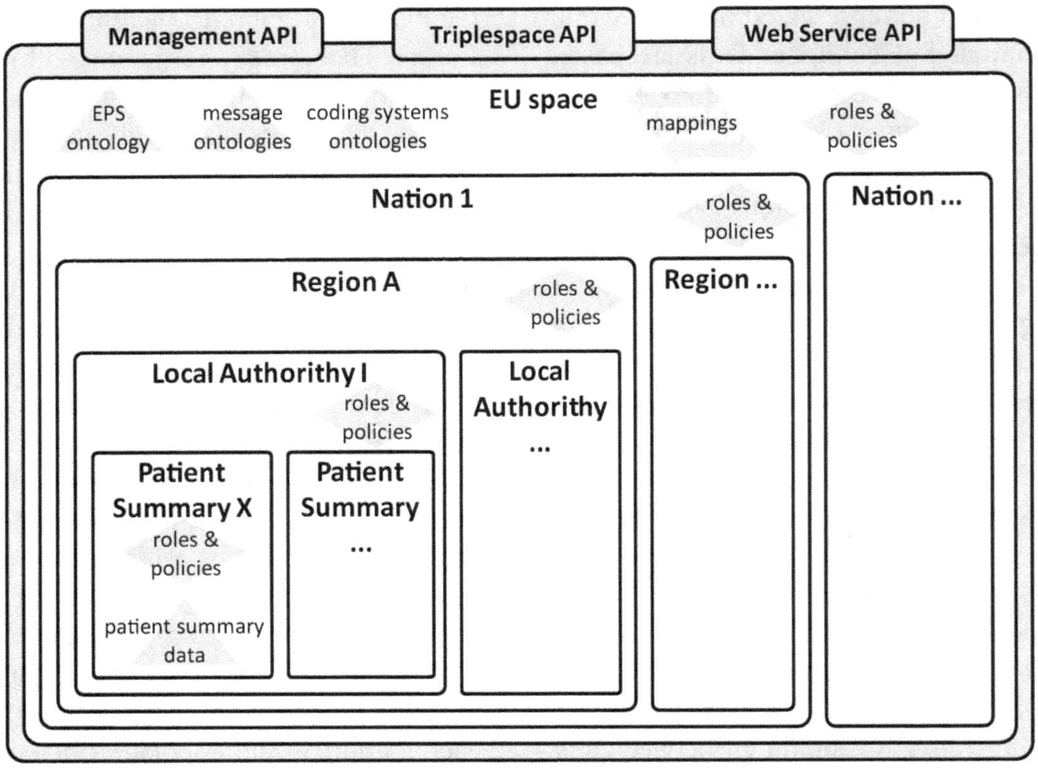

semantic technologies. Having one or more virtual spaces per health authority emphasises the desired local scalability. Since a major share of all EPS interactions are bound to the geographical area of one authority, grouping the resulting coordination to a particular set of virtual spaces makes distribution and discovery more scalable. Having individual patient summary spaces guarantees at least local completeness, local to a particular patient record (see Krummenacher, Simperl & Fensel (2008) for further discussion on scalable information spaces).

Comparison with Current National Solutions for Patient Summaries

In a previous section we showed that existing national solutions for patient summaries are not suitable for crossing the boundaries of a single nation, and thus cannot be used to solve the same problem at the European level. We also discussed how triplespace technology can be effectively used to realise a multilateral and distributed infrastructure for the European Patient Summary. We now look at our EPS realisation from the point of view of the three aspects we considered for existing national systems, i.e. data distribution, security, and communication standards.

Regarding data distribution, triplespaces can effectively enforce the requirements coming from real-world systems, allowing sub-hierarchies of spaces to be hosted on different kernels maintained by different health authorities. The triplespace-based EPS is a distributed infrastructure where there is no central node that controls all the medical records and patients. The triplespace infrastructure allows health authorities to organise their spaces following the natural structure of healthcare authorities in Europe, i.e., according to the existing European and national hierarchies of responsibility. Even if in this way the data is hosted on different kernels, the retrieval mechanisms make this completely transparent to users, which can thus retrieve data (if allowed by relevant security policies) independently from the number of health authorities that are in charge of those data.

Regarding security, our solution allows a security policy to be associated to each space in the hierarchy, and provides a means to control the order (and thus the priority) with which they are evaluated in the hierarchy of spaces. This mechanism allows each health authority to define its own policies on its own spaces, if this is allowed by higher level authorities/policies. Moreover, the attribute mapping mechanism avoids the need for a centralised management of users' identities, roles and access rights, which would be impractical at a European level. Roles and policies can be flexibly defined at each level, and inherited along the space (and authority) hierarchy.

Regarding standards, our solution decouples data representation and data interpretation. As we chose to use RDF as data representation language, each party involved in the European Patient Summary is able to access the system with a unique standard. The interpretation of the triples contained in a patient summary is then left to the participating system. The incorporation of semantic technology in the middleware helps to overcome the heterogeneity challenges that arise from the usage of different terminologies, reducing the efforts necessary to ensure interoperability between different systems. A semantic interoperability module attached to the local system can obtain the ontologies used to model data directly from the space, and can exploit the explicit references to those models contained in the triples, in order to implement a system where data is aligned using concepts similarities and explicit domain-dependant rules.

Finally, it is important to note that our proposed architecture would not be meant to replace existing national solutions, but rather to integrate with them. Triplespace technology can support different existing data distribution strategies, security schemes and messaging standards, thus a European Patient Summary solution adopting triplespaces would allow integrating existing healthcare solutions without the need of radically modifying them. The integration of such solutions would require a coherent space hierarchy to store data respecting national privacy laws, a data translator to convert to and from RDF and to interpret the different semantics of the messages used by different national solutions, and the formalisation of the permissions granted to actors coming from different European countries.

FUTURE RESEARCH DIRECTIONS

According to the 2009 Innovative Medicines Initiative call for research (Innovative Medicine Initiative, 2009), future directions in health record management mainly cover the application of patient information in drug and disease research. The argumentation is that medical records can have a much wider impact in eHealth, far beyond the optimisation of health services, as it was mostly the topic in the scenarios above. Interoperability of patient data between patient records and medical research can improve the drug discovery, development and commercialisation process and enable faster and more secure access for patients to effective new medications through better signal detection and personalised medicines and therapy. Incremental and future research on top of the work presented in this chapter should thus take care of bridging the gap between primary care and medical research in order to leverage aggregated patient data to research, to achieve safer diagnoses and treatments for patients, to speed up the discovery and time to market of new drugs, or to ensure cross-border exchange of knowledge and experience. In particular, the latest point yields an application scenario for which triplespaces offer an interesting solution. The use of RDF, per se already, encourages data sharing and preservation of knowledge across projects and institutions. This notion of globalisation in research is further supported by the shared memory and coordination principles that underlie our triplespace middleware. The use of semantic technology for the coordination and communication of eHealth data allows moreover for integration of knowledge on demand, without the need for reworking when new data sources become relevant, or new types of reports and analyses are needed. This adds a whole new dimension of agility to the medical and pharmaceutical research procedures.

The triplespace infrastructure presented in this chapter, and subsequent achievements thereof, can provide the fundamental building blocks for future research scenarios in eHealth. Notably, it offers a technological baseline for collaborative research over medical data and ensures open access to, and discovery of large volumes of semantic data sources. In this respect we emphasise the synergies with Linked Open Data (n. d.) which already include many of the public life science and bioinformatics data sets such as UniProt (n. d.), OMIM (Online Mendelian Inheritance in Man, n. d.), or the Gene Ontology (n. d.). In order to activate this wealth of information, the development of a secure Web-enabled middleware, e.g. through service technology, is suggested for the publishing and querying of knowledge in combination with potentially proprietary data. A corresponding triplespace-driven solution would not only improve healthcare or accelerate clinical research, but allow for more knowledge-intensive proposals to drug validation and diagnostics tools, or for machine-supported identification of appropriate therapies at the right dose to reduce extensive exposure to side-effects of treatments, as for example in oncology. Consequently, the work presented in this chapter provides a valuable baseline for future work that addresses the eminent lack of platforms for the analysis of large amounts of information in an integrated and predictive way. This lack is still a major barrier in current biomedical and life science research, and prevents the delivery of many scientific and technological advances that would foster the development of safe and more effective medicines and remove the bottlenecks in the drug development process.

First investigations in this direction were conducted with a life science research institute to realise knowledge-intensive collaborative research activities around the discovery of relations between drugs, proteins and diseases (Cerri et al., 2008). Drug discovery is an interdisciplinary and data-driven research domain involving scientists from different communities and pharmaceutical companies. The research is mainly based on public data resources that are openly available for commercial exploitation. The discovery process requires the assumption making on pathomechanisms involved in a given disease. Pharmaceutical companies focus their research on specific domains (e.g., treatment of pain or rheumathoid arthritis), but want to use the existing data infrastructure without any restrictions to any disease. In other words, the different data sources have to be integrated into a common interface that enables researchers to retrieve hypothetical facts for a pathomechanism of a given disease but should be able to assess the same pathomechamisms under a different disease hypothesis. There is thus a particular interest in the integration of knowledge across different phases of drug development. For this purpose, a public and freely available infrastructure for the storage and retrieval of drug/disease models is required, confirming the aforementioned research agenda.

CONCLUSION

Amongst other things, we pointed out in this chapter that there is a general lack of legal and technical standards to realise an integrated and coordinated European eHealth infrastructure. As shown, this situation has been recognised by many EU member states – about half of them are working on national eHealth solutions – and has triggered various implementations that shall ensure faster and more secure access to patient information. Three particularly interesting examples were discussed in the background section. These national efforts continue however to evolve in separation, as accepted standards for basic IT concepts and specific technical standards are still missing. In order to suggest a coordination framework that acknowledges these natural issues of heterogeneity, we presented in this chapter an approach that applies semantics and publicly shared triplespaces to foster interoperability and integration between different eHealth systems. Conceptually, the presented work offers a very promising start, but in order for seamless and collaborative care across organisational and political boundaries to become a reality, all those involved in health services must understand and act on the shared information on a much wider scale. Significantly more work is thus required to realise interoperable multinational eHealth solutions for the management of patient information. The implementation of cost-effective platforms and sustainable business models is required for establishing credible healthcare information systems that will be linked to and leveraged through many diverse sources at regional and national levels. Without comprehensive connectivity, continuous duplication of work will hamper medical services, and limit the access to knowledge for healthcare providers and research bodies that may be able to use it in innovative ways.

REFERENCES

Booth, N. (2003). Sharing patient information electronically throughout the NHS. *British Medical Journal, 327*(7407), 114–115. doi:10.1136/bmj.327.7407.114 PMID:12869425

Cerri, D., & Corcoglioniti, F. (2009). Bridging the gap between user attributes and service policies with attribute mapping. In *Proceedings of the 2009 IEEE Conference on Commerce and Enterprise Computing* (pp. 154-161). IEEE Computer Society.

Cerri, D., Della Valle, E., de Francisco Marcos, D., Giunchiglia, F., Naor, D., Nixon, L., et al. (2008). Towards knowledge in the cloud. In On the move to meaningful internet systems: OTM 2008 Workshops, LNCS 5333 (pp. 986–995). Springer.

Cohen, U. (n. d.). *Inside Gigaspaces XAP – Technical overview and value proposition* (GigaSpaces Technical White Paper). Retrieved from http://www.gigaspaces.com/WhitePapers.

Commission of the European Communities. (2004). *e-Health - Making healthcare better for European citizens: An action plan for a European e-Health area.* Communication from the Commission to the Council, the European Parliament, the European Economic and Social Committee and the Committee of the Regions. COM (2004) 356 final. Retrieved from http://eur-lex.europa.eu/LexUriServ/LexUriServ.do?uri=CELEX:52004DC0356:EN:NOT

CRS-SISS. (n. d.). *Carta regionale dei servizi – Sistema informativo socio-sanitario.* Retrieved from http://www.crs.lombardia.it/

epSOS. (n. d.). Retrieved from http://www.epsos.eu/

European Interoperability Framework for Pan-European eGovernment Services. (2004). Version 1.0. Retrieved from http://ec.europa.eu/idabc.

Fensel, D. (2004). Triple-space computing: Semantic Web services based on persistent publication of information. In *IFIP International Conference on Intelligence in Communication Systems, LNCS 3283* (pp. 43-53). Springer.

Freeman, E., Hupfer, S., & Arnold, K. (1999). *JavaSpaces principles, patterns, and practice.* Prentice Hall PTR.

Gelernter, D. (1985). Generative communication in Linda. *ACM Transactions on Programming Languages and Systems, 7*(1), 80–112. doi:10.1145/2363.2433

Gene Ontology. (n. d.). Retrieved from http://www.geneontology.org/

Innovative Medicine Initiative. (2009). *Innovative Medicines Joint Undertaking (IMI JU) 2009 Call for proposals.* Retrieved from http://www.imi.europa.eu.

Krummenacher, R., Simperl, E., & Fensel, D. (2008). Scalability in semantic computing: Semantic middleware. In *Proceedings of the 2008 IEEE International Conference on Semantic Computing* (pp. 538-545). IEEE Computer Society.

Linked Open Data. (n. d.). Retrieved from http://www.linkeddata.org/

NHS. (n. d.). *NHS Connecting for Health.* Retrieved from http://www.connectingforhealth.nhs.uk/

NICTIZ. (n. d.). *AORTA.* Retrieved from http://www.nictiz.nl/

Online Mendelian Inheritance in Man. (n. d.). Retrieved from http://www.ncbi.nlm.nih.gov/omim/

UniProt. (n. d.). Retrieved from http://www.uniprot.org/

Wyckoff, P., McLaughry, S. W., Lehman, T. J., & Ford, D. A. (1998). T Spaces. *IBM Systems Journal, 37*(3), 454–474. doi:10.1147/sj.373.0454

ADDITIONAL READING

Alonso, G., Casati, F., Kuno, H., & Machiraju, V. (2003). *Web Services – Concepts, Architectures and Applications*. Springer.

Beeler, G. (1998). HL7 version 3: An object-oriented methodology for collaborative standards development. *International Journal of Medical Informatics*, *48*(1-3), 151–161. doi:10.1016/S1386-5056(97)00121-4 PMID:9600415

Berners-Lee, T., Hendler, J., & Lassila, O. (2001). The Semantic Web. *Scientific American*, *284*(5), 34–43. doi:10.1038/scientificamerican0501-34 PMID:11396337

Brickley, D., & Guha, R. V. (Eds.). (2004). *RDF Vocabulary Description Language 1.0: RDF Schema*. W3C Recommendation. Retrieved from http://www.w3.org/TR/2004/REC-rdf-schema-20040210/.

Cardoso, J., & Sheth, A. P. (Eds.). (2006). *Semantic Web Services, Processes and Applications*. Springer. doi:10.1007/978-0-387-34685-4

Centers for Disease Control and Prevention. (n.d.). *International Classification of Diseases, Ninth Revision, Clinical Modification (ICD-9-CM)*. Retrieved from http://www.cdc.gov/nchs/icd/icd9cm.htm.

Dolin, R., Alschuler, L., Boyer, S., Beebe, C., Behlen, F., Biron, P., & Shabo, A. (2006). HL7 clinical document architecture, release 2. *Journal of the American Medical Informatics Association*, *13*(1), 30–39. doi:10.1197/jamia.M1888 PMID:16221939

Forrey, A. W., McDonald, C. J., DeMoor, G., Huff, S. M., Leavelle, D., & Leland, D. et al. (1996). Logical observation identifier names and codes (LOINC) database: a public use set of codes and names for electronic reporting of clinical laboratory test results. *Clinical Chemistry*, *42*(1), 81–90. PMID:8565239

Manola, F., & Miller, E. (Eds.). (2004). *RDF Primer*. W3C Recommendation. Retrieved from http://www.w3.org/TR/2004/REC-rdf-primer-20040210/.

McGuinness, D. L., & van Harmelen, F. (Eds.). (2004). *OWL Web Ontology Language Overview*. W3C Recommendation. Retrieved from http://www.w3.org/TR/2004/REC-owl-features-20040210/.

Prud'hommeaux, E., & Seaborne, A. (Eds.). (2008). *SPARQL Query Language for RDF*. W3C Recommendation. Retrieved from http://www.w3.org/TR/2008/REC-rdf-sparql-query-20080115/.

Roman, D., Keller, U., Lausen, H., de Bruijn, J., Lara, R., & Stollberg, M. et al. (2005). Web Service Modeling Ontology. *Applied Ontology*, *1*(1), 77–106.

Shadbolt, N., Berners-Lee, T., & Hall, W. (2006). The Semantic Web Revisited. [IEEE Computer Society.]. *IEEE Intelligent Systems*, *21*(3), 96–101. doi:10.1109/MIS.2006.62

Wang, A., Sable, J., & Spackman, K. (2002). The SNOMED clinical terms development process: refinement and analysis of content. In *Proceedings of the AMIA Symposium* (pp. 845-9). American Medical Informatics Association.

Chapter 10

Semantic Integration of Patient Data for Clinical Decision Support in Breast Cancer Care

Leonardo Lezcano
University of Alcalá, Spain

Miguel-Ángel Sicilia
University of Alcalá, Spain

Eydel Rivero
University of Alcalá, Spain

ABSTRACT

Achieving semantic interoperability between heterogeneous healthcare systems and integrating clinical guidelines in the automatic decision support of healthcare institutions are two key priorities of current medical informatics. They can lead to a significant improvement on patient safety by reducing medical risks and delays in diagnosis, facilitating continuity of care and preventing life threatening adverse events. The present chapter describes a project that addresses those two priorities in the field of Breast Cancer for which effective clinical guidelines are available, as well as the clinical data to apply them. However, the deployment of semantic interoperability techniques based on clinical terminologies such as SNOMED-CT and EHR exchange models such as openEHR and HL7 is required to meaningfully combine the available data. Then data mining techniques are capable of automatically adapting the parameters of clinical guidelines to the particular conditions of each healthcare environment.

1. INTRODUCTION

Like many other fields that heavily rely on the capabilities of information and communication technologies, healthcare and biomedical environments are rapidly increasing the demand for widely accepted agreements on data, information and knowledge exchange. Such needs for compatibility or interoperability go beyond syntactical and structural issues as semantic interoperability is also required. Semantic interoperability (Stroetmann et al.,

DOI: 10.4018/978-1-4666-3000-0.ch010

2009) is essential to facilitate the computerized support for alerts, workflow management and evidence-based healthcare across heterogeneous Electronic Health Record (EHR) systems.

The model of clinical archetypes supported by the CEN/ISO EN13606 standard and the openEHR foundation (Beale, 2002) provides a mechanism to express data structures in a shared and interoperable way. It has acquired considerable acceptance in the last years by allowing the definition of clinical concepts based on a common Reference Model while low level storage implementation can keep its heterogeneity across EHR systems. However, archetype languages do not provide direct support neither for clinical rules nor mappings to formal ontologies, which are both key elements of full semantic interoperability as they allow exploiting reasoning on clinical knowledge (Lezcano et al., 2011).

It has been acknowledged that the World Wide Web demands analogous capabilities to those mentioned above, leading to the development of the Semantic Web extension. The progress made in that field, regarding reasoning and knowledge representation, is combined in this chapter with EHR models in order to enhance the archetype approach and to support features that correspond to a richer level of semantic interoperability.

The present section introduces a research carried out during the last 3 years to increase patient safety and improve outcomes in the particular context of breast cancer treatment. Most of this work is part of the HEDECAMA project, which stands for "Semantic Model and Data Mining Algorithms applied to Breast Cancer Treatment in Specialized Care Centers." The general goal is to develop a series of complementary technology components and applications in order to obtain a clinical decisions support system (CDSS) for breast cancer treatment at care centers (i.e., hospitals, oncology centers, etc.). As a result, the end-user or breast cancer specialist receives relevant information to certain situations and clinical episodes, allowing him/her to access and process in real-time all current and historical information related to the patient's clinical case. This would be an extremely time consuming task if accomplished manually.

The developed solution is configurable and extensible as the integrated technological elements follows commonly accepted standards. They can collect and interpret a wide range of data from the heterogeneous clinical information systems currently available in healthcare institutions, and at different stages of the clinical diagnosis and treatment of breast cancer.

This chapter is structured according to Figure 1. The workflow first includes an Integration stage, based on a Data Integration Framework that is described in Section 2 and a Terminology Server introduced in Section 3. Then the Storage and Classification stage, whose main component is presented in Section 4 interacts with the Knowledge and Machine Learning components described in sections 5 and 6. A visualization stage, the features of which are not covered in the chapter, offers the results to the end-user. Although all the stages will be explained, the current chapter is oriented to put more emphasis on the Data Integration Framework, whose details are provided in the subsections of Section 2. Finally, Section 7 provides the conclusions of the research and its impact from a clinical perspective.

Figure 1. The breast cancer CDSS global architecture

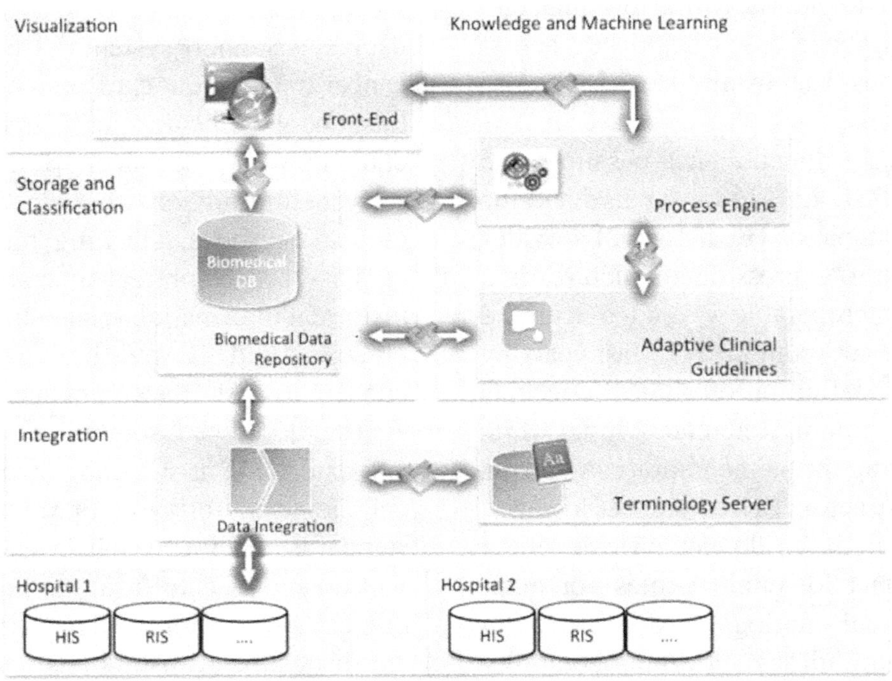

2. THE DATA INTEGRATION FRAMEWORK

The interoperability between heterogeneous healthcare systems is essential to improve the management and continuity of patient care. Several norms and specifications have been proposed to facilitate such interoperability at different levels. The openEHR initiative (Beale & Heard, 2007) is oriented to the definition and distribution of flexible specifications of medical concepts as clinical archetypes.

As part of the HEDECAMA project, a Data Integration Framework has been designed and developed to allow the flow of information between heterogeneous healthcare systems. The implementation of this framework is based on the use of open source software and tools, according to the GNU/GPL license, which makes it possible for the framework itself to be also available for open use. In addition, the facility of the framework components to seamlessly interact with future developed tools has been addressed. This way, the scope of the Integration Framework goes beyond the limits of the HEDECAMA project.

In general terms, the Integration Framework makes use of its integration capabilities to synchronize the available databases in the current hospitals healthcare systems with the Biomedical Data Repository shown in Figure 1 and introduced in Section 4. For that purpose, the following features have been included in the framework:

- Semi-online processing of the clinical information
- ETL/EAI information treatment
- Process planning

Figure 2 shows the architecture of the Data Integration Framework and its connec-

Figure 2. Architecture of the data integration framework

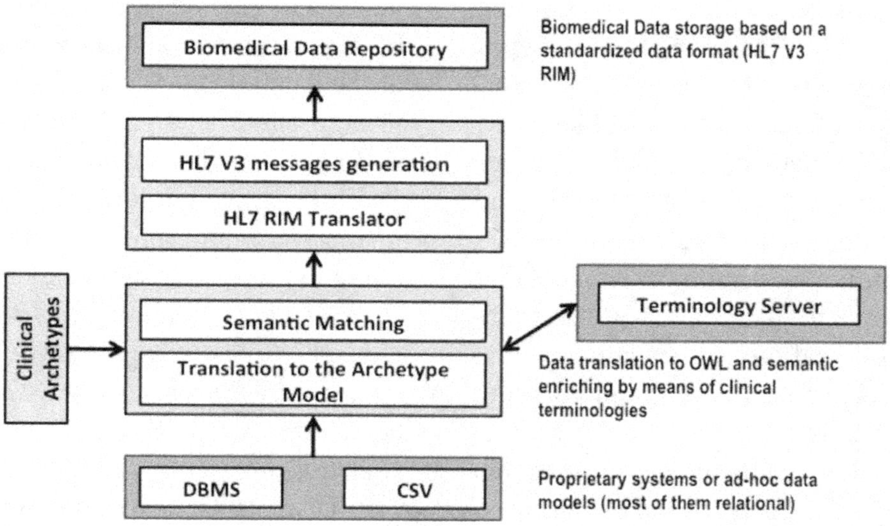

tions to the rest of the CDSS. In a bottom up traversing of the integration process, the first step includes the codification and structuring of the information retrieved from the source databases by means of the openEHR model. Then the resulting instances of clinical archetypes are translated to OWL (W3C OWL Working Group, 2012) following the method described in (Lezcano et al., 2008), which supports higher levels of interoperability, ultimately encouraging the achievement of semantic interoperability.

It should be noted that the interaction between the different components of the integration framework, and with the external systems, requires the internal generation of translation catalogues for the local and proprietary nomenclatures available in the source systems. In order to reduce the time consumed by this task, a connection to an external system providing terminological service based on SNOMED-CT facilitates the generation of such catalogues and the translation between heterogeneous nomenclatures.

The OWL files obtained in the above-described step are provided as input for the generation of messages based on the HL7 V3 RIM international standard (Health Level Seven) (Dolin et al., 2006). Such messages deliver the integrated data to the Biomedical Data Repository on the top of Figure 2. The structure of the repository itself is also based on the reference model (RIM) of HL7 V3.

2.1 Translation of Heterogeneous Relational Models to the openEHR Archetype Model

The openEHR Archetype Definition Language (ADL) (Beale & Heard, 2008) is oriented to formalize the transfer of clinical information between different EHR systems so that the exchange information can be interpreted with the ad-hoc development of a parser for every clinical concept. Therefore, it is based on the Reference Model (RM) that defines the data structures and types required to represent the health record information. The contextual data needed to fulfil the legal and ethical requirements of the health record are also defined in the RM. In order to further constrain the information in the RM, clinical archetypes are specifically defined for each clinical concept in a way that restrain the RM hierarchy, combine certain data structures and further reduce the domain of each datatype. Inside the ADL definition, each RM element receives a name according to the clinical concept that is being described. In contrast with the more stable RM, clinical archetypes are designed to be frequently modified without carrying out significant source code modifications to the underlying healthcare systems. In this manner, they can cope with the evolution of clinical knowledge and practices.

The transfer to the Archetype Model is supported by the HedecamaCSV2ADL tool that has been developed as part of the Hedecama project and allows the generation of an archetype according to the specifications, in Comma Separated Values (CSV) files, that were previously defined for each dataset that must be integrated. A fragment of the Breast Cancer Diagnosis archetype, for the transfer of the data related to such concept, is shown in Figure 3. The larger fragment is included as Annex 2 of this chapter:

Eight archetypes have been defined so far in the Hedecama project, representing key clinical concepts in the Breast Cancer domain: *Breast Cancer Medication*, *History of Breast Cancer*, *Breast Cancer Diagnosis*, *Breast Cancer Evolution*, *Breast Cancer Physical Examination*, *Breast Cancer Response*, *Breast Cancer Treatment* and *Breast Cancer Last Contact*. Once an archetype is defined, the data extraction begins by anonymizing the patient sensitive coming from the source relational databases or CSV files. Finally, the classes in the RM are instantiated for each record or row according to their corresponding archetype (ADL). At this point the workflow

Figure 3. Fragment of the breast cancer diagnosis archetype

```
definition
    OBSERVATION[at0000] matches {        -- Diagnóstico cáncer de mama
        data matches {
            HISTORY[at0001] matches {      -- Event Series
                events cardinality matches {1..*; unordered} matches {
                    EVENT[at0002] occurrences matches {0..1} matches {      -- Any Event
                        data matches {
                            ITEM_TREE[at0003] matches {    -- Item Tree
                                items cardinality matches {1..*; unordered} matches {
                                    CLUSTER[at0004] occurrences matches {0..1} matches {  -- Clínico
                                        items cardinality matches {1..*; unordered} matches {
                                            ELEMENT[at0005] occurrences matches {0..1} matches {  -- Síntoma_inicial_predominante_mama_derecha
                                                value matches {
                                                    DV_CODED_TEXT matches {
                                                        defining_code matches {
                                                            [local::
                                                            at0006, -- Asintomática
                                                            at0007, -- Desconocido
                                                            at0008, -- Fiebre
                                                            at0009, -- Dolor mamario
                                                            at0010, -- Dolor óseo
                                                            at0011, -- Dolor extramamario y extraóseo
                                                            at0012, -- Inflamación
                                                            at0013, -- Palpación de nódulo
                                                            at0014, -- Sangrado
                                                            at0015, -- Retracción del pezón
                                                            at0016, -- Cambios en la piel
                                                            at0017, -- Cefalea
                                                            at0018, -- Mareo
                                                            at0019, -- Síndrome de vena cava
                                                            at0020, -- Compresión medular
                                                            at0021] -- Otros (especificar)
```

continues through the ADL to OWL translation, introduced in the next subsection.

2.2 Archetypes Translation from ADL to the OWL Ontology Language

The ADL to OWL translation process is carried out by the *Archetype Ontologizer* tool, developed in a previous project by the Information Engineering Research Unit (IERU) at the University of Alcalá. Nevertheless, the tool has been further enhanced in the HEDECAMA project to better suit its context. The content of the archetypes is originally conceived by experts in the Breast Cancer field, which is then translated to the ADL language as explained in the previous section. Clinical terminologies such as SNOMED-CT are involved as they provide a common clinical language that prevents ambiguity and increases accuracy (Jiang & Chute, 2009). Figure 3 summarizes the knowledge acquisition method applied in Hedecama, where in the developed HedecamaCSV2ADL tool is playing the role of the Archetype Editor.

As illustrated in Figure 4, an OWL version of the openEHR RM participates in the clinical data integration, in addition to the archetypes and SNOMED-CT. The RM to OWL mapping was accomplished using the Protégé ontology editor (Horridge, 2011). The fact that the RM is expected to be the stable part of the two-level modelling approach proposed by openEHR allows the RM to OWL to be a manual, one time operation, while the more dynamic archetypes require an automatic translation tool or Archetype Ontologizer. It takes ADL file as inputs and fusion them with the RM ontology in order to create classes that specialize the base RM classes. The resulting specialized classes are stored in a separate OWL file to improve modularization and foster the reusability of the generated OWL content. An OWL version of an archetype not only captures all the semantic constrains to the RM defined in its ADL file, but also allows its instantiation with concrete patient data for inference, classification and further semantic activities.

Figure 4. Data integration technique based on clinical archetypes and OWL representation

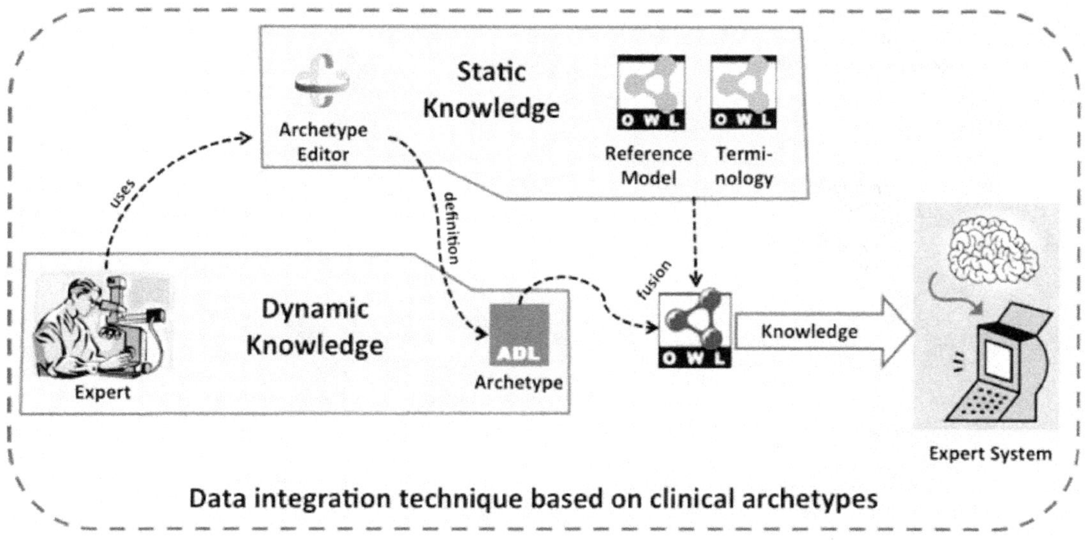

The OWL/XML code below is a fragment of the OWL archetype resulting from translation of the Breast Cancer ADL file, a fragment of which is shown in the previous subsection.

Once the archetypes ADL definitions have been translated to OWL, the actual patient data is extracted from the source databases as instances of the archetype OWL version. The Archetype Mapper tool has been designed and developed for this task. In this manner, not only the archetype definitions but also the clinical data they constrain are both expressed under the same OWL context. Furthermore, the archetype OWL instances fulfil the following properties:

- Rules expressed in the Semantic Web Rule Language (SWRL) can be applied on them.
- The mappings to clinical terminologies allow to take advantage of the logic descriptions available in them (e.g. mappings to SNOMED-CT)
- The abstraction of the OWL model makes it completely independent for the implementation details of particular database systems (Figure 5).

2.3 HL7 RIM V3 Messages Generation

The communication between the Integration Framework and the Biomedical Data Repository is accomplished by exchanging messages based on the Reference Information Model (RIM) from HL7 V3. The process is supported by the HL7 RIM Translator tool that takes the OWL archetype instances (i.e. the patient data) as starting point, and utilizes the API developed by Java SIG (Freter, 2003) to perform the translation (Figure 6).

That API acts as wrapper to a HL7 V3 messaging framework, based on the object oriented RIM model, as well as in unambiguous and standardized data types. The messaging framework al provides access to metadata files that formally describe how the messages according to the RIM model are translated to

Figure 5. Archetype OWL

```
<!-- http://www.cc.uah.es/ie/ont/CISEPonto.owl#Clínico -->

<owl:Class rdf:about="http://www.cc.uah.es/ie/ont/CISEPonto.owl#Clínico">
    <rdfs:subClassOf rdf:resource="http://klt.inf.um.es/~cati/ontologies/OpenEHR-SP-v2.0.owl#CLUSTER"/>
    <rdfs:subClassOf>
        <owl:Restriction>
            <owl:onProperty rdf:resource="http://klt.inf.um.es/~cati/ontologies/OpenEHR-SP-v2.0.owl#items"/>
            <owl:onClass rdf:resource="http://www.cc.uah.es/ie/ont/CISEPonto.owl#Síntoma_inicial_predominante_mama_derecha"/>
            <owl:maxQualifiedCardinality rdf:datatype="http://www.w3.org/2001/XMLSchema#nonNegativeInteger">1</owl:maxQualifiedCardinality>
        </owl:Restriction>
    </rdfs:subClassOf>
    <rdfs:subClassOf>
        <owl:Restriction>
            <owl:onProperty rdf:resource="http://klt.inf.um.es/~cati/ontologies/OpenEHR-SP-v2.0.owl#items"/>
            <owl:onClass rdf:resource="http://www.cc.uah.es/ie/ont/CISEPonto.owl#Localización"/>
            <owl:maxQualifiedCardinality rdf:datatype="http://www.w3.org/2001/XMLSchema#nonNegativeInteger">1</owl:maxQualifiedCardinality>
        </owl:Restriction>
```

Figure 6. Translation

```xml
<observationEvent>
    <id root="2.16.840.1.113883.2.19.4522.4"  extension="4375816"
     assigningAuthorityName="FISEVI LAB"/>
    <code code="404684003"  codeSystemName="SNOMED CT"
     codeSystem="2.16.840.1.113883.6.96"
     displayName="Clinical finding">
                <originalText>
                       Paget's disease of nipple
                </originalText>
                <qualifier>
                       <name code="403946000"  displayName="Paget's disease of nipple"/>
                       <value code="410515003"  displayName="Known present"/>
                </qualifier>
         </code>

    <statusCode code="completed"/>
    <effectiveTime value="201205200730"/>
    <priorityCode code="R"/>
    <confidentialityCode code="N"
     codeSystem="2.16.840.1.113883.5.25"/>

    <author>
    <time value="201205200730"/>
    <modeCode code="WRITTEN"/>
    <signatureCode code="S"/>
     <assignedEntity>
     <id root="2.16.840.1.113883.2.19.4522.3"  extension="327544"/>
     </assignedEntity>
    </author>
    ...
</observationEvent>
```

XML messages and vice versa. The fragment above belongs to a HL7 V3 message that was produced by the component described in the present subsection.

3. TERMINOLOGY SERVER

In addition to the Data Integration Framework, the Terminology Server is the other main component of the Integration stage as it can be appreciated in Figure 1. The Terminology Server is an all-in-one solution to address the tasks related terminologies and classifications. It ensures consistency in all clinical and administrative systems which process information from a single source. By being based on the HL7 CTS 2 standard (Common Terminology Services) it provides a conceptual information model where the most common clinical terminologies (e.g. SNOMED-CT) can fit. Its service layer allows representing, accessing and maintaining the information through a uniform interface. The following key functionalities are provided:

- **Subsets generation:** Creation, maintenance and supervision of defined terminology subsets which can be automatically generated from a given clinical terminology as proposed by Lezcano and Sicilia (2011).

- **Edition**: Creation, edition and validation of new terminology concepts and terms, required by the CDSS.
- **Terms Translation:** A translation workflow allows creating, sharing, maintaining and validating terms translations.
- **Concept Mapping:** Support the establishment of crossmaps between terminologies. They may be: 1-1, 1-n, or n-n relations.
- **Distribution:** Web services based on HL7 CTS2 allow the exploitation of the terms in the Terminology Server.

4. BIOMEDICAL DATA REPOSITORY

As the main component of the Storage and Classification stage the Repository of Biomedical Data shown in Figure 2 stores the EHR history data specifically oriented to breast cancer diagnosis and treatment. Its built on data model standards that support a clear separation between data and the way they are related (i.e., based on meta-information models or abstract patterns such as the RIM HL7 V3). The repository acts as a centralized data access point whose content is enriched by each clinical case and the results of diagnosis and treatments recommended by the inference rules located in the Knowledge and Machine Learning stage (Figure 1).

Healthcare information presents some specific characteristics that have been taken into account in the design and construction of the repository, for example, the large number of dimensions. The diagnostic and procedure coding systems contain tens of thousands of different codes for various items of medical information associated to a patient, in addition to the laboratory codes. Non aggregated variables and rapid expansion of the set of attributes are another two key factors to be considered. For measures that cannot be aggregated the repository stores all their information in detail so that further analytical and decision support components may take advantage of them. Also it is capable of evolving as new scientific advances appear for the diagnosis and treatment of breast cancer and therefore larger sets of attributes are required.

Finally it is worth mentioning the importance of information security when developing decision support platforms. The Biomedical Data Repository mechanisms of security comply with the Spanish Data Protection Law (LOPD) from the Spanish National Data Protection Authority (AEPD). In addition, the systems has been adapted to meet the ethical requirements of each involved hospital and the related bioethics committees.

5. ADAPTIVE CLINICAL GUIDELINES

As one of the two main components of the Knowledge and Machine Learning stage (see Figure 1), Adaptive Clinical Guidelines is based on biomedical data mining techniques, which provide the ability to extract patterns that reside implicitly in the cases and medical knowledge available. The component provides improved medical pilots rules of breast cancer through predictive models for medical decisions. It is capable of re-learning through incremental learning methods, which allow adapting the predictive models to the specific characteristics of the medical environment where the platform is deployed.

To provide analytical capabilities to the medical personal using the platform as a whole (e.g. service chief, multidisciplinary diagnostic group, etc.), the component audits the performance of rules and predictive models deployed in the medical environment, thus offering a dashboard to select the ones that will be shown to the service doctors. The component is based on international standards for knowledge sharing, such as the Predictive Model Markup Language (PMML) defined by the Data Mining Group (DMG, http://www.dmg.org/).

6. PROCESS ENGINE

The Process Engine is the other main component of the Knowledge and Machine Learning stage, in addition to Adaptive Clinical Guidelines. It orchestrates the treatment and monitoring of patients with breast cancer, based on existing tools for Business Process Management Systems (BPMS). Based on the free distribution openCDS (founded by Dr. Kensaku Kawamoto, a co-chair of the HL7 CDS Work Group), the Process Engine works on a correspondence between process rules and clinical guidelines in order to improve the viability of a BPMS in a healthcare environment. It should be noted though, that the main objective of clinical guidelines, i.e., to maximize the quality of care, is preserved at all times.

Once the diagnosis of the patient has been accomplished, the component evaluates the patient to determine the next stage in a breast cancer guideline. Then the recommended actions to be carried out may include "future visits," "medication reviews," "dispensing of new drugs," "view of nursing," "referral to other hospitals," etc. The representation of these possible steps is based on standard networking modelling, where key elements include: action nodes (i.e., tasks that can be medical, internal of the process itself, or external in the form of calls to other systems for performing further actions), decision nodes (decision criteria for forks in the guides), synchronization nodes (i.e., they allow the confluence of several alternative paths within the guideline) and patient state nodes (i.e., initial, intermediate or final checkpoints in the guideline).

7. CONCLUSION

The functional coverage of existing hospital clinical systems has been expanded with advanced modules, which are aligned with the overall objectives of clinical oncology services in hospitals. The clinical process and procedures for each type of diagnosis have been automated, providing control and monitoring capabilities over standards execution and clinical processes for the medical staff. This results in the presence of accountability mechanisms and increased transparency that generate a climate of confidence in the system. The completeness, consistency and continuity of the healthcare data recorded from the actions performed on each patient have been improved. Thus, reducing the risk of medical errors. The registration, incorporation, storage and use of patient essential information allow strengthening the consistency and traceability of the management cycle that patients go through.

Ultimately this is expected to improve the rate of effectiveness of treatments for breast cancer through the provision of health professionals support mechanisms, monitoring, control and monitoring of clinical trials undertaken. The processes and protocols applied to breast cancer will continuously evolve and improve thanks to the ongoing evaluation of the clinical results obtained by applying rules and algorithms derived from the clinical guidelines and practices available nowadays.

ACKNOWLEDGMENT

This research has been supported by the project titled "Semantic Model and Data Mining Algorithms applied to Breast Cancer Treatment in Specialized Care Centers" (HEDECAMA), code CIN/699/2011, funded by the Spanish Ministry of Science and Innovation.

REFERENCES

AECC. (2011). *Estrategia contra el cáncer del Sistema Nacional de Salud. Ministerio de Sanidad y Consumo*. Retrieved from https://www.aecc.es/SobreElCancer/bibliotecadedocumentos/Paginas/estrategiacontraelcancer.aspx

Beale, T. (2002). Archetypes, constraint–based domain models for future–proof information systems. In *Proceedings of the OOPSLA 2002 Conference* (pp. 16–32). Seattle, WA. Boston: Northeastern University.

Beale, T., & Heard, S. (2007). *Archetype definitions and principles*. The openEHR Foundation. Retrieved from http://www.openehr.org/releases/1.0.2/architecture/am/archetype_principles.pdf

Beale, T., & Heard, S. (2008). *The openEHR archetype definition language*. The openEHR Foundation. Retrieved from http://www.openehr.org/releases/1.0.2/architecture/am/adl.pdf

Dolin, R. H., Alschuler, L., Boyer, S., Beebe, C., Behlen, F. M., Biron, P. V., & Shvo, A. S. (2006). HL7 clinical document architecture, release 2. *Journal of the American Medical Informatics Association*, *13*(1), 30–39. doi:10.1197/jamia.M1888 PMID:16221939

Freter, T. (2003). *A Java API for HL7 Version 3 RIM*. Health Level Seven International. Retrieved November 16, 2013, from http://www.hl7.org/documentcenter/public/wg/java/HL7-java.pdf

Horridge, M. (2011). *A practical guide to building OWL ontologies using Protégé 4 and CO-ODE tools (Ed. 1.3)*. University Of Manchester. Retrieved December 20, 2013, from http://130.88.198.11/tutorials/protegeowltutorial/

Jiang, G., & Chute, C. G. (2009). Auditing the semantic completeness of SNOMED CT using formal concept analysis. *Journal of the American Medical Informatics Association*, *16*(1), 89–102. doi:10.1197/jamia.M2541 PMID:18952949

Lezcano, L., & Sicilia, M. A. (2011). Connectivity and semantic patterns in automatically generated SNOMED-CT subsets. In *Metadata and semantic research* (pp. 117–125). Berlin, Heidelberg: Springer. doi:10.1007/978-3-642-24731-6_11

Lezcano, L., Sicilia, M. A., & Rodríguez-Solano, C. (2011). Integrating reasoning and clinical archetypes using OWL ontologies and SWRL rules. *Journal of Biomedical Informatics*, *44*(2), 343–353. doi:10.1016/j.jbi.2010.11.005 PMID:21118725

Lezcano, L., Sicilia, M. A., & Serrano-Balazote, P. (2008). Combining OpenEHR archetype definitions with SWRL rules–A translation approach. In *Emerging technologies and information systems for the knowledge society* (pp. 79–87). Berlin, Heidelberg: Springer. doi:10.1007/978-3-540-87781-3_9

Stroetmann, V. N., Kalra, D., Lewalle, P., Rodrigues, J. M., Stroetmann, K. A., & Surjan, G. et al. (2009). *Semantic interoperability for better health and safer healthcare (Project report)*. Luxembourg: Office for Official Publications of the European Communities: European Commission.

W3C OWL Working Group. (2012). *OWL 2 Web ontology language document overview* (Second Ed.). Retrieved January 10, 2014, from http://www.w3.org/TR/owl2-overview/

APPENDIX A

The following is a set of clinical variables used to improve the treatment of breast cancer:

1. Patient characteristics and demographics;
2. Family and personal history. Genetic studies;
3. Specific clinical situation and presence of comorbidities that affect their health and the feasibility of certain treatments or actions;
4. Oncological disease facts;
5. Diagnostic or therapeutic surgical procedures;
6. Nursing: teaching, exercises, prevention of lymphedema;
7. Psychological care;
8. Tolerance and toxicity of treatments that may condition modifications;
9. Scheduled monitoring and types of studies to be performed;
10. Decisions on relapse;
11. Number of consultations;
12. Time between diagnosis and start of treatment (difference between the time recommended by clinical Guideline and the actual time spent on the case-control);
13. Number of patients reviewed in the Breast Cancer Multidisciplinary Committee of year 2010 (AECC, 2011);
14. Number of patients reviewed in the Breast Cancer Multidisciplinary Committee using the CDSS system;
15. Satisfaction of professionals and patients

APPENDIX B

```
archetype (adl_version=1.4)
 openEHR-EHR-OBSERVATION.Diagnostico_cancer_de_mama.v1
concept
 [at0000] -- Diagnostico cancer de mama
language
 original_language = <[ISO_639-1::es]>
description
 original_author = <
 ["name"] = <"Eydel Rivero Ruíz">
 ["organisation"] = <"University of Alcalá">
 ["email"] = <"eydel.rivero@uah.es">
 ["date"] = <"08/04/2013 01:24:31">
 >
 details = <
 ["es"] = <
```

```
 language = <[ISO_639-1::es]>
 purpose = <"Para registrar información detallada sobre el diagnóstico de
cáncer de mama.">
 use = <"Se utiliza para registrar cualquier diagnóstico, presente o pasado so-
bre cáncer de mama. Se recoge información sobre síntomas clínicos, radiología,
anatomía, genética y clasificación.">
 keywords = <"tumour", "cancer", "breast">
 misuse = <"No está diseñado para utilizar en otro arquetipo distinto de
openEHR-EHR-OBSERVATION.Diagnostico_cancer_de_mama.v1.adl.">
 copyright = <"HEDECAMA project">
 >
 >
 lifecycle_state = <"AuthorDraft">
 other_contributors = <>
 other_details = <
 ["MD5-CAM-1.0.1"] = <"C98294B415C1FF5FD4D84AF20A3A814F">
 >

definition
 OBSERVATION[at0000] matches { -- Diagnostico cancer de mama
 data matches {
 HISTORY[at0001] matches { -- Event Series
  events cardinality matches {1..*; unordered} matches {
  EVENT[at0002] occurrences matches {0..1} matches { -- Any Event
   data matches {
   ITEM_TREE[at0003] matches { -- Item Tree
    items cardinality matches {1..*; unordered} matches {
    CLUSTER[at0004] occurrences matches {0..1} matches { -- Clínico
     items cardinality matches {1..*; unordered} matches {
     ELEMENT[at0005] occurrences matches {0..1} matches { -- Síntoma_inicial_
predominante_mama_derecha
      value matches {
      DV_CODED_TEXT matches {
       defining_code matches {
       [local::
       at0006, -- Asintomática
       at0007, -- Desconocido
       at0008, -- Fiebre
       at0009, -- Dolor mamario
       at0010, -- Dolor óseo
       at0011, -- Dolor extramamario y extraóseo
       at0012, -- Inflamación
       at0013, -- Palpación de nódulo
```

```
        at0014, -- Sangrado
        at0015, -- Retracción del pezón
        at0016, -- Cambios en la piel
        at0017, -- Cefalea
        at0018, -- Mareo
        at0019, -- Síndrome de vena cava
        at0020, -- Compresión medular
        at0021] -- Otros (especificar)
        }
       }
       }
      }
      ELEMENT[at0022] occurrences matches {0..1} matches { -- Síntoma_inicial_
predominante_mama_izquierda
       value matches {
       DV_CODED_TEXT matches {
        defining_code matches {
        [local::
        at0023, -- Asintomática
        at0024, -- Desconocido
        at0025, -- Fiebre
        at0026, -- Dolor mamario
        at0027, -- Dolor óseo
        at0028, -- Dolor extramamario y extraóseo
        at0029, -- Inflamación
        at0030, -- Palpación de nódulo
        at0031, -- Sangrado
        at0032, -- Retracción del pezón
        at0033, -- Cambios en la piel
        at0034, -- Cefalea
        at0035, -- Mareo
        at0036, -- Síndrome de vena cava
        at0037, -- Compresión medular
        at0038] -- Otros (especificar)
        }
       }
       }
      }
      ELEMENT[at0039] occurrences matches {0..1} matches { -- Localización
       value matches {
       DV_CODED_TEXT matches {
        defining_code matches {
        [local::
```

```
at0040, -- Mama izquierda
at0041, -- Mama derecha
at0042] -- Ambas mamas
}
}
}
}
ELEMENT[at0043] occurrences matches {0..1} matches { -- Mama_con_signos_
de_inflamación_al_diagnóstico_inicial
value matches {
DV_CODED_TEXT matches {
defining_code matches {
[local::
at0044, -- En la mama izquierda
at0045, -- En la mama derecha
at0046, -- En ambas mamas
at0047, -- No
at0048] -- Desconocido
}
}
}
}
}
}
CLUSTER[at0049] occurrences matches {0..1} matches { -- Radiológicos
items cardinality matches {1..*; unordered} matches {
CLUSTER[at0050] occurrences matches {0..1} matches { -- Ecografía
items cardinality matches {1..*; unordered} matches {
ELEMENT[at0051] occurrences matches {0..1} matches { -- Fecha_Ecografía
value matches {
DV_DATE_TIME matches {*}
}
}
ELEMENT[at0052] occurrences matches {0..1} matches { -- Ecografía_mama_
izquierda
value matches {
DV_CODED_TEXT matches {
defining_code matches {
[local::
at0053, -- Sospechosa
at0054, -- No sospechosa
at0055, -- No realizada
at0056] -- Desconocido
```

```
        }
       }
       }
      }
      ELEMENT[at0057] occurrences matches {0..1} matches { -- Localización_
eco_mama_izquierda
       value matches {
       DV_CODED_TEXT matches {
        defining_code matches {
        [local::
        at0058, -- Pezón
        at0059, -- Retroareolar
        at0060, -- Porción central de la mama
        at0061, -- CSI
        at0062, -- CII
        at0063, -- CSE
        at0064, -- CIE
        at0065, -- Parte axilar de la mama
        at0066, -- Desconocido
        at0067] -- Otras (especificar)
        }
       }
       }
      }
      ELEMENT[at0068] occurrences matches {0..1} matches { -- Bi-rads_eco_
mama_izquierda
       value matches {
       DV_CODED_TEXT matches {
        defining_code matches {
        [local::
        at0069, -- 0
        at0070, -- 1
        at0071, -- 2
        at0072, -- 3
        at0073, -- 4
        at0074, -- 5
        at0075, -- 6
        at0076] -- Desconocido
        }
       }
       }
      }
      ELEMENT[at0077] occurrences matches {0..1} matches { -- Ecografía_mama_
```

```
derecha
       value matches {
       DV_CODED_TEXT matches {
        defining_code matches {
        [local::
        at0078, -- Sospechosa
        at0079, -- No sospechosa
        at0080, -- No realizada
        at0081] -- Desconocido
        }
       }
       }
      }
      ELEMENT[at0082] occurrences matches {0..1} matches { -- Localización_
eco_mama_derecha
       value matches {
       DV_CODED_TEXT matches {
        defining_code matches {
        [local::
        at0083, -- Pezón
        at0084, -- Retroareolar
        at0085, -- Porción central de la mama
        at0086, -- CSI
        at0087, -- CII
        at0088, -- CSE
        at0089, -- CIE
        at0090, -- Parte axilar de la mama
        at0091, -- Desconocido
        at0092] -- Otras (especificar)
        }
       }
       }
      }
```

Related References

To continue our tradition of advancing medical information science and technology research, we have compiled a list of recommended IGI Global readings. These references will provide additional information and guidance to further enrich your knowledge and assist you with your own research and future publications.

Abu-Faraj, Z. O. (2012). Handbook of research on biomedical engineering education and advanced bioengineering learning: Interdisciplinary concepts (2 Volumes) (pp. 1-1122). doi: doi:10.4018/978-1-4666-0122-2

Al-Fedaghi, S. (2008). Scrutinizing the rule: Privacy realization in HIPAA. *International Journal of Healthcare Information Systems and Informatics*, *3*(2), 32–47. doi:10.4018/jhisi.2008040104

Al-Hakim, L. (2007). *Web mobile-based applications for healthcare management* (pp. 1-450). doi:10.4018/978-1-59140-658-7

Al-Kadi, A., & Chatterjee, S. (2012). Tapping the wisdom of crowd phenomenon in healthcare social networks. *International Journal of Business Data Communications and Networking*, *8*(3), 42–56. doi:10.4018/jbdcn.2012070103

Allard, T., Anciaux, N., Bouganim, L., Pucheral, P., & Thion, R. (2009). seamless access to healthcare folders with strong privacy guarantees. *International Journal of Healthcare Delivery Reform Initiatives*, *1*(4), 82–107. doi:10.4018/jhdri.2009100106

Allard, T., Anciaux, N., Bouganim, L., Pucheral, P., & Thion, R. (2010). Trustworthiness of pervasive healthcare folders. In A. Coronato, & G. De Pietro (Eds.), *Pervasive and smart technologies for healthcare: Ubiquitous methodologies and tools* (pp. 172–196). Hershey, PA: Medical Information Science Reference. doi:10.4018/978-1-61520-765-7.ch009

Allen, P., Bartlett, W., Pérotin, V., Matchaya, G., Turner, S., & Zamora, B. (2011). Healthcare providers in the english national health service: Public, private or hybrids? *International Journal of Public and Private Healthcare Management and Economics*, *1*(3), 1–18. doi:10.4018/ijpphme.2011070101

Arling, P. A., Doebbeling, B. N., & Fox, R. L. (2011). Improving the implementation of evidence-based practice and information systems in healthcare: A social network approach. *International Journal of Healthcare Information Systems and Informatics*, *6*(2), 37–59. doi:10.4018/jhisi.2011040104

Armoni, A. (2000). *Healthcare information systems: Challenges of the new millennium* (pp. 1-243). doi:10.4018/978-1-878289-62-9

Armoni, A. (2002). *Effective healthcare information systems* (pp. 1-340). doi:10.4018/978-1-93177-701-8

Association, I. R. (2014). Assistive technologies: Concepts, methodologies, tools, and applications (3 Volumes) (pp. 1-1794). doi: doi:10.4018/978-1-4666-4422-9

Au, S., & Gupta, A. (2008). Gastrointestinal motility online educational endeavor. *International Journal of Healthcare Information Systems and Informatics*, *3*(1), 24–43. doi:10.4018/jhisi.2008010102

Augustyniak, P., & Tadeusiewicz, R. (2009). *Ubiquitous cardiology: Emerging wireless telemedical applications* (pp. 1-430). doi:10.4018/978-1-60566-080-6

Azari, A., Janeja, V. P., & Mohseni, A. (2012). Healthcare data mining: Predicting hospital length of stay (PHLOS). *International Journal of Knowledge Discovery in Bioinformatics, 3*(3), 44–66. doi:10.4018/jkdb.2012070103

Baker, L., Greco, M. J., & Narayanan, A. (2010). Doctors using patient feedback to establish professional learning goals: Results from a communication skill development program. In W. Pease, M. Cooper, & R. Gururajan (Eds.), *Biomedical knowledge management: Infrastructures and processes for E-Health systems* (pp. 303–314). Hershey, PA: Medical Information Science Reference. doi:10.4018/978-1-60566-266-4.ch022

Bali, R. K. (2005). *Clinical knowledge management: Opportunities and challenges* (pp. 1-334). doi:10.4018/978-1-59140-300-5

Banderker, N., & Van Belle, J. (2009). Adoption of mobile technology by public healthcare doctors: A developing country perspective. *International Journal of Healthcare Delivery Reform Initiatives, 1*(3), 38–54. doi:10.4018/jhdri.2009070103

Barnet, R. J. (2010). Biobanking: Justice, social consensus, and the marginalized. In S. Kabene (Ed.), *Healthcare and the effect of technology: Developments, challenges and advancements* (pp. 216–232). Hershey, PA: Medical Information Science Reference. doi:10.4018/978-1-61520-733-6.ch013

Battini, D., Faccio, M., Persona, A., & Sgarbossa, F. (2013). Modelling the growing process of integrated healthcare supply networks. *International Journal of System Dynamics Applications, 2*(1), 1–13. doi:10.4018/ijsda.2013010101

Belfi, M. M., & Jones, K. E. (2010). assistive technology for teacher education: from research to curriculum. In S. Seok, E. Meyen, & B. DaCosta (Eds.), Handbook of research on human cognition and assistive technology: Design, accessibility and transdisciplinary perspectives (pp. 325-338). Hershey, PA: Medical Information Science Reference. doi: doi:10.4018/978-1-61520-817-3.ch023

Belsis, P., Skourlas, C., & Gritzalis, S. (2011). Secure electronic healthcare records management in wireless environments. *Journal of Information Technology Research, 4*(4), 1–17. doi:10.4018/jitr.2011100101

Ben Elhadj, H., Chaari, L., & Kamoun, L. (2012). A survey of routing protocols in wireless body area networks for healthcare applications. *International Journal of E-Health and Medical Communications, 3*(2), 1–18. doi:10.4018/jehmc.2012040101

Bielenia-Grajewska, M. (2011). Actor-network-theory in medical e-communication – The role of websites in creating and maintaining healthcare corporate online identity. *International Journal of Actor-Network Theory and Technological Innovation, 3*(1), 39–53. doi:10.4018/jantti.2011010104

Bilotta, E., & Pantano, P. (2010). *Cellular automata and complex systems: Methods for modeling biological phenomena* (pp. 1-502). doi:10.4018/978-1-61520-787-9

Bircher, N. G. (2010). The electronic patient record: A practicing physician's perspective. In S. Kabene (Ed.), *Healthcare and the effect of technology: Developments, challenges and advancements* (pp. 84–100). Hershey, PA: Medical Information Science Reference. doi:10.4018/978-1-61520-733-6.ch006

Biswas, R. (2011). [IJUDH]. *International Journal of User-Driven Healthcare*. doi: doi:10.4018/IJUDH

Biswas, R. (2013). *Clinical solutions and medical progress through user-driven healthcare* (pp. 1-216). doi:10.4018/978-1-4666-1876-3

Biswas, R., & Martin, C. M. (2011). *User-driven healthcare and narrative medicine: Utilizing collaborative social networks and technologies* (pp. 1-642). doi:10.4018/978-1-60960-097-6

Biswas, R., Sturmberg, J., Martin, C. M., Ganesh, A. U., Umakanth, S., & Lee, E. W. (2010). Persistent clinical encounters in user driven E-Health care. In W. Pease, M. Cooper, & R. Gururajan (Eds.), *Biomedical knowledge management: Infrastructures and processes for E-Health systems* (pp. 101–117). Hershey, PA: Medical Information Science Reference. doi:10.4018/978-1-60566-266-4.ch008

Blake, J., & Kerr, D. (2010). Development of an online sleep diary. In W. Pease, M. Cooper, & R. Gururajan (Eds.), *Biomedical knowledge management: Infrastructures and processes for E-Health systems* (pp. 289–302). Hershey, PA: Medical Information Science Reference. doi:10.4018/978-1-60566-266-4.ch021

Borycki, E. M., & Kushniruk, A. W. (2010). Use of clinical simulations to evaluate the impact of health information systems and ubiquitous computing devices upon health professional work. In S. Mohammed, & J. Fiaidhi (Eds.), *Ubiquitous health and medical informatics: The ubiquity 2.0 trend and beyond* (pp. 552–573). Hershey, PA: Medical Information Science Reference. doi:10.4018/978-1-61520-777-0.ch026

Bottazzi, D., Montanari, R., & Taleb, T. (2010). Integrating supports for ubiquitous eldercare. In S. Kabene (Ed.), *Healthcare and the effect of technology: Developments, challenges and advancements* (pp. 252–268). Hershey, PA: Medical Information Science Reference. doi:10.4018/978-1-61520-733-6.ch015

Breas, R., & Guah, M. W. (2009). Preparing healthcare organizations for new IT systems adoption: A readiness framework. *International Journal of Healthcare Delivery Reform Initiatives*, *1*(2), 25–38. doi:10.4018/jhdri.2009040102

Brown, M. R., & Fitzpatrick, M. (2010). Digital inequity: Understanding the divide as it relates to culture and disability. In S. Seok, E. Meyen, & B. DaCosta (Eds.), *Handbook of research on human cognition and assistive technology: Design, accessibility and transdisciplinary perspectives* (pp. 374–387). Hershey, PA: Medical Information Science Reference. doi:10.4018/978-1-61520-817-3.ch026

Bryant, B., Seok, S., & Bryant, D. (2010). assistive technology solutions for individuals with learning problems: Conducting assessments using the functional evaluation for assistive technology (FEAT). In S. Seok, E. Meyen, & B. DaCosta (Eds.), Handbook of research on human cognition and assistive technology: Design, accessibility and transdisciplinary perspectives (pp. 264-285). Hershey, PA: Medical Information Science Reference. doi: doi:10.4018/978-1-61520-817-3.ch018

Buyurgan, N., Hardgrave, B. C., Lo, J., & Walker, R. T. (2009). RFID in healthcare: A framework of uses and opportunities. *International Journal of Advanced Pervasive and Ubiquitous Computing*, *1*(1), 1–25. doi:10.4018/japuc.2009010101

Buyurgan, N., Rardin, R. L., Jayaraman, R., Varghese, V. M., & Burbano, A. (2011). A novel GS1 data standard adoption roadmap for healthcare providers. *International Journal of Healthcare Information Systems and Informatics*, *6*(4), 42–59. doi:10.4018/jhisi.2011100103

Cannataro, M. (2009). *Handbook of research on computational grid technologies for life sciences, biomedicine, and healthcare* (pp. 1–960). doi:10.4018/978-1-60566-374-6

Carlucci, D., & Schiuma, G. (2012). Assessing and managing organizational climate in healthcare organizations: An intellectual capital based perspective. *International Journal of Information Systems in the Service Sector*, *4*(4), 49–61. doi:10.4018/jisss.2012100103

Caruana, C. J. (2012). The ongoing crisis in medical device education for healthcare professionals: Breaking the vicious circle through online learning. *International Journal of Reliable and Quality E-Healthcare*, *1*(2), 29–40. doi:10.4018/ijrqeh.2012040103

Cashin, A., & Cook, R. (2011). *Evidence-based practice in nursing informatics: Concepts and applications* (pp. 1-320). doi:10.4018/978-1-60960-034-1

Cassim, M. (2010). TACMIS: A total access care and medical information system. In W. Pease, M. Cooper, & R. Gururajan (Eds.), *Biomedical knowledge management: Infrastructures and processes for E-Health systems* (pp. 315–326). Hershey, PA: Medical Information Science Reference. doi:10.4018/978-1-60566-266-4.ch023

Castro, E. A., & Haghi, A. K. (2012). *Advanced methods and applications in chemoinformatics: Research progress and new applications* (pp. 1-512). doi:10.4018/978-1-60960-860-6

Cerrito, P. (2010). *Cases on health outcomes and clinical data mining: Studies and frameworks* (pp. 1-464). doi:10.4018/978-1-61520-723-7

Cerrito, P., & Cerrito, J. (2010). *Clinical data mining for physician decision making and investigating health outcomes: Methods for prediction and analysis* (pp. 1-370). doi:10.4018/978-1-61520-905-7

Cerrito, P., & Cerrito, J. (2010). Preprocessing the data. In P. Cerrito, & J. Cerrito (Eds.), *Clinical data mining for physician decision making and investigating health outcomes: Methods for prediction and analysis* (pp. 1–10). Hershey, PA: Medical Information Science Reference. doi:10.4018/978-1-61520-905-7.ch001

Cerrito, P., & Cerrito, J. (2010). Errors and missing values in the dataset. In P. Cerrito, & J. Cerrito (Eds.), *Clinical data mining for physician decision making and investigating health outcomes: Methods for prediction and analysis* (pp. 11–18). Hershey, PA: Medical Information Science Reference. doi:10.4018/978-1-61520-905-7.ch002

Cerrito, P., & Cerrito, J. (2010). Introduction to the use of MEPS (medical expenditure panel survey). In P. Cerrito, & J. Cerrito (Eds.), *Clinical data mining for physician decision making and investigating health outcomes: Methods for prediction and analysis* (pp. 19–56). Hershey, PA: Medical Information Science Reference. doi:10.4018/978-1-61520-905-7.ch003

Cerrito, P., & Cerrito, J. (2010). Preprocessing Medpar data. In P. Cerrito, & J. Cerrito (Eds.), *Clinical data mining for physician decision making and investigating health outcomes: Methods for prediction and analysis* (pp. 57–68). Hershey, PA: Medical Information Science Reference. doi:10.4018/978-1-61520-905-7.ch004

Cerrito, P., & Cerrito, J. (2010). Extracting data from the national inpatient sample. In P. Cerrito, & J. Cerrito (Eds.), *Clinical data mining for physician decision making and investigating health outcomes: Methods for prediction and analysis* (pp. 69–93). Hershey, PA: Medical Information Science Reference. doi:10.4018/978-1-61520-905-7.ch005

Cerrito, P., & Cerrito, J. (2010). Creating a one-to-one relationship in the data from a many-to-many. In P. Cerrito, & J. Cerrito (Eds.), *Clinical data mining for physician decision making and investigating health outcomes: Methods for prediction and analysis* (pp. 94–115). Hershey, PA: Medical Information Science Reference. doi:10.4018/978-1-61520-905-7.ch006

Cerrito, P., & Cerrito, J. (2010). Merging different datasets to allow for a complete analysis (inpatient, outpatient, physician visits, medications). In P. Cerrito, & J. Cerrito (Eds.), *Clinical data mining for physician decision making and investigating health outcomes: Methods for prediction and analysis* (pp. 116–153). Hershey, PA: Medical Information Science Reference. doi:10.4018/978-1-61520-905-7.ch007

Cerrito, P., & Cerrito, J. (2010). Introduction to analysis using time components. In P. Cerrito, & J. Cerrito (Eds.), *Clinical data mining for physician decision making and investigating health outcomes: Methods for prediction and analysis* (pp. 154–192). Hershey, PA: Medical Information Science Reference. doi:10.4018/978-1-61520-905-7.ch008

Cerrito, P., & Cerrito, J. (2010). More survival data mining of multiple time of endpoints. In P. Cerrito, & J. Cerrito (Eds.), *Clinical data mining for physician decision making and investigating health outcomes: Methods for prediction and analysis* (pp. 193–214). Hershey, PA: Medical Information Science Reference. doi:10.4018/978-1-61520-905-7.ch009

Cerrito, P., & Cerrito, J. (2010). Using the data to define patient compliance. In P. Cerrito, & J. Cerrito (Eds.), *Clinical data mining for physician decision making and investigating health outcomes: Methods for prediction and analysis* (pp. 215–233). Hershey, PA: Medical Information Science Reference. doi:10.4018/978-1-61520-905-7.ch010

Cerrito, P., & Cerrito, J. (2010). Compression of diagnosis and procedure codes. In P. Cerrito, & J. Cerrito (Eds.), *Clinical data mining for physician decision making and investigating health outcomes: Methods for prediction and analysis* (pp. 234–248). Hershey, PA: Medical Information Science Reference. doi:10.4018/978-1-61520-905-7.ch011

Cerrito, P., & Cerrito, J. (2010). Comparisons of patient severity indices. In P. Cerrito, & J. Cerrito (Eds.), *Clinical data mining for physician decision making and investigating health outcomes: Methods for prediction and analysis* (pp. 249–286). Hershey, PA: Medical Information Science Reference. doi:10.4018/978-1-61520-905-7.ch012

Cerrito, P., & Cerrito, J. (2010). Decision trees and their development: Use of data to determine the quality of care. In P. Cerrito, & J. Cerrito (Eds.), *Clinical data mining for physician decision making and investigating health outcomes: Methods for prediction and analysis* (pp. 287–304). Hershey, PA: Medical Information Science Reference. doi:10.4018/978-1-61520-905-7.ch013

Cerrito, P., & Cerrito, J. (2010). Example of diabetes using CMS data. In P. Cerrito, & J. Cerrito (Eds.), *Clinical data mining for physician decision making and investigating health outcomes: Methods for prediction and analysis* (pp. 305–317). Hershey, PA: Medical Information Science Reference. doi:10.4018/978-1-61520-905-7.ch014

Cerrito, P., & Cerrito, J. (2010). Example of breathing illnesses, asthma and COPD using MEPS data. In P. Cerrito, & J. Cerrito (Eds.), *Clinical data mining for physician decision making and investigating health outcomes: Methods for prediction and analysis* (pp. 318–328). Hershey, PA: Medical Information Science Reference. doi:10.4018/978-1-61520-905-7.ch015

Cerrito, P., & Cerrito, J. (2010). Example of wound care using Medpar data. In P. Cerrito, & J. Cerrito (Eds.), *Clinical data mining for physician decision making and investigating health outcomes: Methods for prediction and analysis* (pp. 329–345). Hershey, PA: Medical Information Science Reference. doi:10.4018/978-1-61520-905-7.ch016

Cerrito, P., & Cerrito, J. (2010). Discussion. In P. Cerrito, & J. Cerrito (Eds.), *Clinical data mining for physician decision making and investigating health outcomes: Methods for prediction and analysis* (pp. 346–351). Hershey, PA: Medical Information Science Reference. doi:10.4018/978-1-61520-905-7.ch017

Chaari, L., & Kamoun, L. (2011). QoS concepts and architecture over wireless body area networks for healthcare applications. *International Journal of E-Health and Medical Communications*, *2*(4), 50–66. doi:10.4018/jehmc.2011100104

Chan, L. L., Celler, B. G., Zhang, J. Z., & Lovell, N. H. (2010). Pervasive networks and ubiquitous monitoring for wellness monitoring in residential aged care. In A. Coronato, & G. De Pietro (Eds.), *Pervasive and smart technologies for healthcare: Ubiquitous methodologies and tools* (pp. 1–24). Hershey, PA: Medical Information Science Reference. doi:10.4018/978-1-61520-765-7.ch001

Charles, D., Fyfe, C., Livingstone, D., & McGlinchey, S. (2008). *Biologically inspired artificial intelligence for computer games* (pp. 1-278). doi:10.4018/978-1-59140-646-4

Chen, W., Oetomo, S. B., & Feijs, L. (2012). *Neonatal monitoring technologies: Design for integrated solutions* (pp. 1-536). doi:10.4018/978-1-4666-0975-4

Chermin, B., Frey, I., Reijers, H., & Smeets, H. (2012). On predicting the results of applying workflow management in a healthcare context. *International Journal of Knowledge-Based Organizations*, *2*(4), 20–34. doi:10.4018/ijkbo.2012100102

Chiong, R. (2010). *Nature-inspired informatics for intelligent applications and knowledge discovery: implications in business, science, and engineering* (pp. 1-450). doi:10.4018/978-1-60566-705-8

Chiu, D. K., Kwok, B. W., Wong, R. L., Kafeza, M., Cheung, S., Kafeza, E., & Hung, P. C. (2009). Alerts in healthcare applications: Process and data integration. *International Journal of Healthcare Information Systems and Informatics*, *4*(2), 36–56. doi:10.4018/jhisi.2009040103

Chiu, D. K., Wang, Y., Hung, P., Cheng, V. S., Chan, K., & Kafeza, E., & Tung. (2011). Governance of cross-organizational healthcare document exchange through watermarking services and alerts. *International Journal of Systems and Service-Oriented Engineering*, *2*(4), 83–108. doi:10.4018/jssoe.2011100105

Chorbev, I., & Joksimoski, B. (2010). An integrated system for E-Medicine (E-Health, telemedicine and medical expert systems). In S. Mohammed, & J. Fiaidhi (Eds.), *Ubiquitous health and medical informatics: The ubiquity 2.0 trend and beyond* (pp. 104–126). Hershey, PA: Medical Information Science Reference. doi:10.4018/978-1-61520-777-0.ch006

Chryssanthou, A., Varlamis, I., Sarivougioukas, J. C., & Apostolakis, I. (2012). Hospital information systems replacement and healthcare quality. *International Journal of Reliable and Quality E-Healthcare*, *1*(3), 1–12. doi:10.4018/ijrqeh.2012070101

Ciulla, C. (2009). *Improved signal and image interpolation in biomedical applications: The case of magnetic resonance imaging* (pp. 1–640). MRI. doi:10.4018/978-1-60566-202-2.ch001

Clark, J. M. (2014). Implementation of electronic records in a medical practice setting. In J. Krueger (Ed.), *Cases on electronic records and resource management implementation in diverse environments* (pp. 211–225). Hershey, PA: Information Science Reference.

Claster, W., Ghotbi, N., & Shanmuganathan, S. (2010). The use of artificial intelligence systems for support of medical decision-making. In W. Pease, M. Cooper, & R. Gururajan (Eds.), *Biomedical knowledge management: Infrastructures and processes for E-Health systems* (pp. 18–30). Hershey, PA: Medical Information Science Reference. doi:10.4018/978-1-60566-266-4.ch002

Claster, W., Ghotbi, N., & Shanmuganathan, S. (2010). Data-mining techniques for an analysis of non-conventional methodologies: Deciphering of alternative medicine. In W. Pease, M. Cooper, & R. Gururajan (Eds.), *Biomedical knowledge management: Infrastructures and processes for E-Health systems* (pp. 82–91). Hershey, PA: Medical Information Science Reference. doi:10.4018/978-1-60566-266-4.ch006

Constantinides, P. (2010). Managing crises in the healthcare service chain: Lessons from the past and future directions. *International Journal of Information Systems for Crisis Response and Management*, *2*(4), 33–47. doi:10.4018/jiscrm.2010100103

Cooper, G. J. (2010). Mental health management in New Zealand: The pathways model for client-based treatment. In W. Pease, M. Cooper, & R. Gururajan (Eds.), *Biomedical knowledge management: Infrastructures and processes for E-Health systems* (pp. 253–266). Hershey, PA: Medical Information Science Reference. doi:10.4018/978-1-60566-266-4.ch018

Coronato, A., & De Pietro, G. (2010). *Pervasive and smart technologies for healthcare: Ubiquitous methodologies and tools* (pp. 1-408). doi:10.4018/978-1-61520-765-7

Cruz-Cunha, M. M., Miranda, I. M., & Gonçalves, P. (2013). *Handbook of research on ICTs for human-centered healthcare and social care services* (pp. 1–978). doi:10.4018/978-1-4666-3986-7

Cruz-Cunha, M. M., Tavares, A., & Simoes, R. (2010). Handbook of research on developments in E-Health and telemedicine: Technological and social perspectives (2 Volumes) (pp. 1-1486). doi: doi:10.4018/978-1-61520-670-4

D'Ulizia, A., Ferri, F., Grifoni, P., & Guzzo, T. (2010). Smart homes to support elderly people: Innovative technologies and social impacts. In A. Coronato, & G. De Pietro (Eds.), *Pervasive and smart technologies for healthcare: Ubiquitous methodologies and tools* (pp. 25–38). Hershey, PA: Medical Information Science Reference. doi:10.4018/978-1-61520-765-7.ch002

DaCosta, B., & Seok, S. (2010). Human cognition in the design of assistive technology for those with learning disabilities. In S. Seok, E. Meyen, & B. DaCosta (Eds.), *Handbook of research on human cognition and assistive technology: Design, accessibility and transdisciplinary perspectives* (pp. 1–20). Hershey, PA: Medical Information Science Reference. doi:10.4018/978-1-61520-817-3.ch001

DaCosta, B., & Seok, S. (2010). Managing cognitive load in the design of assistive technology for those with learning disabilities. In S. Seok, E. Meyen, & B. DaCosta (Eds.), *Handbook of research on human cognition and assistive technology: Design, accessibility and transdisciplinary perspectives* (pp. 21–42). Hershey, PA: Medical Information Science Reference. doi:10.4018/978-1-61520-817-3.ch002

DaCosta, B., & Seok, S. (2010). Multimedia Design of assistive technology for those with learning disabilities. In S. Seok, E. Meyen, & B. DaCosta (Eds.), *Handbook of research on human cognition and assistive technology: Design, accessibility and transdisciplinary perspectives* (pp. 43–60). Hershey, PA: Medical Information Science Reference. doi:10.4018/978-1-61520-817-3.ch003

DaCosta, B., & Seok, S. (2014). *Assistive technology research, practice, and theory* (pp. 1-282). doi:10.4018/978-1-4666-5015-2

Das, S., Caragea, D., Welch, S., & Hsu, W. H. (2010). *Handbook of research on computational methodologies in gene regulatory networks* (pp. 1–740).

Daskalaki, A. (2009). *Handbook of research on systems biology applications in medicine* (pp. 1–982).

Daskalaki, A. (2009). Dental computing and applications: Advanced techniques for clinical dentistry (pp. 1-406). doi:10.4018/978-1-60566-292-3

Daskalaki, A. (2010). *Informatics in oral medicine: Advanced techniques in clinical and diagnostic technologies* (pp. 1-346). doi:10.4018/978-1-60566-733-1

Daskalaki, A. (2013). *Medical advancements in aging and regenerative technologies: Clinical tools and applications* (pp. 1-333). doi:10.4018/978-1-4666-2506-8

Davis, E. (2010). Technology transforming healthcare: Tipping points, strange attractors, and a singularity. In S. Kabene (Ed.), *Healthcare and the effect of technology: Developments, challenges and advancements* (pp. 290–306). Hershey, PA: Medical Information Science Reference. doi:10.4018/978-1-61520-733-6.ch017

de la Torre Díez, I., Sánchez, R. H., Coronado, M. L., & López Gálvez, M. I. (2010). Electronic health records system using HL7 and DICOM in ophthalmology. In W. Pease, M. Cooper, & R. Gururajan (Eds.), *Biomedical knowledge management: Infrastructures and processes for E-Health systems* (pp. 42–60). Hershey, PA: Medical Information Science Reference. doi:10.4018/978-1-60566-266-4.ch004

Delgosha, M. S., Ojaki, A. A., & Farhadi, H. (2013). The business values of patient knowledge management (PKM) in the healthcare industry. *International Journal of Healthcare Information Systems and Informatics*, *8*(2), 70–79. doi:10.4018/jhisi.2013040106

Demirbilek, M. (2010). Cognitive load and disorientation issues in hypermedia as assistive technology. In S. Seok, E. Meyen, & B. DaCosta (Eds.), *Handbook of research on human cognition and assistive technology: Design, accessibility and transdisciplinary perspectives* (pp. 109–120). Hershey, PA: Medical Information Science Reference. doi:10.4018/978-1-61520-817-3.ch007

Dimitrovski, I., & Loskovska, S. (2010). Feature evaluation and classification for content-based medical image retrieval system. In S. Mohammed, & J. Fiaidhi (Eds.), *Ubiquitous health and medical informatics: The ubiquity 2.0 trend and beyond* (pp. 509–531). Hershey, PA: Medical Information Science Reference. doi:10.4018/978-1-61520-777-0.ch024

Dohan, M., Xenodemetropoulos, T., & Tan, J. (2012). The RCQ model: Conceptualizing inter-clinician relationships, communities of practice and quality improvement in healthcare. *International Journal of Healthcare Information Systems and Informatics*, *7*(2), 29–45. doi:10.4018/jhisi.2012040103

Dotterer, G. (2010). Effects of assistive technologies combined with desktop virtual reality in instructional procedures. In S. Seok, E. Meyen, & B. DaCosta (Eds.), *Handbook of research on human cognition and assistive technology: Design, accessibility and transdisciplinary perspectives* (pp. 299–305). Hershey, PA: Medical Information Science Reference. doi:10.4018/978-1-61520-817-3.ch020

Dotterer, G. (2010). Effects of assistive technologies combined with desktop virtual reality in instructional procedures. In S. Seok, E. Meyen, & B. DaCosta (Eds.), *Handbook of research on human cognition and assistive technology: Design, accessibility and transdisciplinary perspectives* (pp. 306–312). Hershey, PA: Medical Information Science Reference. doi:10.4018/978-1-61520-817-3.ch021

Dunn, M. W. (2010). Response to intervention: assistive technologies which can help teachers with intervention programming and assessment. In S. Seok, E. Meyen, & B. DaCosta (Eds.), *Handbook of research on human cognition and assistive technology: Design, accessibility and transdisciplinary perspectives* (pp. 313–324). Hershey, PA: Medical Information Science Reference. doi:10.4018/978-1-61520-817-3.ch022

Duquenoy, P., George, C., & Kimppa, K. (2008). *Ethical, legal and social issues in medical informatics* (pp. 1-320). doi:10.4018/978-1-59904-780-5

Dwivedi, A. N. (2009). *Handbook of Research on information technology management and clinical data administration in healthcare* (pp. 1–1072). doi:10.4018/978-1-60566-356-2

Eades, J. S. (2010). Sun, surgery and cyberspace: The role of the Internet in the rise of medical tourism. In W. Pease, M. Cooper, & R. Gururajan (Eds.), *Biomedical knowledge management: Infrastructures and processes for E-Health systems* (pp. 217–231). Hershey, PA: Medical Information Science Reference. doi:10.4018/978-1-60566-266-4.ch015

Echarte, F., Astrain, J. J., Córdoba, A., & Villadangos, J. (2010). A semantic model to address health questions to professionals in healthcare social networks. In S. Mohammed, & J. Fiaidhi (Eds.), *Ubiquitous health and medical informatics: The ubiquity 2.0 trend and beyond* (pp. 84–103). Hershey, PA: Medical Information Science Reference. doi:10.4018/978-1-61520-777-0.ch005

Eder, L. B. (2000). *Managing healthcare information systems with Web-enabled technologies* (pp. 1-278). doi:10.4018/978-1-878289-65-0

El Morr, C. (2010). Mobile virtual communities in healthcare: The chronic disease management case. In S. Mohammed, & J. Fiaidhi (Eds.), *Ubiquitous health and medical informatics: The ubiquity 2.0 trend and beyond* (pp. 258–274). Hershey, PA: Medical Information Science Reference. doi:10.4018/978-1-61520-777-0.ch013

El Morr, C. (2014). *Research perspectives on the role of informatics in health policy and management* (pp. 1-351). doi:10.4018/978-1-4666-4321-5

El Naqa, I., Wei, L., & Yang, Y. (2010). Content-based image retrieval for digital mammography. In S. Mohammed, & J. Fiaidhi (Eds.), *Ubiquitous health and medical informatics: The ubiquity 2.0 trend and beyond* (pp. 485–508). Hershey, PA: Medical Information Science Reference. doi:10.4018/978-1-61520-777-0.ch023

Ervin, K. (2014). Legal and ethical considerations in the implementation of electronic health records. In J. Krueger (Ed.), *Cases on electronic records and resource management implementation in diverse environments* (pp. 193–210). Hershey, PA: Information Science Reference.

Esmahi, L., Badidi, E., & Edwards, J. W. (2010). Managing demographic data inconsistencies in healthcare information systems. *International Journal of Information Systems and Social Change, 1*(1), 56–72. doi:10.4018/jissc.2010092905

Estrada-Hernández, N., & Stachowiak, J. R. (2010). Evaluating systemic assistive technology needs. In S. Seok, E. Meyen, & B. DaCosta (Eds.), *Handbook of research on human cognition and assistive technology: Design, accessibility and transdisciplinary perspectives* (pp. 239–250). Hershey, PA: Medical Information Science Reference. doi:10.4018/978-1-61520-817-3.ch016

Exarchos, T. P., Papadopoulos, A., & Fotiadis, D. I. (2009). *Handbook of research on advanced techniques in diagnostic imaging and biomedical applications* (pp. 1–598). doi:10.4018/978-1-60566-314-2

Falan, S. L., Han, B., Zoeller, L. H., Tarn, J. M., & Roach, D. M. (2011). Sustaining healthcare through waste elimination: A taxonomic analysis with case illustrations. *International Journal of Healthcare Information Systems and Informatics, 6*(4), 1–22. doi:10.4018/jhisi.2011100101

Falchuk, B., Famolari, D., Fischer, R., Loeb, S., & Panagos, E. (2010). The mHealth stack: Technology enablers for patient-centric mobile healthcare. *International Journal of E-Health and Medical Communications, 1*(1), 1–17. doi:10.4018/jehmc.2010010101

Favela, J., Tentori, M., Segura, D., & Berzunza, G. (2009). Adaptive awareness of hospital patient information through multiple sentient displays. *International Journal of Ambient Computing and Intelligence, 1*(1), 27–38. doi:10.4018/jaci.2009010103

Federici, T., & Resca, A. (2009). Managing E-Procurement in public healthcare: A knowledge management perspective. *International Journal of Healthcare Delivery Reform Initiatives, 1*(1), 1–15. doi:10.4018/jhdri.2009010101

Feiser, J., Raghavan, V. V., & Cata, T. (2011). A risk-based classification of mobile applications in healthcare. *International Journal of Healthcare Delivery Reform Initiatives, 3*(2), 28–39. doi:10.4018/jhdri.2011040103

Fernández, D. R. (2010). An agent-based architecture to ubiquitous health. In S. Mohammed, & J. Fiaidhi (Eds.), *Ubiquitous health and medical informatics: The ubiquity 2.0 trend and beyond* (pp. 213–232). Hershey, PA: Medical Information Science Reference. doi:10.4018/978-1-61520-777-0.ch011

Fiaidhi, J., Mohammed, S., & Wei, Y. (2010). Implications of Web 2.0 technology on healthcare: A biomedical semantic blog case study. In S. Kabene (Ed.), *Healthcare and the effect of technology: Developments, challenges and advancements* (pp. 269–289). Hershey, PA: Medical Information Science Reference. doi:10.4018/978-1-61520-733-6.ch016

Fitzpatrick, M., & Theoharis, R. (2010). Assistive technology for deaf and hard of hearing students. In S. Seok, E. Meyen, & B. DaCosta (Eds.), *Handbook of research on human cognition and assistive technology: Design, accessibility and transdisciplinary perspectives* (pp. 179–191). Hershey, PA: Medical Information Science Reference. doi:10.4018/978-1-61520-817-3.ch012

Gangopadhyay, A. (2013). *Methods, models, and computation for medical informatics* (pp. 1-345). doi:10.4018/978-1-4666-2653-9

Gasmelseid, T. M. (2012). *Pharmacoinformatics and drug discovery technologies: Theories and applications* (pp. 1-442). doi:10.4018/978-1-4666-0309-7

Georgiadis, D., Germanakos, P., Mourlas, C., Samaras, G., & Christodoulou, E. (2010). Dynamic business processes and virtual communities in wireless eHealth environments. In S. Mohammed, & J. Fiaidhi (Eds.), *Ubiquitous health and medical informatics: The ubiquity 2.0 trend and beyond* (pp. 431–456). Hershey, PA: Medical Information Science Reference. doi:10.4018/978-1-61520-777-0.ch021

Ghotbi, N., & Claster, W. (2010). The use of public health surveillance data for preventive control of diseases that depend on individual risky behavior: The case of HIV infection in Japan. In W. Pease, M. Cooper, & R. Gururajan (Eds.), *Biomedical knowledge management: Infrastructures and processes for E-Health systems* (pp. 232–241). Hershey, PA: Medical Information Science Reference. doi:10.4018/978-1-60566-266-4.ch016

Glascock, A. P., & Kutzik, D. M. (2009). Embrace the chaos, it's not noise: Lessons learned from non-traditional environments. *International Journal of Mobile Human Computer Interaction*, *1*(2), 22–36. doi:10.4018/jmhci.2009040102

Gligorov, N., & Krieger, S. C. (2010). Functional neuroimaging, free will, and privacy. In S. Kabene (Ed.), *Healthcare and the effect of technology: Developments, challenges and advancements* (pp. 233–251). Hershey, PA: Medical Information Science Reference. doi:10.4018/978-1-61520-733-6.ch014

Glusker, A., & Hoelscher, E. (2014). Transitioning from print to online-only resources: the experience of a medium-sized healthcare organization library. In J. Krueger (Ed.), *cases on electronic records and resource management implementation in diverse environments* (pp. 226–242). Hershey, PA: Information Science Reference.

Grandison, T., & Bhatti, R. (2010). Regulatory compliance and the correlation to privacy protection in healthcare. *International Journal of Computational Models and Algorithms in Medicine*, *1*(2), 37–52. doi:10.4018/jcmam.2010040103

Grütter, R. (2002). *Knowledge media in healthcare: Opportunities and challenges* (pp. 1-296). doi:10.4018/978-1-930708-13-6

Guah, M. (2011). *Healthcare delivery reform and new technologies: Organizational initiatives* (pp. 1-462). doi:10.4018/978-1-60960-183-6

Guah, M. W. (2009). [IJHDRI]. *International Journal of Healthcare Delivery Reform Initiatives*. doi: doi:10.4018/IJHDRI

Gulla, V., Mori, A. R., Gabbrielli, F., & Lanzafame, P. (2013). *Telehealth networks for hospital services: New methodologies* (pp. 1-428). doi:10.4018/978-1-4666-2979-0

Gupta, A., Goyal, R. K., Joiner, K. A., & Saini, S. (2008). Outsourcing in the healthcare industry: Information technology, intellectual property, and allied aspects. *Information Resources Management Journal*, *21*(1), 1–26. doi:10.4018/irmj.2008010101

Gururajan, R. (2009). Drivers for wireless technology acceptance in Indian healthcare. *International Journal of Healthcare Delivery Reform Initiatives*, *1*(1), 48–52. doi:10.4018/jhdri.2009010104

Gururajan, R., Gurney, T., & Hafeez-Baig, A. (2009). confirmatory factor analysis to establish determinants of wireless technology in the Indian healthcare. *International Journal of Healthcare Delivery Reform Initiatives*, *1*(3), 19–37. doi:10.4018/jhdri.2009070102

Hackbarth, G., & McQuade, J. (2009). Information completeness: A qualitative analysis of indoor air quality (IAQ). *International Journal of Healthcare Delivery Reform Initiatives*, *1*(2), 1–24. doi:10.4018/jhdri.2009040101

Hafeez-Baig, A., & Gururajan, R. (2010). An exploratory study to understand the drivers and inhibitors for the successful adoption of wireless technology in Australian healthcare systems. In W. Pease, M. Cooper, & R. Gururajan (Eds.), *Biomedical knowledge management: Infrastructures and processes for E-Health systems* (pp. 267–278). Hershey, PA: Medical Information Science Reference. doi:10.4018/978-1-60566-266-4.ch019

Haghi, A. K. (2013). *Methodologies and applications for chemoinformatics and chemical engineering* (pp. 1-500). doi:10.4018/978-1-4666-4010-8

Hajiheydari, N., Khakbaz, S. B., & Farhadi, H. (2013). Proposing a business model in healthcare industry: E-Diagnosis. *International Journal of Healthcare Information Systems and Informatics*, *8*(2), 41–57. doi:10.4018/jhisi.2013040104

Hammond, W. (2010). Semantic interoperability issue of standardizing medical vocabularies. In S. Mohammed, & J. Fiaidhi (Eds.), *Ubiquitous health and medical informatics: The ubiquity 2.0 trend and beyond* (pp. 19–42). Hershey, PA: Medical Information Science Reference. doi:10.4018/978-1-61520-777-0.ch002

Harno, K. (2010). Healthcare Information exchange in advancing shared care regionally. *International Journal of Healthcare Delivery Reform Initiatives*, *2*(1), 43–58. doi:10.4018/jhdri.2010010103

Heilman, G. E., Cain, M., & Morton, R. S. (2008). Predicting voluntary participation in a public health program using a neural network. *International Journal of Healthcare Information Systems and Informatics*, *3*(2), 1–11. doi:10.4018/jhisi.2008040101

Helms, M. M., Moore, R., & Ahmadi, M. (2008). Information technology (IT) and the healthcare industry: A SWOT analysis. *International Journal of Healthcare Information Systems and Informatics*, *3*(1), 75–92. doi:10.4018/jhisi.2008010105

Hine, M. J., Farion, K. J., Michalowski, W., & Wilk, S. (2009). Decision making by emergency room physicians and residents: Implications for the design of clinical decision support systems. *International Journal of Healthcare Information Systems and Informatics*, *4*(2), 17–35. doi:10.4018/jhisi.2009040102

Hines, E. L., & Leeson, M. S. (2011). *Intelligent systems for machine olfaction: tools and methodologies* (pp. 1-354). doi:10.4018/978-1-61520-915-6

Ho, K. (2010). Health in the digital world: transformational trends. In S. Kabene (Ed.), *Healthcare and the effect of technology: Developments, challenges and advancements* (pp. 1–12). Hershey, PA: Medical Information Science Reference. doi:10.4018/978-1-61520-733-6.ch001

Hodapp, J. B., & Rachow, C. (2010). Impact of text-to-speech software on access to print: A longitudinal study. In S. Seok, E. Meyen, & B. DaCosta (Eds.), *Handbook of research on human cognition and assistive technology: Design, accessibility and transdisciplinary perspectives* (pp. 199–219). Hershey, PA: Medical Information Science Reference. doi:10.4018/978-1-61520-817-3.ch014

Hodapp, J. B., & Rachow, C. (2010). Measure it, monitor it: Tools for monitoring implementation of text-to-speech software. In S. Seok, E. Meyen, & B. DaCosta (Eds.), *Handbook of research on human cognition and assistive technology: Design, accessibility and transdisciplinary perspectives* (pp. 220–238). Hershey, PA: Medical Information Science Reference. doi:10.4018/978-1-61520-817-3.ch015

Hongladarom, S. (2011). *Genomics and bioethics: Interdisciplinary perspectives, technologies and advancements* (pp. 1-332). doi:10.4018/978-1-61692-883-4

Hsu, H. (2006). *Advanced data mining technologies in bioinformatics* (pp. 1-342). doi:10.4018/978-1-59140-863-5

Hu, J., & Peyton, L. (2010). A framework for privacy assurance and ubiquitous knowledge discovery in health 2.0 data mashups. In S. Mohammed, & J. Fiaidhi (Eds.), *ubiquitous health and medical informatics: The ubiquity 2.0 trend and beyond* (pp. 64–83). Hershey, PA: Medical Information Science Reference. doi:10.4018/978-1-61520-777-0.ch004

Hughes, B. (2010). Managing E-Health in the age of Web 2.0: The impact on E-Health evaluation. In S. Mohammed, & J. Fiaidhi (Eds.), *Ubiquitous health and medical informatics: The ubiquity 2.0 trend and beyond* (pp. 329–349). Hershey, PA: Medical Information Science Reference. doi:10.4018/978-1-61520-777-0.ch016

Hung, W., Chang, L., & Lee, M. (2012). Factors influencing the success of national healthcare services information systems: An empirical study in Taiwan. *Journal of Global Information Management*, *20*(3), 84–108. doi:10.4018/jgim.2012070104

Ilie, V., Van Slyke, C., Courtney, J. F., & Styne, P. (2009). Challenges associated with physicians' usage of electronic medical records. *International Journal of Healthcare Information Systems and Informatics*, *4*(3), 38–54. doi:10.4018/jhisi.2009070103

Isern, D., Sánchez, D., Solé-Ribalta, A., Moreno, A., & Varga, L. Z. (2010). The K4Care platform design and implementation. In S. Mohammed, & J. Fiaidhi (Eds.), *Ubiquitous health and medical informatics: The ubiquity 2.0 trend and beyond* (pp. 370–389). Hershey, PA: Medical Information Science Reference. doi:10.4018/978-1-61520-777-0.ch018

Jean-Jules, J., & Villeneuve, A. O. (2009). Toward a better understanding of the assimilation of telehealth systems. *International Journal of E-Services and Mobile Applications*, *1*(2), 20–37. doi:10.4018/jesma.2009040102

Johnson, V., & Price, C. (2010). A longitudinal case study on the use of assistive technology to support cognitive processes across formal and informal educational settings. In S. Seok, E. Meyen, & B. DaCosta (Eds.), *Handbook of research on human cognition and assistive technology: Design, accessibility and transdisciplinary perspectives* (pp. 192–198). Hershey, PA: Medical Information Science Reference. doi:10.4018/978-1-61520-817-3.ch013

Jordanova, M. (2010). Closing the gap: E-Health and optimization of patient care. In S. Kabene (Ed.), *Healthcare and the effect of technology: Developments, challenges and advancements* (pp. 38–59). Hershey, PA: Medical Information Science Reference. doi:10.4018/978-1-61520-733-6.ch003

Juzwishin, D. W. (2010). Enabling Technologies and challenges for the future of ubiquitous health The interoperability framework. In S. Mohammed, & J. Fiaidhi (Eds.), *Ubiquitous health and medical informatics: The ubiquity 2.0 trend and beyond* (pp. 596–622). Hershey, PA: Medical Information Science Reference. doi:10.4018/978-1-61520-777-0.ch028

Kabene, S., & Wolfe, M. (2010). Risks and benefits of technology in health care. In S. Kabene (Ed.), *Healthcare and the effect of technology: Developments, challenges and advancements* (pp. 60–71). Hershey, PA: Medical Information Science Reference. doi:10.4018/978-1-61520-733-6.ch004

Kabene, S. M. (2010). *Healthcare and the effect of technology: Developments, challenges and advancements* (pp. 1-392). doi:10.4018/978-1-61520-733-6

Kabene, S. M. King, Lisa, & Gibson, C. J. (2010). Technology and human resources management in health care. In S. Mohammed & J. Fiaidhi (Eds.), Ubiquitous health and medical informatics: The ubiquity 2.0 trend and beyond (pp. 574-595). Hershey, PA: Medical Information Science Reference. doi: doi:10.4018/978-1-61520-777-0.ch027

Kaldoudi, E., Konstantinidis, S., & Bamidis, P. D. (2010). Web 2.0 approaches for active, collaborative learning in medicine and health. In S. Mohammed, & J. Fiaidhi (Eds.), *Ubiquitous health and medical informatics: The ubiquity 2.0 trend and beyond* (pp. 127–149). Hershey, PA: Medical Information Science Reference. doi:10.4018/978-1-61520-777-0.ch007

Kapoor, B., & Kleinbart, M. (2012). Building an integrated patient information system for a healthcare network. *Journal of Cases on Information Technology*, *14*(2), 27–41. doi:10.4018/jcit.2012040103

Kapoor, B., & Mullen, T. (2012). Integration of just in time (JIT) inventory in outpatient pharmacy information systems. *Journal of Cases on Information Technology*, *14*(4), 27–40. doi:10.4018/jcit.2012100103

Kastania, A. N., & Moumtzoglou, A. (2012). [IJRQEH]. *International Journal of Reliable and Quality E-Healthcare*. doi: doi:10.4018/IJRQEH

Kazandjian, V. A. (2012). Quality is not an accident: The planning for a safe journey through the healthcare system. *International Journal of Reliable and Quality E-Healthcare*, *1*(2), 1–11. doi:10.4018/ijrqeh.2012040101

Kellam, H., MacDonald, C. J., Archibald, D., & Puddester, D. (2012). Designing digital video to support learner outcomes: A study in an online learning resource for healthcare professionals and students. *International Journal of Online Pedagogy and Course Design*, *2*(3), 45–66. doi:10.4018/ijopcd.2012070104

Khan, K. M. (2012). State of sharing clinical information in a healthcare system in the gulf. *International Journal of Reliable and Quality E-Healthcare*, *1*(3), 27–42. doi:10.4018/ijrqeh.2012070104

Khetrapal, N. (2010). Cognition meets assistive technology: Insights from load theory of selective attention. In S. Seok, E. Meyen, & B. DaCosta (Eds.), *Handbook of research on human cognition and assistive technology: Design, accessibility and transdisciplinary perspectives* (pp. 96–108). Hershey, PA: Medical Information Science Reference. doi:10.4018/978-1-61520-817-3.ch006

Khoumbati, K., Dwivedi, Y. K., Srivastava, A., & Lal, B. (2010). Handbook of research on advances in health informatics and electronic healthcare applications: Global adoption and impact of information communication technologies (pp. 1-628). doi: doi:10.4018/978-1-60566-030-1

King, K. P. (2012). The mind–body-spirit learning model transformative learning connections to holistic perspectives: Seizing control of your healthcare - The relationship among self-agency, transformative learning, and wellness. *International Journal of Adult Vocational Education and Technology*, *3*(3), 37–51. doi:10.4018/javet.2012070104

Kinsell, C. (2010). Investigating assistive technologies using computers to simulate basic curriculum for individuals with cognitive impairments. In S. Seok, E. Meyen, & B. DaCosta (Eds.), *Handbook of research on human cognition and assistive technology: Design, accessibility and transdisciplinary perspectives* (pp. 61–75). Hershey, PA: Medical Information Science Reference. doi:10.4018/978-1-61520-817-3.ch004

Kitsios, F., Papadopoulos, T., & Angelopoulos, S. (2010). A roadmap to the introduction of pervasive information systems in healthcare. *International Journal of Advanced Pervasive and Ubiquitous Computing*, *2*(3), 21–32. doi:10.4018/japuc.2010070102

Kock, N., & Verville, J. (2012). Exploring free questionnaire data with anchor variables: An illustration based on a study of IT in healthcare. *International Journal of Healthcare Information Systems and Informatics*, *7*(1), 46–63. doi:10.4018/jhisi.2012010104

Kolker, A., & Story, P. (2012). *Management engineering for effective healthcare delivery: Principles and applications* (pp. 1-512). doi:10.4018/978-1-60960-872-9

Kossida, S., & Kastania, A. (2012). [IJSBBT]. *International Journal of Systems Biology and Biomedical Technologies*. doi: doi:10.4018/IJSBBT

Kouba, B. J., & Newberry, B. (2010). Assistive technology's past, present and future. In S. Seok, E. Meyen, & B. DaCosta (Eds.), *Handbook of research on human cognition and assistive technology: Design, accessibility and transdisciplinary perspectives* (pp. 360–373). Hershey, PA: Medical Information Science Reference. doi:10.4018/978-1-61520-817-3.ch025

Koufi, V., Malamateniou, F., & Vassilacopoulos, G. (2010). Pervasive process-based healthcare systems on a grid environment. In A. Coronato, & G. De Pietro (Eds.), *Pervasive and smart technologies for healthcare: Ubiquitous methodologies and tools* (pp. 130–154). Hershey, PA: Medical Information Science Reference. doi:10.4018/978-1-61520-765-7.ch007

Kouroupetroglou, G. (2014). *Assistive technologies and computer access for motor disabilities* (pp. 1-351). doi:10.4018/978-1-4666-4438-0

Kouroupetroglou, G. (2014). *Disability informatics and Web accessibility for motor limitations* (pp. 1-443). doi:10.4018/978-1-4666-4442-7

Krontiris, I. (2010). Sensor networks security for pervasive healthcare. In A. Coronato, & G. De Pietro (Eds.), *Pervasive and smart technologies for healthcare: Ubiquitous methodologies and tools* (pp. 155–171). Hershey, PA: Medical Information Science Reference. doi:10.4018/978-1-61520-765-7.ch008

Kudyba, S., & Perry, T. L. (2008). Informatics application challenges for managed care organizations: The three faces of population segmentation and a proposed classification system. *International Journal of Healthcare Information Systems and Informatics*, *3*(2), 21–31. doi:10.4018/jhisi.2008040103

Kurschl, W., Mitsch, S., & Schoenboeck, J. (2010). Model-driven prototyping support for pervasive healthcare applications. In A. Coronato, & G. De Pietro (Eds.), *pervasive and smart technologies for healthcare: Ubiquitous methodologies and tools* (pp. 251–281). Hershey, PA: Medical Information Science Reference. doi:10.4018/978-1-61520-765-7.ch012

Kushniruk, A., & Borycki, E. (2008). *Human, social, and organizational aspects of health information systems* (pp. 1-422). doi:10.4018/978-1-59904-792-8

Laffey, J., Stichter, J., & Schmidt, M. (2010). Social orthotics for youth with ASD to learn in a collaborative 3D VLE. In S. Seok, E. Meyen, & B. DaCosta (Eds.), *Handbook of research on human cognition and assistive technology: Design, accessibility and transdisciplinary perspectives* (pp. 76–95). Hershey, PA: Medical Information Science Reference. doi:10.4018/978-1-61520-817-3.ch005

Laskowski, M. (2011). A prototype agent based model and machine learning hybrid system for healthcare decision support. *International Journal of E-Health and Medical Communications*, *2*(4), 67–90. doi:10.4018/jehmc.2011100105

Lazakidou, A., & Daskalaki, A. (2012). *Quality assurance in healthcare service delivery, nursing and personalized medicine: technologies and processes* (pp. 1-302). doi:10.4018/978-1-61350-120-7

Lazakidou, A., Siassiakos, K., & Ioannou, K. (2011). *Wireless technologies for ambient assisted living and healthcare: Systems and applications* (pp. 1-270). doi:10.4018/978-1-61520-805-0

Lazakidou, A. A. (2006). *Handbook of research on informatics in healthcare and biomedicine* (pp. 1–479). doi:10.4018/978-1-59140-982-3

Lazakidou, A. A. (2010). *Biocomputation and biomedical informatics: Case studies and applications* (pp. 1-356). doi:10.4018/978-1-60566-768-3

Lazakidou, A. A., & Siassiakos, K. (2009). *Handbook of research on distributed medical informatics and E-Health* (pp. 1–600).

Lecca, P., Tulpan, D., & Rajaraman, K. (2012). *Systemic approaches in bioinformatics and computational systems biology: Recent advances* (pp. 1-471). doi:10.4018/978-1-61350-435-2

Lee, E., & Chang, P. (2010). [IJALR]. *International Journal of Artificial Life Research.* doi: doi:10.4018/IJALR

Lee, O. F., & Guster, D. C. (2010). Virtualized disaster recovery model for large scale hospital and healthcare systems. *International Journal of Healthcare Information Systems and Informatics*, *5*(3), 69–81. doi:10.4018/jhisi.2010070105

Lemma, F., Denko, M. K., Tan, J. K., & Kassegne, S. K. (2008). Envisioning a national e-medicine network architecture in a developing country: A case study. *International Journal of Healthcare Information Systems and Informatics*, *3*(1), 44–62. doi:10.4018/jhisi.2008010103

Li, X., & Ng, S. (2009). *Biological data mining in protein interaction networks* (pp. 1-450). doi:10.4018/978-1-60566-398-2

Li, X., & Ng, S. (2010). [IJKDB]. *International Journal of Knowledge Discovery in Bioinformatics.* doi: doi:10.4018/IJKDB

Li, X., & Ng, S. (2012). *Computational knowledge discovery for bioinformatics research* (pp. 1-463). doi:10.4018/978-1-4666-1785-8

Lin, L., Chen, H., Chen, P., & Tennyson, R. D. (2012). Critical managerial activity and competency of healthcare management: A study of eighteen hospitals. *International Journal of Asian Business and Information Management*, *3*(1), 11–20. doi:10.4018/jabim.2012010102

Linnavuo, M., & Rimminen, H. (2010). Localization and monitoring of people with a near-field imaging system: Boosting the elderly care. In A. Coronato, & G. De Pietro (Eds.), *Pervasive and smart technologies for healthcare: Ubiquitous methodologies and tools* (pp. 78–96). Hershey, PA: Medical Information Science Reference. doi:10.4018/978-1-61520-765-7.ch004

Lio, P., & Verma, D. (2012). *Biologically inspired networking and sensing: Algorithms and architectures* (pp. 1-312). doi:10.4018/978-1-61350-092-7

Liu, L. A., Wei, D., & Li, Y. (2011). *Interdisciplinary research and applications in bioinformatics, computational biology, and environmental sciences* (pp. 1-396). doi:10.4018/978-1-60960-064-8

Liu, L. A., Wei, D., Li, Y., & Lei, H. (2011). Handbook of research on computational and systems biology: Interdisciplinary applications (pp. 1-776). doi: doi:10.4018/978-1-60960-491-2

Liu, S. Y. (2010). Personal health records status-quo and future perspectives. In S. Mohammed, & J. Fiaidhi (Eds.), *Ubiquitous health and medical informatics: The ubiquity 2.0 trend and beyond* (pp. 43–63). Hershey, PA: Medical Information Science Reference. doi:10.4018/978-1-61520-777-0.ch003

Lodhi, H., & Yamanishi, Y. (2011). *Chemoinformatics and advanced machine learning perspectives: Complex computational methods and collaborative techniques* (pp. 1-418). doi:10.4018/978-1-61520-911-8

Lowe, M. A. (2010). Developing electronic portfolios. In S. Seok, E. Meyen, & B. DaCosta (Eds.), *Handbook of research on human cognition and assistive technology: Design, accessibility and transdisciplinary perspectives* (pp. 251–263). Hershey, PA: Medical Information Science Reference. doi:10.4018/978-1-61520-817-3.ch017

Lueth, T. C., D'Angelo, L. T., & Czabke, A. (2010). TUM-AgeTech: A new framework for pervasive medical devices. In A. Coronato, & G. De Pietro (Eds.), *Pervasive and smart technologies for healthcare: Ubiquitous methodologies and tools* (pp. 295–321). Hershey, PA: Medical Information Science Reference. doi:10.4018/978-1-61520-765-7.ch014

M., K. (2014). *International Journal of Pharmacology and Pharmaceutical Technology (IJPPT).* doi:10.4018/IJPPT

Macdonald, A. S., Loudon, D., & Li, C. S. (2010). User-centric and inclusive design methods: Implications for E-Healthcare. In W. Pease, M. Cooper, & R. Gururajan (Eds.), *Biomedical knowledge management: Infrastructures and processes for E-Health systems* (pp. 134–153). Hershey, PA: Medical Information Science Reference. doi:10.4018/978-1-60566-266-4.ch010

Maliapen, M., & Gillies, A. (2010). The integration of systems dynamics and balanced scorecards in strategic healthcare policy simulation analysis. *International Journal of Healthcare Delivery Reform Initiatives*, *2*(2), 10–34. doi:10.4018/jhdri.2010040102

Management Association. I. (2011). Clinical technologies: Concepts, methodologies, tools and applications (3 Volumes) (pp. 1-2366). doi: doi:10.4018/978-1-60960-561-2

Management Association. I. (2013). User-driven healthcare: Concepts, methodologies, tools, and applications (3 Volumes) (pp. 1-1512). doi: doi:10.4018/978-1-4666-2770-3

Management Association. I. (2013). Bioinformatics: Concepts, methodologies, tools, and applications (3 Volumes) (pp. 1-1246). doi: doi:10.4018/978-1-4666-3604-0

Martinho, R., Rijo, R., Cruz-Cunha, M. M., & Varajão, J. (2013). *Information systems and technologies for enhancing health and social care* (pp. 1-421). doi:10.4018/978-1-4666-3667-5

Masaud-Wahaishi, A., & Ghenniwa, H. (2010). Privacy-based multiagent brokering architecture for ubiquitous healthcare systems. In S. Mohammed, & J. Fiaidhi (Eds.), *Ubiquitous health and medical informatics: The ubiquity 2.0 trend and beyond* (pp. 296–328). Hershey, PA: Medical Information Science Reference. doi:10.4018/978-1-61520-777-0.ch015

McGrady, E., & Nelms, L. W. (2010). Ethical issues of health management predictive modeling. In W. Pease, M. Cooper, & R. Gururajan (Eds.), *Biomedical knowledge management: Infrastructures and processes for E-Health systems* (pp. 92–100). Hershey, PA: Medical Information Science Reference. doi:10.4018/978-1-60566-266-4.ch007

McLeod, A. J. Jr, & Clark, J. G. (2009). Using stakeholder analysis to identify users in healthcare information systems research: Who is the real user? *International Journal of Healthcare Information Systems and Informatics*, *4*(3), 1–15. doi:10.4018/jhisi.2009070101 PMID:20523757

Meglic, M., & Brodnik, A. (2010). Electronic Environments for integrated care management case of depression treatment. In S. Mohammed, & J. Fiaidhi (Eds.), *Ubiquitous health and medical informatics: The ubiquity 2.0 trend and beyond* (pp. 390–411). Hershey, PA: Medical Information Science Reference. doi:10.4018/978-1-61520-777-0.ch019

Meyers, T. W. (2012). Literature synthesis on evaluative measures in healthcare simulation. *International Journal of Gaming and Computer-Mediated Simulations*, *4*(3), 38–48. doi:10.4018/jgcms.2012070103

Michell, V., Gulliver, S. R., Rosenorn-Lanng, D. J., & Currie, W. (2014). *Patient safety and quality care through health informatics* (pp. 1-357). doi:10.4018/978-1-4666-4546-2

Miller, T. W., Morgan, R. D., & Woods, J. A. (2009). Tele-practice technology: A model for healthcare delivery to underserved populations. *International Journal of Healthcare Delivery Reform Initiatives*, *1*(3), 55–69. doi:10.4018/jhdri.2009070104

Mo, H. (2009). Handbook of research on artificial immune systems and natural computing: Applying complex adaptive technologies (pp. 1-634). doi: doi:10.4018/978-1-60566-310-4

Mohammed, S., & Fiaidhi, J. (2010). *Ubiquitous health and medical informatics: The ubiquity 2.0 trend and beyond* (pp. 1-728). doi:10.4018/978-1-61520-777-0

Mohammed, S., & Fiaidhi, J. (2010). Identifying the emerging e-Health technologies to ubiquity 2.0 and beyond. In S. Mohammed, & J. Fiaidhi (Eds.), *Ubiquitous health and medical informatics: The ubiquity 2.0 trend and beyond* (pp. 1–18). Hershey, PA: Medical Information Science Reference. doi:10.4018/978-1-61520-777-0.ch001

Moloney, C. (2010). The role of wireless technology in addressing sleeping disorders in aged care. In W. Pease, M. Cooper, & R. Gururajan (Eds.), *Biomedical knowledge management: Infrastructures and processes for E-Health systems* (pp. 279–288). Hershey, PA: Medical Information Science Reference. doi:10.4018/978-1-60566-266-4.ch020

Moumtzoglou, A., & Kastania, A. (2011). *E-Health systems quality and reliability: Models and standards* (pp. 1-398). doi:10.4018/978-1-61692-843-8

Moumtzoglou, A., & Kastania, A. (2013). *E-Health technologies and improving patient safety: Exploring organizational factors* (pp. 1-372). doi:10.4018/978-1-4666-2657-7

Muhammad, I., Moghimi, F. H., Taylor, N. J., Redley, B., Nguyen, L., & Stein, M. et al. (2013). Using ANT to uncover the full potential of an intelligent operational planning and support tool (IOPST) for acute healthcare contexts. *International Journal of Actor-Network Theory and Technological Innovation*, *5*(2), 29–49. doi:10.4018/jantti.2013040103

Nakamoto, T. (2013). Human Olfactory Displays and Interfaces: Odor Sensing and Presentation (pp. 1-555). doi:10.4018/978-1-4666-2521-1

Nankee, C. (2010). Switch technologies. In S. Seok, E. Meyen, & B. DaCosta (Eds.), *Handbook of research on human cognition and assistive technology: Design, accessibility and transdisciplinary perspectives* (pp. 157–168). Hershey, PA: Medical Information Science Reference. doi:10.4018/978-1-61520-817-3.ch010

Neumann, C. P., & Lenz, R. (2012). The alpha-flow approach to inter-institutional process support in healthcare. *International Journal of Knowledge-Based Organizations*, *2*(4), 52–68. doi:10.4018/ijkbo.2012100104

Niazi, M. A. (2013). [IJPHIM]. *International Journal of Privacy and Health Information Management.* doi: doi:10.4018/IJPHIM

Nunes de Castro, L. (2010). [IJNCR]. *International Journal of Natural Computing Research.* doi: doi:10.4018/IJNCR

Nunes de Castro, L. (2012). *Nature-inspired computing design, development, and applications* (pp. 1-435). doi:10.4018/978-1-4666-1574-8

Nunes de Castro, L. (2014). *Natural computing for simulation and knowledge discovery* (pp. 1-326). doi:10.4018/978-1-4666-4253-9

Nunes de Castro, L., & Von Zuben, F. (2005). *Recent developments in biologically inspired computing* (pp. 1-456). doi:10.4018/978-1-59140-312-8

O'Flaherty, B., & O'Donoghue, J. (2010). The Development of emerging medical devices: The lead-user method in practice. In S. Becker, & R. Niebuhr (Eds.), *Cases on technology innovation: Entrepreneurial successes and pitfalls* (pp. 121–133). Hershey, PA: Business Science Reference. doi:10.4018/978-1-61520-609-4.ch006

Oinas-Kukkonen, H., Raisanen, T., Leiviska, K., Seppanen, M., & Kallio, M. (2009). Physicians' user experiences of mobile pharmacopoeias and evidence-based medical guidelines. *International Journal of Healthcare Information Systems and Informatics*, *4*(2), 57–68. doi:10.4018/jhisi.2009040104

Okrigwe, B. N. (2010). Cognition and learning. In S. Seok, E. Meyen, & B. DaCosta (Eds.), *Handbook of research on human cognition and assistive technology: Design, accessibility and transdisciplinary perspectives* (pp. 388–400). Hershey, PA: Medical Information Science Reference. doi:10.4018/978-1-61520-817-3.ch027

Okun, O. (2011). *Feature selection and ensemble methods for bioinformatics: Algorithmic classification and implementations* (pp. 1-460). doi:10.4018/978-1-60960-557-5

Olla, P., & Tan, J. (2009). *Mobile health solutions for biomedical applications* (pp. 1-366). doi:10.4018/978-1-60566-332-6

Omachonu, V. K., & Shatlock, K. (2012). Implementation of electronic health record system at a community healthcare organization. *International Journal of Innovation in the Digital Economy, 3*(2), 27–39. doi:10.4018/jide.2012040103

Omar, W. M. (2010). Healthcare collaborative framework based on Web 2.0, grid computing and SOA. In S. Mohammed, & J. Fiaidhi (Eds.), *Ubiquitous health and medical informatics: The ubiquity 2.0 trend and beyond* (pp. 190–212). Hershey, PA: Medical Information Science Reference. doi:10.4018/978-1-61520-777-0.ch010

Ozcelik, Y., Carter, C. H., Clark, M., & Martinez, A. (2010). Digitizing healthcare: Electronic medication administration record (eMAR) and bedside medication verification (BMV). In W. Pease, M. Cooper, & R. Gururajan (Eds.), *Biomedical knowledge management: Infrastructures and processes for E-Health systems* (pp. 31–41). Hershey, PA: Medical Information Science Reference. doi:10.4018/978-1-60566-266-4.ch003

Paavola, T. (2008). Exploiting process thinking in health care. *International Journal of Healthcare Information Systems and Informatics, 3*(2), 12–20. doi:10.4018/jhisi.2008040102

Pak, R., Fink, N., Price, M., & Battisto, D. (2010). Two case studies in human factors in healthcare: The nurse and older patient. *International Journal of Healthcare Delivery Reform Initiatives*, *2*(4), 17–38. doi: doi:10.4018/978-1-60960-177-5.ch012

Paolucci, F., Ergas, H., Hannan, T., & Aarts, J. (2010). The effectiveness of health informatics. In S. Kabene (Ed.), *Healthcare and the effect of technology: Developments, challenges and advancements* (pp. 13–37). Hershey, PA: Medical Information Science Reference. doi:10.4018/978-1-61520-733-6.ch002

Parry, D., & Parry, E. (2009). *Medical informatics in obstetrics and gynecology* (pp. 1-428). doi:10.4018/978-1-60566-078-3

Pasupathy, K. S. (2010). Systems engineering and health informatics: Context, content, and implementation. In S. Kabene (Ed.), *Healthcare and the effect of technology: Developments, challenges and advancements* (pp. 123–144). Hershey, PA: Medical Information Science Reference. doi:10.4018/978-1-61520-733-6.ch009

Pasupathy, K. S. (2010). Transforming healthcare: Leveraging the complementarities of health informatics and systems engineering. *International Journal of Healthcare Delivery Reform Initiatives, 2*(2), 35–55. doi:10.4018/jhdri.2010040103

Pate, C. L., & Turner-Ferrier, J. E. (2010). Exploring linkages between quality, E-Health and healthcare education. *International Journal of Healthcare Delivery Reform Initiatives*, *2*(4), 66–81. doi: doi:10.4018/978-1-61692-843-8.ch013

Pease, W., Cooper, M., & Gururajan, R. (2010). *Biomedical knowledge management: Infrastructures and processes for E-Health systems* (pp. 1-412). doi:10.4018/978-1-60566-266-4

Pereira, J. (2011). *Handbook of research on personal autonomy technologies and disability informatics* (pp. 1–462).

Pereira, M., & Freire, M. (2011). *Biomedical diagnostics and clinical technologies: Applying high-performance cluster and grid computing* (pp. 1-396). doi:10.4018/978-1-60566-280-0

Peruš, M., & Loo, C. K. (2011). *Biological and quantum computing for human vision: Holonomic models and applications* (pp. 1-314). doi:10.4018/978-1-61520-785-5

Petoukhov, S., & He, M. (2010). *Symmetrical analysis techniques for genetic systems and bioinformatics: Advanced patterns and applications* (pp. 1-290). doi:10.4018/978-1-60566-124-7

Pino, E., Curtis, D., Stair, T., & Ohno-Machado, L. (2010). SMART: mobile patient monitoring in an emergency department. In A. Coronato, & G. De Pietro (Eds.), *Pervasive and smart technologies for healthcare: Ubiquitous methodologies and tools* (pp. 97–113). Hershey, PA: Medical Information Science Reference. doi:10.4018/978-1-61520-765-7.ch005

Plunkett, D., Banerjee, R., & Horn, E. (2010). Supporting early childhood outcomes through assistive technology. In S. Seok, E. Meyen, & B. DaCosta (Eds.), *Handbook of research on human cognition and assistive technology: Design, accessibility and transdisciplinary perspectives* (pp. 339–359). Hershey, PA: Medical Information Science Reference. doi:10.4018/978-1-61520-817-3.ch024

Porto Pazos, A., Pazos Sierra, A., & Buño Buceta, W. (2009). *Advancing artificial intelligence through biological process applications* (pp. 1-460). doi:10.4018/978-1-59904-996-0

Prematilleke, M. N. (2010). The use of laboratory test results in health care management. In W. Pease, M. Cooper, & R. Gururajan (Eds.), *Biomedical knowledge management: Infrastructures and processes for E-Health systems* (pp. 204–216). Hershey, PA: Medical Information Science Reference. doi:10.4018/978-1-60566-266-4.ch014

Prince, V., & Roche, M. (2009). *Information retrieval in biomedicine: Natural language processing for knowledge integration* (pp. 1-460). doi:10.4018/978-1-60566-274-9

Puustjärvi, J., & Puustjärvi, L. (2010). Integrating medicinal learning objects with daily duties. In S. Mohammed, & J. Fiaidhi (Eds.), *Ubiquitous health and medical informatics: The ubiquity 2.0 trend and beyond* (pp. 150–165). Hershey, PA: Medical Information Science Reference. doi:10.4018/978-1-61520-777-0.ch008

Rada, R. (2008). *Information systems and healthcare enterprises* (pp. 1-380). doi:10.4018/978-1-59904-651-8

Ranerup, A. (2008). In what ways does Web technology support the individual in choice reforms in health care? A comparison among Norway, Denmark, and Sweden. *International Journal of Healthcare Information Systems and Informatics*, *3*(2), 48–68. doi:10.4018/jhisi.2008040105

Rao, P., Chandra, S., & Theng, Y. (2011). Adoption and usage of healthcare portals: Examining the factors influencing consumers' decisions. *International Journal of Organizational and Collective Intelligence*, *2*(3), 50–73. doi:10.4018/joci.2011070104

Rastogi, A., Daim, T., & Tan, J. (2008). Charting health information technology futures for healthcare services organizations. *International Journal of Healthcare Information Systems and Informatics*, *3*(1), 1–23. doi:10.4018/jhisi.2008010101

Reardon, J. L. (2009). Perceptions of an organizing vision for electronic medical records by independent physician practices. *International Journal of Healthcare Information Systems and Informatics*, *4*(3), 16–37. doi:10.4018/jhisi.2009070102

Reibling, N., & Wendt, C. (2011). Regulating patients' access to healthcare services. *International Journal of Public and Private Healthcare Management and Economics*, *1*(2), 1–16. doi:10.4018/ijpphme.2011040101

Reina, R., Cetani, T., Lacroce, A., & Ventura, M. (2012). A healthcare project: managing knowledge through electronic medical record -empirical cases. *International Journal of Information Systems in the Service Sector*, *4*(4), 1–19. doi:10.4018/jisss.2012100101

Rennard, J. (2007). *Handbook of research on nature-inspired computing for economics and management* (pp. 1–1066).

Rocha, Á. (2011). Evolution of information systems and technologies maturity in healthcare. *International Journal of Healthcare Information Systems and Informatics*, *6*(2), 28–36. doi:10.4018/jhisi.2011040103

Röcker, C., & Ziefle, M. (2011). *Smart healthcare applications and services: Developments and practices* (pp. 1-384). doi:10.4018/978-1-60960-180-5

Röcker, C., & Ziefle, M. (2011). *E-Health, assistive technologies and applications for assisted living: challenges and solutions* (pp. 1-392). doi:10.4018/978-1-60960-469-1

Rodrigues, J. J. (2010). Health information systems: Concepts, methodologies, tools, and applications (4 Volumes) (pp. 1-2456). doi: doi:10.4018/978-1-60566-988-5

Rodrigues, J. J. (2010). [IJEHMC]. *International Journal of E-Health and Medical Communications*. doi: doi:10.4018/IJEHMC

Rodrigues, J. J. (2012). Emerging communication technologies for E-. *Health & Medicine*, 1–378. doi: doi:10.4018/978-1-4666-0909-9

Rodrigues, J. J. (2013). *Digital advances in medicine, E-Health, and communication technologies* (pp. 1-348). doi:10.4018/978-1-4666-2794-9

Rodrigues, J. J. (2014). *Advancing medical practice through technology: Applications for healthcare delivery, management, and quality* (pp. 1-361). doi:10.4018/978-1-4666-4619-3

Rodrigues, J. J., de la Torre Díez, I., & Sainz de Abajo, B. (2012). *Telemedicine and E-Health services, policies, and applications: Advancements and developments* (pp. 1-572). doi:10.4018/978-1-4666-0888-7

Rodrigues-Filho, J., & Gomes, N. P. (2010). E-Health in Brazil: Less care for the poor? In W. Pease, M. Cooper, & R. Gururajan (Eds.), *Biomedical knowledge management: Infrastructures and processes for E-Health systems* (pp. 242–252). Hershey, PA: Medical Information Science Reference. doi:10.4018/978-1-60566-266-4.ch017

Rojo, M. G., & Daniel, C. (2010). Digital pathology and virtual microscopy integration in E-Health records. In S. Mohammed, & J. Fiaidhi (Eds.), *Ubiquitous health and medical informatics: The ubiquity 2.0 trend and beyond* (pp. 457–484). Hershey, PA: Medical Information Science Reference. doi:10.4018/978-1-61520-777-0.ch022

Rosiek, A. B. (2010). Integration of business and healthcare delivery processes: Case study on quality and clinical effectiveness of performance measurement in Polish healthcare. *International Journal of Healthcare Delivery Reform Initiatives*, *2*(3), 20–28. doi:10.4018/jhdri.2010070103

Rosiek, A. B., & Leksowski, K. (2011). Quality assurance and evaluation of healthcare reform initiatives: Strategy for improving the quality of health care services in public health care units, management model that allows the providing of high quality health care and efficient brand-building. *International Journal of Healthcare Delivery Reform Initiatives*, *3*(3), 42–53. doi:10.4018/jhdri.2011070104

Ross, S. (2011). A lexicon for user driven healthcare. *International Journal of User-Driven Healthcare*, *1*(1), 50–54. doi:10.4018/ijudh.2011010107

Sadr, S. S., Sadr, S. M., & Farahani, Y. G. (2013). Implication of E-Health and IT governance on healthcare expenditure: An econometrics approach (case study Middle East countries). *International Journal of Healthcare Information Systems and Informatics*, *8*(2), 58–69. doi:10.4018/jhisi.2013040105

Saito, M., Wickramasinghe, N., Fuji, M., & Geisler, E. (2010). Redesigning Innovative Healthcare Operation and the Role of Knowledge Management (pp. 1-322). doi:10.4018/978-1-60566-284-8

Sarnikar, S., Bennett, D., & Gaynor, M. (2013). *Cases on healthcare information technology for patient care management* (pp. 1-349). doi:10.4018/978-1-4666-2671-3

Sarnikar, S., & Murphy, M. (2012). A usability analysis framework for healthcare information technology. *International Journal of Technology Diffusion*, *3*(4), 20–28. doi:10.4018/jtd.2012100102

Seok, S., Meyen, E., & DaCosta, B. (2010). Handbook of research on human cognition and assistive technology: Design, accessibility and transdisciplinary perspectives (pp. 1-484). doi: doi:10.4018/978-1-61520-817-3

Shaban-Nejad, A., & Haarslev, V. (2010). Human factors in dynamic E-Health systems and digital libraries. In W. Pease, M. Cooper, & R. Gururajan (Eds.), *Biomedical knowledge management: Infrastructures and processes for E-Health systems* (pp. 192–203). Hershey, PA: Medical Information Science Reference. doi:10.4018/978-1-60566-266-4.ch013

Shachak, A., & Reis, S. (2010). The Computer-assisted patient consultation: Promises and challenges. In S. Kabene (Ed.), *Healthcare and the effect of technology: Developments, challenges and advancements* (pp. 72–83). Hershey, PA: Medical Information Science Reference. doi:10.4018/978-1-61520-733-6.ch005

Shah, G. H., Lertwachara, K., & Ayanso, A. (2010). New technology and implications for healthcare and public health: The Case of probabilistic record linkage. In S. Kabene (Ed.), *Healthcare and the effect of technology: Developments, challenges and advancements* (pp. 197–215). Hershey, PA: Medical Information Science Reference. doi:10.4018/978-1-61520-733-6.ch012

Shah, G. H., Lertwachara, K., & Ayanso, A. (2010). Record linkage in healthcare: Applications, opportunities, and challenges for public health. *International Journal of Healthcare Delivery Reform Initiatives*, *2*(3), 29–47. doi:10.4018/jhdri.2010070104

Shanmuganathan, S. (2010). A stroke information system (SIS), critical issues and solutions. In W. Pease, M. Cooper, & R. Gururajan (Eds.), *Biomedical knowledge management: Infrastructures and processes for E-Health systems* (pp. 177–191). Hershey, PA: Medical Information Science Reference. doi:10.4018/978-1-60566-266-4.ch012

Shukla, A., & Tiwari, R. (2010). *Intelligent medical technologies and biomedical engineering: Tools and applications* (pp. 1-376). doi:10.4018/978-1-61520-977-4

Shukla, A., & Tiwari, R. (2011). *Biomedical engineering and information systems: Technologies, tools and applications* (pp. 1-384). doi:10.4018/978-1-61692-004-3

Sicilia, M. Á., & Balazote, P. (2013). *Interoperability in healthcare information systems: Standards, management, and technology* (pp. 1-355). doi:10.4018/978-1-4666-3000-0

Siddiqi, S., & Lee, R. E. (2010). Building virtual communities for health promotion emerging best practices through an analysis of the international health challenge & related literature in second life. In S. Mohammed, & J. Fiaidhi (Eds.), *Ubiquitous health and medical informatics: The ubiquity 2.0 trend and beyond* (pp. 412–430). Hershey, PA: Medical Information Science Reference. doi:10.4018/978-1-61520-777-0.ch020

Slotznick, B. (2010). Point-and-Chat®: Instant messaging for AAC users. In S. Seok, E. Meyen, & B. DaCosta (Eds.), *Handbook of research on human cognition and assistive technology: Design, accessibility and transdisciplinary perspectives* (pp. 169–178). Hershey, PA: Medical Information Science Reference. doi:10.4018/978-1-61520-817-3.ch011

Smith, A. C., & Edirippulige, S. (2010). Extending health services to rural communities: Telepediatrics in Queensland. In S. Kabene (Ed.), *Healthcare and the effect of technology: Developments, challenges and advancements* (pp. 101–111). Hershey, PA: Medical Information Science Reference. doi:10.4018/978-1-61520-733-6.ch007

Smith, A. D. (2012). RFID practices for competitive inventory management systems: Case studies in healthcare and voice-recognition industries. *International Journal of Knowledge-Based Organizations, 2*(3), 47–62. doi:10.4018/ijkbo.2012070103

Sobol, M., & Prater, E. (2011). Adoption, usage and efficiency: Benchmarking healthcare IT in private practices. *International Journal of Healthcare Information Systems and Informatics, 6*(1), 36–50. doi:10.4018/jhisi.2011010103

Sorwar, G., & Murugesan, S. (2010). Electronic medical prescription: An overview of current status and issues. In W. Pease, M. Cooper, & R. Gururajan (Eds.), *Biomedical knowledge management: Infrastructures and processes for E-Health systems* (pp. 61–81). Hershey, PA: Medical Information Science Reference. doi:10.4018/978-1-60566-266-4.ch005

Spil, A. M., Le, T., Rouge, C., Trimmer, K., & Wiggins, C. (2009). IT adoption and evaluation in healthcare: Evolutions and insights in theory, methodology, and practice. *International Journal of Healthcare Information Systems and Informatics, 4*(3), 69–96. doi:10.4018/jhisi.2009070105

Spil, T., & Schuring, R. (2006). *E-Health systems diffusion and use: The innovation, the user and the use IT model* (pp. 1-342). doi:10.4018/978-1-59140-423-1

Spil, T., & Stegwee, R. (2001). *Strategies for healthcare information systems* (pp. 1-232). doi:10.4018/978-1-878289-89-6

Sriraam, N. (2012). [IJBCE]. *International Journal of Biomedical and Clinical Engineering*. doi: doi:10.4018/IJBCE

Stachowiak, J. R., & Estrada-Hernández, N. (2010). Improving assistive technology training in teacher education programs: The Iowa model. In S. Seok, E. Meyen, & B. DaCosta (Eds.), *Handbook of research on human cognition and assistive technology: Design, accessibility and transdisciplinary perspectives* (pp. 286–298). Hershey, PA: Medical Information Science Reference. doi:10.4018/978-1-61520-817-3.ch019

Staudinger, B., Höß, V., & Ostermann, H. (2009). *Nursing and clinical informatics: Socio-technical approaches* (pp. 1-340). doi:10.4018/978-1-60566-234-3

Stingl, C., & Slamanig, D. (2010). Privacy enhancing technologies in electronic health records. In S. Mohammed, & J. Fiaidhi (Eds.), *Ubiquitous health and medical informatics: The ubiquity 2.0 trend and beyond* (pp. 275–295). Hershey, PA: Medical Information Science Reference. doi:10.4018/978-1-61520-777-0.ch014

Suganuma, T., Sugawara, K., Kinoshita, T., Hattori, F., & Shiratori, N. (2009). Concept of symbiotic computing and its agent-based application to a ubiquitous care-support service. *International Journal of Cognitive Informatics and Natural Intelligence*, *3*(1), 34–56. doi:10.4018/jcini.2009010103

Szewczak, E. J., & Snodgrass, C. R. (2009). business associates in the national health information network: Implications for medical information privacy. *International Journal of E-Business Research*, *5*(2), 48–62. doi:10.4018/jebr.2009040103

Tafa, Z. (2010). Sensor networks in pervasive healthcare computing. *International Journal of Advanced Pervasive and Ubiquitous Computing*, *2*(3), 1–20. doi:10.4018/japuc.2010070101

Tamura, T., Mizukura, I., Kimura, Y., & Tatsumi, H. (2010). Designing pervasive healthcare applications in the home. In A. Coronato, & G. De Pietro (Eds.), *Pervasive and smart technologies for healthcare: Ubiquitous methodologies and tools* (pp. 282–294). Hershey, PA: Medical Information Science Reference. doi:10.4018/978-1-61520-765-7.ch013

Tan, J. (2006). [IJHISI]. *International Journal of Healthcare Information Systems and Informatics*. doi: doi:10.4018/IJHISI

Tan, J. (2008). *Healthcare information systems and informatics: Research and practices* (pp. 1-448). doi:10.4018/978-1-59904-690-7

Tan, J. (2009). Medical informatics: Concepts, methodologies, tools, and applications (4 Volumes) (pp. 1-2772). doi: doi:10.4018/978-1-60566-050-9

Tan, J. (2011). *Developments in healthcare information systems and technologies: Models and methods* (pp. 1-398). doi:10.4018/978-1-61692-002-9

Tan, J. (2011). *New technologies for advancing healthcare and clinical* practices (pp. 1-472). doi:10.4018/978-1-60960-780-7

Tan, J. (2012). *Advancing technologies and intelligence in healthcare and clinical environments breakthroughs* (pp. 1-382). doi:10.4018/978-1-4666-1755-1

Tan, J. (2013). *Healthcare information technology innovation and sustainability: Frontiers and adoption* (pp. 1-355). doi:10.4018/978-1-4666-2797-0

Tara, M. (2010). Semantic Web architecture to provide E-Health content and services. In S. Mohammed, & J. Fiaidhi (Eds.), *Ubiquitous health and medical informatics: The ubiquity 2.0 trend and beyond* (pp. 233–257). Hershey, PA: Medical Information Science Reference. doi:10.4018/978-1-61520-777-0.ch012

Tashiro, J. S. (2009). Ethical analysis of publisher and faculty roles in building and using electronic educational products. *Journal of Electronic Commerce in Organizations*, *7*(1), 1–17. doi:10.4018/jeco.2009010101

Temel, T. (2011). *System and circuit design for biologically-inspired intelligent learning* (pp. 1-412). doi:10.4018/978-1-60960-018-1

Tentori, M., González, V. M., & Favela, J. (2010). Lessons from evaluating ubiquitous applications in support of hospital work. In A. Coronato, & G. De Pietro (Eds.), *Pervasive and smart technologies for healthcare: Ubiquitous methodologies and tools* (pp. 228–250). Hershey, PA: Medical Information Science Reference. doi:10.4018/978-1-61520-765-7.ch011

Tong, C. K., & Wong, E. T. (2009). Governance of picture archiving and communications systems: Data security and quality management of filmless radiology (pp. 1-366). doi:10.4018/978-1-59904-672-3

Topacan, U., Basoglu, A. N., & Daim, T. U. (2010). exploring the adoption of technology driven services in the healthcare industry. *International Journal of Information Systems in the Service Sector*, *2*(1), 71–93. doi:10.4018/jisss.2010093005

Topps, D. (2010). Academic family health teams collaborative lessons from the far flung north. In S. Mohammed, & J. Fiaidhi (Eds.), *Ubiquitous health and medical informatics: The ubiquity 2.0 trend and beyond* (pp. 350–369). Hershey, PA: Medical Information Science Reference. doi:10.4018/978-1-61520-777-0.ch017

Torkestani, S. S., Sahuguede, S., Julien-Vergonjanne, A., Cances, J., & Daviet, J. C. (2012). Infrared communication technology applied to indoor mobile healthcare monitoring system. *International Journal of E-Health and Medical Communications*, *3*(3), 1–11. doi:10.4018/jehmc.2012070101

Turchetti, G., & Geisler, E. (2010). Economic and organizational factors in the future of telemedicine and home care. In A. Coronato, & G. De Pietro (Eds.), *Pervasive and smart technologies for healthcare: Ubiquitous methodologies and tools* (pp. 322–335). Hershey, PA: Medical Information Science Reference. doi:10.4018/978-1-61520-765-7.ch015

Übeyli, E. D. (2010). Telemedicine and biotelemetry for E-Health systems: Theory and applications. In W. Pease, M. Cooper, & R. Gururajan (Eds.), *Biomedical knowledge management: Infrastructures and processes for E-Health systems* (pp. 1–17). Hershey, PA: Medical Information Science Reference. doi:10.4018/978-1-60566-266-4.ch001

Ukwandu, E., & Iro, S. (2013). E-Health solutions in rural healthcare in the Mbaise area of Imo state: Nigeria. *International Journal of E-Planning Research*, *2*(2), 40–44. doi:10.4018/ijepr.2013040103

van Ooijen, P., & Broekema, A. (2010). Incorporating radiological patient data acquired at other hospitals into the local workflow. In W. Pease, M. Cooper, & R. Gururajan (Eds.), *Biomedical knowledge management: Infrastructures and processes for E-Health systems* (pp. 118–133). Hershey, PA: Medical Information Science Reference. doi:10.4018/978-1-60566-266-4.ch009

von Lubitz, D. (2010). Healthcare among the people: Teams of leaders concept (ToL) and the world of technology-oriented global healthcare. In S. Kabene (Ed.), *Healthcare and the Effect of Technology: Developments, Challenges and Advancements* (pp. 145–177). Hershey, PA: Medical Information Science Reference. doi:10.4018/978-1-61520-733-6.ch010

Vouyioukas, D., & Maglogiannis, I. (2010). Communication issues in pervasive healthcare systems and applications. In A. Coronato, & G. De Pietro (Eds.), *Pervasive and smart technologies for healthcare: Ubiquitous methodologies and tools* (pp. 197–227). Hershey, PA: Medical Information Science Reference. doi:10.4018/978-1-61520-765-7.ch010

Wager, K. A. (2008). Assessing physician and nurse satisfaction with an ambulatory care EMR: One facility's approach. *International Journal of Healthcare Information Systems and Informatics*, *3*(1), 63–74. doi:10.4018/jhisi.2008010104

Wagner, C. L., & Delisi, J. (2010). Multi-sensory environments and augmentative communication tools. In S. Seok, E. Meyen, & B. DaCosta (Eds.), *Handbook of research on human cognition and assistive technology: design, accessibility and transdisciplinary perspectives* (pp. 121–131). Hershey, PA: Medical Information Science Reference. doi:10.4018/978-1-61520-817-3.ch008

Walczak, S., & Mann, R. (2010). Utilization and perceived benefit for diverse users of communities of practice in a healthcare organization. *Journal of Organizational and End User Computing*, *22*(4), 24–50. doi:10.4018/joeuc.2010100102

Wall, W. P. (2009). Developing global competitiveness in healthcare: A Thai healthcare organization's perspective. *International Journal of Information Systems in the Service Sector*, *1*(4), 61–72. doi:10.4018/jisss.2009062905

Walsh, M. J., Barton, J., O'Flynn, B., Hayes, M. J., O'Mathuna, C., & Alavi, S. M. (2011). An antiwindup approach to power controller switching in an ambient healthcare network. *International Journal of Ambient Computing and Intelligence*, *3*(2), 35–55. doi:10.4018/jaci.2011040103

Wan, Y., & Evans-Mueller, S. (2010). Health service quality information comparison: A preliminary investigation. In S. Kabene (Ed.), *Healthcare and the effect of technology: Developments, challenges and advancements* (pp. 112–122). Hershey, PA: Medical Information Science Reference. doi:10.4018/978-1-61520-733-6.ch008

Wang, J., Zhou, B., & Yan, R. (2012). Benefits and barriers in mining the healthcare industry data. *International Journal of Strategic Decision Sciences*, *3*(4), 51–67. doi:10.4018/jsds.2012100103

Wang, W., Zhao, M., Wang, H., & Hua, K. (2012). Exploring region of interest (ROI) to support quality of service in unreliable wireless electronic healthcare communications. *International Journal of Healthcare Information Systems and Informatics*, *7*(4), 1–12. doi:10.4018/jhisi.2012100101

Watfa, M. K. (2012). *E-Healthcare systems and wireless communications: Current and future challenges* (pp. 1-462). doi:10.4018/978-1-61350-123-8

Wei, J., Lin, B., & Loho-Noya, M. (2013). Development of an E-Healthcare information security risk assessment method. *Journal of Database Management*, *24*(1), 36–57. doi:10.4018/jdm.2013010103

West, G., Lazarescu, M., & Ou, M. (2010). Telederm: A Web-based decision support system for medical practitioners. In W. Pease, M. Cooper, & R. Gururajan (Eds.), *Biomedical knowledge management: Infrastructures and processes for E-Health systems* (pp. 154–176). Hershey, PA: Medical Information Science Reference. doi:10.4018/978-1-60566-266-4.ch011

Whitaker, R. (2011). securing health-effective medicine in practice: A critical perspective on user-driven healthcare. *International Journal of User-Driven Healthcare*, *1*(2), 1–15. doi:10.4018/ijudh.2011040101

Wickramasinghe, N. (2010). The role for knowledge management in modern healthcare delivery. *International Journal of Healthcare Delivery Reform Initiatives*, *2*(2), 1–9. doi:10.4018/jhdri.2010040101

Wickramasinghe, N., & Bali, R. K. (2009). The S'ANT imperative for realizing the vision of healthcare network centric operations. *International Journal of Actor-Network Theory and Technological Innovation*, *1*(1), 45–58. doi:10.4018/jantti.2009010103

Wickramasinghe, N., Chalasani, S., Goldberg, S., & Koritala, S. (2012). The benefits of wireless enabled applications to facilitate superior healthcare delivery: The case of DiaMonD. *International Journal of E-Health and Medical Communications*, *3*(4), 15–30. doi:10.4018/jehmc.2012100102

Wickramasinghe, N., & Geisler, E. (2008). *Encyclopedia of healthcare information systems* (pp. 1–1566). doi:10.4018/978-1-59904-889-5

Wickramasinghe, N., Gupta, J. N., & Sharma, S. (2005). *Creating knowledge-based healthcare organizations* (pp. 1-388). doi:10.4018/978-1-59140-459-0

Wickramasinghe, N., Troshani, I., & Goldberg, S. (2010). An investigation into the use of pervasive wireless technologies to support diabetes self-care. In A. Coronato, & G. De Pietro (Eds.), *Pervasive and smart technologies for healthcare: Ubiquitous methodologies and tools* (pp. 114–129). Hershey, PA: Medical Information Science Reference. doi:10.4018/978-1-61520-765-7.ch006

Wiljer, D., Urowitz, S., & Jones, E. (2010). Personal health information in the age of ubiquitous health. In S. Mohammed, & J. Fiaidhi (Eds.), *Ubiquitous health and medical informatics: The ubiquity 2.0 trend and beyond* (pp. 166–189). Hershey, PA: Medical Information Science Reference. doi:10.4018/978-1-61520-777-0.ch009

Wilson, E. (2009). *Patient-centered E-Health* (pp. 1-300). doi:10.4018/978-1-60566-016-5

Wilson, M. S., & Pascoe, J. (2010). Using software to deliver language intervention in inclusionary settings. In S. Seok, E. Meyen, & B. DaCosta (Eds.), *Handbook of research on human cognition and assistive technology: Design, accessibility and transdisciplinary perspectives* (pp. 132–156). Hershey, PA: Medical Information Science Reference. doi:10.4018/978-1-61520-817-3.ch009

Woodside, J. M., & Sikder, I. U. (2009). Space-time cluster analysis: Application of healthcare service data in epidemiological studies. *International Journal of Healthcare Information Systems and Informatics*, *4*(4), 69–82. doi:10.4018/jhisi.2009071005

Wu, J. (2011). *Early detection and rehabilitation technologies for dementia: Neuroscience and biomedical applications* (pp. 1-480). doi:10.4018/978-1-60960-559-9

Wu, J. (2013). *Biomedical engineering and cognitive neuroscience for healthcare: Interdisciplinary applications* (pp. 1-472). doi:10.4018/978-1-4666-2113-8

Wu, J. (2013). *Technological advancements in biomedicine for healthcare applications* (pp. 1-382). doi:10.4018/978-1-4666-2196-1

Wu, R., Ahn, G., & Hu, H. (2012). Towards HIPAA-compliant healthcare systems in cloud computing. *International Journal of Computational Models and Algorithms in Medicine*, *3*(2), 1–22. doi:10.4018/jcmam.2012040101

Xie, S., Xiao, Y., & Chen, H. (2010). Nursing home. In A. Coronato, & G. De Pietro (Eds.), *Pervasive and smart technologies for healthcare: Ubiquitous methodologies and tools* (pp. 39–77). Hershey, PA: Medical Information Science Reference. doi:10.4018/978-1-61520-765-7.ch003

Yamamoto, S. (2010). IT applications for medical services in Japan. In W. Pease, M. Cooper, & R. Gururajan (Eds.), *Biomedical knowledge management: Infrastructures and processes for E-Health systems* (pp. 327–336). Hershey, PA: Medical Information Science Reference. doi:10.4018/978-1-60566-266-4.ch024

Yu, J., Guo, C., & Kim, M. (2008). Developing a user centered model for ubiquitous healthcare system implementation: An empirical study. *International Journal of Healthcare Information Systems and Informatics*, *3*(3), 58–76. doi:10.4018/jhisi.2008070104

Yu, W. D., Adiga, A. S., Rao, S., & Panakkel, M. J. (2012). A SOA based system development methodology for cloud computing environment: Using uHealthcare as practice. *International Journal of E-Health and Medical Communications*, *3*(4), 42–63. doi:10.4018/jehmc.2012100104

Yu, W. D., Patel, J., Mehta, V., & Joshi, A. (2012). An approach to design a SOA services governance architecture for an u-healthcare system with mobility. *International Journal of E-Health and Medical Communications*, *3*(2), 36–65. doi:10.4018/jehmc.2012040103

Zgodavová, K., & Bourek, A. (2012). Potential of WEB based learning in managing for the sustained success of a healthcare organization based on IMPROHEALTH® Project. *International Journal of Reliable and Quality E-Healthcare*, *1*(2), 12–28. doi:10.4018/ijrqeh.2012040102

Ziefle, M., & Röcker, C. (2011). *Human-centered design of E-Health technologies: Concepts, methods and applications* (pp. 1-426). doi:10.4018/978-1-60960-177-5

Compilation of References

Abbas, A. (2003). *Grid computing: A practical guide to technology and applications*. Hingham, MA: Charles River Media. *AFS file system.* (2013). Retrieved from: http://lxr.linux.no/linux/Documentation/filesystems/afs.txt

AECC. (2011). *Estrategia contra el cáncer del Sistema Nacional de Salud. Ministerio de Sanidad y Consumo*. Retrieved from https://www.aecc.es/SobreElCancer/bibliotecadedocumentos/Paginas/estrategiacontraelcancer.aspx

AHRQ. (n. d.). *Agency for Healthcare Research and Quality*. Retrieved December 20, 2009, from http://www.ahrq.gov/.

Akman, V., & Surav, M. (1996). Steps toward formalizing context. *AI Magazine*, *17*(3), 55–72.

Akyildiz, I. F., Weilian, Su, Sankarasubramaniam, Y., & Cayirci, E. (2002). A survey on sensor network. *IEEE Communications Magazine*, *40*, 102–114. doi:10.1109/MCOM.2002.1024422

Amendolia, S. R. (2007). Mammogrid - A prototype distributed mammographic database for Europe. *Clinical Radiology*, *62*, 1044–1051. doi:10.1016/j.crad.2006.09.032 PMID:17920862

Analyti, A., Antoniou, G., & Damasio, C. V. (2008). A principled framework for modular Web rule bases and its semantics. In G. Brewka & J. Lang (Eds.), *Principles of Knowledge Representation and Reasoning: Proceedings of the Eleventh International Conference, KR 2008*. Sydney, Australia, (pp. 390–400). AAAI Press.

Analyti, A., Antoniou, G., Damasio, C. V., & Wagner, G. (2004). Negation and negative information in the W3C resource description framework. *Annals of Mathematics. Computing and Teleinformatics*, *2*, 25–34.

Analyti, A., Antoniou, G., Damasio, C. V., & Wagner, G. (2008). Extended RDF as a semantic foundation of rule markup languages. *Journal of Artificial Intelligence Research*, *32*, 37–94.

Angulo, C., Crespo, P., Maldonado, J. A., Moner, D., Pérez, D., & Abad, I. et al. (2007). Non-invasive lightweight integration engine for building EHR from autonomous distributed systems. *International Journal of Medical Informatics*, *76*(Suppl 3), S417–S424. doi:10.1016/j.ijmedinf.2007.05.002 PMID:17600763

ANSI American National Standards Institute. (2003). *HL7 messaging standard version 2.5*. Retrieved June, 2010, from http://webstore.ansi.org/FindStandards.aspx?Action=displaydept&DeptID=3104&Acro=HL7&DpName=HL7:%20Health%20Level%20Seven&source=google&adgroup=hl7&keyword=hl7%20standard&gclid=CJ6Vm8Gv_aICFZUA4wode3pXnA

AQL . (n. d.). Retrieved November 2013, from http://www.openehr.org/wiki/display/spec/Archetype+Query+Language+Description

Arcstyler. (n. d.). *Interactive objects*. Retrieved December 20, 2009 from http://www.interactive-objects.com/

Arduini, F., & Morabito, V. (2010). Business continuity and the banking industry. *Communications of the ACM*, *53*(3), 121–125. doi:10.1145/1666420.1666452

Argüello, M., & Des, J. J. (2008). Clinical practice guidelines: A case study of combining OWL-S, OWL, and SWRL. *Knowledge-Based Systems*, *21*(3), 247–255. doi:10.1016/j.knosys.2007.11.008

Ashburner, M., Ball, C. A., Blake, J. A., Botstein, D., Butler, H., & Cherry, J. M. et al. (2000). Gene ontology: Tool for the unification of biology. *Nature Genetics*, *25*(1), 25–29. doi:10.1038/75556 PMID:10802651

Ash, J. S., Sittig, D. F., Poon, E. G., Guappone, K., Campbell, E., & Dykstra, R. H. (2007). The extent and importance of unintended consequences related to computerized provider order entry. *Journal of the American Medical Informatics Association*, *14*, 415–423. doi:10.1197/jamia.M2373 PMID:17460127

Aspden, P. (2004). *Patient safety: Achieving a new standard for care. Committee on Data Standards for Patient Safety, Institute of Medicine*. U.S.: National Academies Press.

Australia National E-Health Transition Authority. (2010). Retrieved June 20, 2010, from http://www.nehta.gov.au/

Avison, D., & Young, T. (2007). Time to rethink health care and ICT? *Communications of the ACM*, *50*(6), 69–74. doi:10.1145/1247001.1247008

Baader, F., Calvanese, D., McGuinness, D., Nardi, D., & Patel-Schneider, P. (2003). *The description logic handbook: Theory, implementation, and applications*. New York, NY: Cambridge University Press.

Bail, S., Parsia, B., & Sattler, U. (2010). JustBench: A framework for OWL benchmarking. *The Semantic Web–ISWC*, *2010*, 32–47.

Bangalore, A., Thorn, K. E., Tilley, C., & Peters, L. (2003). The UMLS knowledge source server: An object model for delivering UMLS data. *AMIA Annual Symposium Proceedings 2003* (Vol. 2003, pp. 51-55). Presented at the AMIA Annual Symposium.

Baseline Services Working Group . (2013). Retrieved from http://lcg.web.cern.ch/LCG/peb/BS

Beale, T. (1999). The GEHR software architecture for a reliable EHR. *Toward an Electronic Health Record Europe*, *99*, 328–339.

Beale, T. (2002). Archetypes: Constraint-based domain models for future-proof information systems. In OOPSLA 2002 workshop on Behavioural Semantics (pp. 1–18).

Beale, T. (2007). *The openEHR archetype object model*. The openEHR Foundation.

Beale, T., & Heard, S. (2007). *Archetype definitions and principles*. The openEHR Foundation. Retrieved from http://www.openehr.org/releases/1.0.2/architecture/am/archetype_principles.pdf

Beale, T., & Heard, S. (2008). *The openEHR archetype definition language*. The openEHR Foundation. Retrieved from http://www.openehr.org/releases/1.0.2/architecture/am/adl.pdf

Beale, T., Heard, S., Kalra, D., & Lloyd, D. (2008). *The openEHR EHR information model*. The openEHR Foundation. Retrieved from http://www.openehr.org/releases/1.0.2/architecture/rm/ehr_im.pdf

Beale, T., Heard, S., Kalra, D., Lloyd, D., & Schloeffel, P. (2006). *Introducing openEHR* (No. Technical Report 1.1). The openEHR Foundation.

Benson, T. (2010). Why interoperability is hard. In *Principles of health interoperability HL7 and SNOMED* (pp. 25–34). London: Springer-Verlag London Ltd. doi:10.1007/978-1-84882-803-2_2

Bergenti, F., & Poggi, A. (2009). *Multi-agent systems for e-Health: Recent projects and initiatives*. Paper presented at the Tenth National Workshop From Objects to Agents (WOA 2009), Parma Italy.

Berg, M., & Toussaint, P. (2003). The mantra of modeling and the forgotten powers of paper: A sociotechnical view on the development of process-oriented ICT in health care. *International Journal of Medical Informatics*, *69*, 223–234. doi:10.1016/S1386-5056(02)00178-8 PMID:12810126

Bergman, M. K. The deep Web: Surfacing hidden value. *Journal of Electronic Publishing*. Retrieved December 8, 2009, from http://www.brightplanet.com/pdf/deepwebwhitepaper.pdf

Berler, D. K. A., & Pavlopoulos, S. (2004). *Design of an interoperability framework in a regional healthcare system*. Paper presented at the 26th Annual International Conference of the IEEE Engineering in Medicine and Biology Society (IEMBS '04), San Francisco, CA.

Berners-Lee, T. B. (2006). *Linked data*. Retrieved February 15, 2011, from http://www.w3.org/DesignIssues/LinkedData.html

Berners-Lee, T., & Kagal, L. (2008). On the semantics of linking and importing in modular ontologies. In I. F. Cruz, S. Decker, D. Allemang, C. Preist, D.Schwabe, P. Mika, M. Uschold, & L. Aroyo (Eds.), *The Semantic Web - ISWC 2006, 5th International Semantic Web Conference, ISWC 2006. Athens, GA, Proceedings (Lecture Notes in Computer Science, 4273).* (pp. 72–86). Germany: Springer-Verlag.

Berners-Lee, T. B., Hendler, J., & Lassila, O. (2001). The semantic web. *Scientific American*, *284*(5), 34–43. doi:10.1038/scientificamerican0501-34 PMID:11396337

Béziau, J.-Y., Carnielli, W., & Gabbay, D. M. (2007). *Handbook of paraconsistency*. College Publications.

Bicer, V., Kilic, O., Dogac, A., & Laleci, G. B. (2005). Archetype-based semantic interoperability of web service messages in the health care domain. *International Journal on Semantic Web and Information Systems*, *1*(4), 1–23. doi:10.4018/jswis.2005100101

Bicer, V., Laleci, G. B., Dogac, A., & Kabak, Y. (2005). Artemis message exchange framework: Semantic interoperability of exchanged messages in the healthcare domain.[ACM Special Interest Group on Management of Data]. *SIGMOD Record*, *34*(3), 71–76. doi:10.1145/1084805.1084819

Bilgic, M., Licamele, L., Getoor, L., & Shneiderman, B. (2006). D-Dupe: an interactive tool for entity resolution in social networks. *Visual Analytics Science and Technology*. Retrieved December 8, 2009 from http://waimea.cs.umd.edu:8080/basilic/web/Publications/2006/bilgic:vast06/

Biomedical Informatics Research Network (USA BIRN). (2013). Retrieved from http://www.nbirn.net

Blobel, B. (2006). Advanced and secure architectural EHR approaches. *International Journal of Medical Informatics*, *75*(3-4), 185–190. doi:10.1016/j.ijmedinf.2005.07.017 PMID:16112891

Bodenreider, O. (2004). The Unified Medical Language System (UMLS), integrating biomedical terminology. *Nucleic Acids Research*, *32*(90001), 267D–270. doi:10.1093/nar/gkh061 PMID:14681409

Booth, N. (2003). Sharing patient information electronically throughout the NHS. *British Medical Journal*, *327*(7407), 114–115. doi:10.1136/bmj.327.7407.114 PMID:12869425

Borgida, A., & Serafini, L. (2003). Distributed description logics: Assimilating information from peer sources. *Journal on Data Semantics*, *1*, 153–184.

Bouquet, P., Giunchiglia, F., van Harmelen, F., Serafini, L., & Stuckenschmidt, H. (2003). C-OWL: contextualizing ontologies. In D. Fensel, K. P. Sycara, & J. Mylopoulos (Eds.), *The Semantic Web - ISWC 2003, Second International Semantic Web Conference, Sanibel Island, FL. Proceedings (Lecture Notes in Computer Science, 2870).* (pp. 164–179). Germany: Springer-Verlag.

Bouquet, P., Giunchiglia, F., van Harmelen, F., Serafini, L., & Stuckenschmidt, H. (2004). Contextualizing ontologies. *Journal of Web Semantics*, *1*(4), 325–343. doi:10.1016/j.websem.2004.07.001

BPMI. (n. d.). *Business Process Management Initiative*. Retrieved December 8, 2009 from http://www.bpmi.org/

Bramley, R., Chiu, K., Huffman, J. C., Huffman, K., & McMullen, D. F. (2003). *Instruments and sensors as network services: Making instruments first class members of the grid* (Technical Report 588). Indiana University Computer Science Department.

Breton, V., Dean, K., & Solomonides, T. (2005). From grid to healthgrid: The healthgrid white paper. In *Proceedings of Healthgrid Conference* (pp. 249-321). Amsterdam, The Netherlands: IOS Press.

Breton, V., Dean, K., Solomonides, T., Blanquer, I., Hernandez, V., & Medico, E. … Herveg, J. A. (2004). The healthgrid white paper. Studies in Health Technology and Informatics, *112*, 249-321.

Brewster, C., & O'Hara, K. (2007). Knowledge representation with ontologies: Present challenges-future possibilities. *Journal of Human-Computer Studies*, *65*(7), 563–688. doi:10.1016/j.ijhcs.2007.04.003

Brickley, D., & Guha, R. V. (2004*). Description Language 1.0: RDF Schema, W3C Recommendation.* Paper presented at the World Wide Web Consortium (W3C).

Brickley, D., & Miller, L. (2007). *The Friend Of A Friend (FOAF) vocabulary specification.* Retrieved from http://xmlns.com/foaf/spec/ http://xmlns.com/foaf/spec/

Browne, E. D. (2005). *Workflow modelling of coordinated inter. health-provider care plans* (Unpublished doctoral dissertation). School of Computer and Information Science, University of South Australia, Adelaide.

Buhler, P. A., & Vidal, J. M. (2005). Towards adaptive workflow enactment using multiagent systems. *Information Technology Management*, *6*(1), 61–87. doi:10.1007/s10799-004-7775-2

Buyya, R., Date, S., Mizuno-Matsumoto, Y., Venugopal, S., & Abramson, D. (2003). Composition and on-demand deployment of distributed brain activity analysis application on global grids. In *10th Proceedings of the International Conference on High Performance Computing (HiPC)* (pp.1-10). New Delhi, India: Elite Publishing House.

Caire, G., Gotta, D., & Banzi, M. (2008). *WADE: A software platform to develop mission critical applications exploiting agents and workflows.* Paper presented at the 7th International Conference on Autonomous Agents and Multiagent Systems - Industry and Applications Track (AAMAS 2008), Estoril, Portugal.

Calvanese, D., Franconi, E., Haarslev, V., Lembo, D., Motik, B., Tessaris, S., & Turhan, A.-Y. (Eds.). (2007). *Proceedings of the 20th International Workshop on Description Logics DL'07.* Brixen/Bressanone, Italy: Bolzano University Press.

Campbell, E. M., Sittig, D. F., Ash, J. S., Guappone, K. P., & Dykstra, R. H. (2006). Types of unintended consequences related to computerized provider order entry. *Journal of the American Medical Informatics Association*, *13*, 547–556. doi:10.1197/jamia.M2042 PMID:16799128

Canada Health Infoway. (2010) Retrieved June 27, 2010, from http://www.infoway-inforoute.ca/lang-en/

CAP. (n. d.). College of American Pathologists. Retrieved December 8, 2009 from http://www.cap.org/apps/cap.portal

Carroll, J. J., Bizer, C., Hayes, P. J., & Stickler, P. (2007). Named graphs, provenance and trust. In A. Ellis & T. Hagino (Eds.), *Proceedings of the 14th International Conference on World Wide Web, WWW 2005,* (pp. 613–622). ACM Press.

Carroll, J. J., & Pan, J. Z. (2006). *XML schema datatypes in RDF and OWL (No. Note NOTE-swbp-xsch-datatypes-20060314).* World Wide Web Consortium.

CEN/ISSS eHealth Focus Group. (2005). *Report from the CEN/ISSS eHealth Standardization Focus Group: Current and Future Standardization Issues in the eHealth Domain: Achieving Interoperability.* Retrieved June, 2010, from ftp://ftp.cen.eu/CEN/Sectors/List/ICT/FocusGroups/eHealthStandardizationExsummaryFinal.pdf.

CEN/TC 251 (TC251). (n. d.). Retrieved November 2013, from http://www.centc251.org

CEN/TC251, (2007). *ISO/CD12967-2-prEN12967-2 HISA information view.* Retrieved February, 2009, from http://www.google.gr/url?sa=t&source=web&cd=1&ved=0CBYQFjAA&url=http%3A%2F%2Fwww.kith.no%2Fupload%2F4120%2FISOTC215_pCD_12967-2_HISA-20070208.doc&ei=XpIzTe2hDYfMswb3_KyTCg&usg=AFQjCNE3OTP0sJou6b04AB3dD5GGg-0zs7g.

Cerri, D., & Corcoglioniti, F. (2009). Bridging the gap between user attributes and service policies with attribute mapping. In *Proceedings of the 2009 IEEE Conference on Commerce and Enterprise Computing* (pp. 154-161). IEEE Computer Society.

Cerri, D., Della Valle, E., de Francisco Marcos, D., Giunchiglia, F., Naor, D., Nixon, L., et al. (2008). Towards knowledge in the cloud. In On the move to meaningful internet systems: OTM 2008 Workshops, LNCS 5333 (pp. 986–995). Springer.

Chen, C., Chen, K., Hsu, C. Y., & Li, Y. C. (2010). Developing guideline-based decision support systems using protégé and jess. Computer Methods and Programs in Biomedicine. In Press, Corrected Proof. doi: doi:10.1016/j.cmpb.2010.05.010

Chen, R., & Klein, G. (2007). The openEHR Java reference implementation project. *Studies in Health Technology and Informatics*, *129*(1), 58–62. PMID:17911678

Chesnevar, C. I., Maguitman, A. G., & Loui, R. P. (2000). Logical models of argument. *ACM Computing Surveys*, *32*(4), 337–383. doi:10.1145/371578.371581

Choi, B. C. K. (2005). Understanding the basic principles of knowledge translation. *Journal of Epidemiology and Community Health*, *59*(2), 93. PMID:15650137

Christiaens, S. 2006. Metadata mechanisms: From ontology to folksonomy..., & back. In OTM Workshops (1), 199-207.

Chute, C. G. (2000). Clinical classification and terminology: Some history and current observations. *Journal of the American Medical Informatics Association*, *7*, 298–303. doi:10.1136/jamia.2000.0070298 PMID:10833167

CLEF-integrating information for the clinical E-Scientist . (2013). Retrieved from: http://www.clinical-escience.org

Cohen, U. (n. d.). *Inside Gigaspaces XAP – Technical overview and value proposition* (GigaSpaces Technical White Paper). Retrieved from http://www.gigaspaces.com/WhitePapers.

Cohen, F. (2002). *Understanding Web service interoperability*. IBM Technical Library.

Coiera, E. 1997. *Guide to Medical informatics, the Internet and telemedicine* (1st ed.). A Hodder Arnold Publication, January 15.

Coiera, E., & Hovenga, E. J. S. (2007). Building a sustainable health system. *IMIA: Yearbook Medical Informatics*, *2*(1), 11–18. PMID:17700898

Collen, M. F., Van Brunt, E. E., & Davis, L. S. (1976). Problems of computerization of large computer medical record systems. *Informatics for Health & Social Care*, *1*(1), 47–53. doi:10.3109/14639237609017803

Commission of the European Communities. (2004). *e-Health - Making healthcare better for European citizens: An action plan for a European e-Health area*. Communication from the Commission to the Council, the European Parliament, the European Economic and Social Committee and the Committee of the Regions. COM (2004) 356 final. Retrieved from http://eur-lex.europa.eu/LexUriServ/LexUriServ.do?uri=CELEX:52004DC0356:EN:NOT

Cormen, T. H., Leiserson, C. E., Rivest, R. L., & Stein, C. (1990). *Introduction to algorithms*. NEw York: McGraw-Hill Companies.

Cristani, M., & Cuel, R. (2005). A survey on ontology creation methodologies. *International Journal on Semantic Web and Information Systems*, *1*(2), 49–69. doi:10.4018/jswis.2005040103

Crossbow Technology, Inc. (2003). Mote in network programming user reference (Technical Report). Berkeley WEbS.

CRS-SISS. (n. d.). *Carta regionale dei servizi – Sistema informativo socio-sanitario*. Retrieved from http://www.crs.lombardia.it/

Czajkowski, K., Ferguson, D., Foster, I., Frey, J., Graham, S., & Maquire, T. et al. (2004). *From open grid services infrastructure to WSResource framework: Refactoring & evolution*. IBM DeveloperWorks.

Day, J. D., Fukushima, T., & Giannotta, S. L. (1997). Cranial base approaches to posterior circulation aneurysms. *Journal of Neurosurgery*, *87*(4), 544–554. doi:10.3171/jns.1997.87.4.0544 PMID:9322845

Dazzi, L., Fassino, C., & Saracco, R. Quaglini, S., & Stefanelli, Mario. (n.d.). A patient workflow management system built on guidelines. *Consorzio di Bioingegneria e Informatica Medica, Pavia, Italy*. Retrieved December 8, 2009 from http://www2.amia.org/pubs/symposia/D004083.PDF

Dogac, A., Bicer, V., & Okcan, A. (2006), Collaborative business process support in IHE XDS through ebXML business processes, In *Proceedings of the 22nd International Conference on Data Engineering ICDE '06*, p. 91.

Dogac, A., Namli, T., Okcan, A., Laleci, G., Kabak, Y., & Eichelberg, M. (n.d.). *Key issues of technical interoperability solutions in eHealth and the RIDE project.* Retrieved July, 2010, from http://ec.europa.eu/idabc/servlets/Doc?id=27836.

Dogac, A., Laleci, G. B., Kirbas, S., Kabak, Y., Sinir, S. S., Yildiz, A., & Gurcan, Y. (2006). Artemis: Deploying semantically enriched Web services in the healthcare domain. *Information Systems*, *31*(4-5), 321–339. doi:10.1016/j.is.2005.02.006

Dolin, H. R., Alschudler, L., Boyer, S., Beebe, C., Behlen, M. F., Biron, P.V., & Shabo, Amnon. (2006). HL7 clinical document, release 2. *Journal of American Informatics Association*. Retrieved November 20, 2009 from http://www.jamia.org/cgi/content/abstract/13/1/30

Dolin, R. H., Alschuler, L., Beebe, C., Biron, P. V., Boyer, S. L., & Essin, D. et al. (2001). The HL7 clinical document architecture. *Journal of the American Medical Informatics Association*, *8*(6), 552–569. doi:10.1136/jamia.2001.0080552 PMID:11687563

Dolin, R. H., Alschuler, L., Boyer, S., Beebe, C., Behlen, F. M., Biron, P. V., & Shvo, A. S. (2006). HL7 clinical document architecture, release 2. *Journal of the American Medical Informatics Association*, *13*(1), 30–39. doi:10.1197/jamia.M1888 PMID:16221939

Donini, F. M., Nardi, D., & Rosati, R. (2002). Description logics of minimal knowledge and negation as failure. *ACM Transactions on Computational Logic*, *3*(2), 177–225. doi:10.1145/505372.505373

Dorr, D. A., Jones, S. S., & Wilcox, A. (2007). A framework for information system usage in collaborative care. *Journal of Biomedical Informatics*, *40*, 282–287. doi:10.1016/j.jbi.2006.10.001 PMID:17097927

Downing, G. (2007). Improving health and accelerating personalized health care through health information technology and genetic information in population-and community-based health care delivery systems. *Personalized Medicine Coalition*. Retrieved December 8, 2009 from http://www.personalizedmedicinecoalition.org/PMC_Response_to_HHS_RFI_on_HIT_final_1_25_071.pdf

Drummond, N., Rector, A. L., Stevens, R., Moulton, G., Horridge, M., Wang, H., & Seidenberg, J. (2006). Putting OWL in order: Patterns for sequences in OWL. In *Proc. 2nd Workshop on OWL: Experiences and Directions*.

EHRflex. (2013). EHRflex project. Retrieved from http://ehrflex.sourceforge.net

Eichelberg, M., Aden, T., Riesmeier, J., Dogac, A., & Laleci, G. B. (2005). A survey and analysis of electronic healthcare record standards. *ACM Computing Surveys*, *37*(4), 277–315. doi:10.1145/1118890.1118891

Eiter, T., Ianni, G., Krennwallner, T., & Polleres, A. (2008). Rules and ontologies for the Semantic Web. In C. Baroglio, P. A. Bonatti, J. Maluszynski, M.Marchiori, A. Polleres, & S. Schaffert (Eds.), Reasoning Web, 4th International Summer School 2008, Venice, Italy, Tutorial Lectures (Lecture Notes in Computer Science, 5224). (pp., 1–53). Germany: Springer-Verlag.

EN13606 - a standard for EHR system communication. (n. d.). Retrieved December 8, 2009 from http://www.openehr.org/standards/cen.html

Enabling grid for E-science (EGEE). (2013). Retrieved from http://www.eu-egee.org

Epic-sun grid engine integration with globus toolkit . (2013). Retrieved from http://www.lesc.ic.ac.uk/projects/epic-gt-sge.html

epSOS. (n. d.). Retrieved from http://www.epsos.eu/

EU mammogrid. (2013). Retrieved from, ftp://ftp.cordis.europa.eu/pub/ist/docs/grids/mammogrid_achievement.pdf

European Community. (2009). *Semantic interoperability for better health and safer healthcare. deployment and research roadmap for Europe*. EC Roadmap.

European data grid (EDG). (2013). Retrieved from http://www.edg.org

European Interoperability Framework for Pan-European eGovernment Services. (2004). Version 1.0. Retrieved from http://ec.europa.eu/idabc.

Euzenat, J., Polleres, A., & Scharffe, F. (2008). SPARQL extensions for processing alignments. *IEEE Intelligent Systems*, *23*(6), 82–84.

Euzenat, J., Scharffe, F., & Zimmermann, A. (2007). *Expressive alignment language and implementation (Deliverable D2.2.10)*. Knowledge Web NoE.

Fagin, R., Kolaitis, P. G., Miller, R. J., & Popa, L. (2005). Data exchange: Semantics and query answering. *Theoretical Computer Science*, *336*, 89–124. doi:10.1016/j.tcs.2004.10.033

Fensel, D. (2004). Triple-space computing: Semantic Web services based on persistent publication of information. In *IFIP International Conference on Intelligence in Communication Systems, LNCS 3283* (pp. 43-53). Springer.

Field, M. J., & Lohr, K. N. (1990). Attributes of good practice guidelines. In *Clinical Practice Guidelines: Directions for a New Program* (pp. 53–77). Washington, DC: The National Academy Press.

Ford, E. W., Menachemi, N., Peterson, L. T., & Huerta, T. R. (2009). Resistance is futile: But it is slowing the pace of EHR adoption nonetheless. *Journal of the American Medical Informatics Association*, *16*, 274–281. doi:10.1197/jamia.M3042 PMID:19261931

Forrey, A. W., McDonald, C. J., DeMoor, G., Huff, S. M., Leavelle, D., & Leland, D. et al. (1996). Logical observation identifier names and codes (LOINC) database: A public use set of codes and names for electronic reporting of clinical laboratory test results. *Clinical Chemistry*, *42*(1), 81–90. PMID:8565239

Foster, I., Kesselman, C., Nick, J., & Tuecke, S. (2002). *The physiology of the grid: An open grid services architecture for distributed systems integration.* Open Grid Service Infrastructure WG, Global Grid Forum.

Foster, I., & Kesselman, C. (1997). Globus: A metacomputing infrastructure toolkit. *The International Journal of Supercomputer Applications*, *11*, 115–128. doi:10.1177/109434209701100205

Foster, I., Kesselman, C., & Tuecke, S. (2001). The anatomy of the grid: Enabling scalable virtual organizations. *The International Journal of Supercomputer Applications*, *15*, 200–222. doi:10.1177/109434200101500302

Fox, R., Sahay, R., & Hauswirth, M. (2008). PPEPR for enterprise healthcare integration. In D. Weerasinghe (Ed.), *Electronic Healthcare, First International Conference, eHealth 2008, London, UK. Revised Selected Papers (Lecture Notes of the Institute for Computer Sciences, Social Informatics and Telecommunications Engineering, 1).* (pp. 130–137). Germany: Springer-Verlag.

Fox, J., Alabassi, A., Patkar, V., Rose, T., & Black, E. (2006). An ontological approach to modelling tasks and goals. *Computers in Biology and Medicine*, *36*(7-8), 837–856. doi:10.1016/j.compbiomed.2005.04.011 PMID:16169546

Freeman, E., Hupfer, S., & Arnold, K. (1999). *JavaSpaces principles, patterns, and practice.* Prentice Hall PTR.

Freter, T. (2003). *A Java API for HL7 Version 3 RIM.* Health Level Seven International. Retrieved November 16, 2013, from http://www.hl7.org/documentcenter/public/wg/java/HL7-java.pdf

Fritschy, J., Horesh, L., Holder, D., & Bayford, R. (2005). Applications of grid in clinical neurophysiology and electrical impedance tomography of brain function. In *Proceedings of Healthgrid from Grid to Healthgrid* (pp. 138–145). Amsterdam, The Netherlands: IOS Press.

Garcia, A. J., & Simari, G. R. (2004). Defeasible logic programming: An argumentative approach. *Theory and Practice of Logic Programming*, *4*(1–2), 95–138. doi:10.1017/S1471068403001674

Garde, S., Knaup, P., Hovenga, E. J. S., & Heard, S. (2007). Towards semantic interoperability for electronic health records: Domain knowledge governance for openEHR archetypes. *Methods of Information in Medicine*, *46*(3), 332–343. PMID:17492120

GEHR – Good European Health Record (n.d.). Retrieved December 8, 2009 from http://www.chime.ucl.ac.uk/work-areas/ehrs/GEHR/.

Gelernter, D. (1985). Generative communication in Linda. *ACM Transactions on Programming Languages and Systems*, *7*(1), 80–112. doi:10.1145/2363.2433

Gene Ontology. (n. d.). Retrieved from http://www.geneontology.org/

Ghidini, C., & Giunchiglia, F. (2001). Local models semantics, or contextual reasoning=locality+compatibilit y. *Artificial Intelligence*, *127*(2), 221–259. doi:10.1016/S0004-3702(01)00064-9

Gil, Y., Motta, E., Benjamins, V. R., & Musen, M. A. (Eds.). (2005). *The Semantic Web - ISWC 2005: 4th International Semantic Web Conference, Galway, Ireland, Proceedings (Lecture Notes in Computer Science 3729).* Germany: Springer-Verlag.

Girosi, F., Meili, R., & Scoville, R. P. (2005). *Extrapolating evidence of health information technology savings and costs.* Santa Monica, CA: Rand Corporation.

Giunchiglia, F. (1993). Contextual reasoning. *Epistemologica, 16*, 345–364.

Golbreich, C., & Imai, A. (2004). Combining SWRL rules and OWL ontologies with Protégé OWL Plugin, Jess, and Racer. In *Proceedings of 7th International Protégé Conference*. Bethesda. Retrieved from http://protege.stanford.edu/conference/2004/abstracts/Golbreich.pdf

Grimson, J., Grimson, W., Berry, D., Stephens, G., Felton, E., Kalra, D., Toussaint, P., et al. (1998). A CORBA-based integration of distributed electronic healthcare records using the synapses approach. *IEEE Transactions on Information Technology in Biomedicine: A Publication of the IEEE Engineering in Medicine and Biology Society, 2*(3), 124-138.

Grimson, J., Grimson, W., & Hasselbring, W. (2000). The SI challenge in health care. *Communications of the ACM, 43*(6), 49–55. doi:10.1145/336460.336474

Grimson, W., Berry, D., Grimson, J., Stephens, G., Felton, E., Given, P., & O'Moore, R. (1998). Federated healthcare record server–The Synapses paradigm. *International Journal of Medical Informatics, 52*(1-3), 3–27. doi:10.1016/S1386-5056(98)00121-X PMID:9848399

Gritzalis, D. A. (1998). Enhancing security and improving interoperability in healthcare information systems. *Informatics for Health & Social Care, 23*(4), 309–323. doi:10.3109/14639239809025367 PMID:9922951

Gruber, T. R. (2009). Ontology. In L. Liu & T. Özsu, (Eds.), *Encyclopedia of database systems*. Retrieved from http://tomgruber.org/writing/ontology-definition-2007.htm

Gruber, T. R. (1993). A translation approach to portable ontology specifications. *Knowledge Acquisition, 5*(2), 199–220. doi:10.1006/knac.1993.1008

Gruber, T. R. (1993). Towards principles for the design of ontologies used for knowledge sharing. *International Journal of Human-Computer Studies, 43*(5-6), 907–928. doi:10.1006/ijhc.1995.1081

Guha, R. V. (1991). *Contexts: A formalization and some applications* (Ph.D. thesis). Stanford University, Stanford, CA.

Guha, R. V., McCool, R., & Fikes, R. (2004). Contexts for the Semantic Web. In F. van Harmelen, S. McIlraith, & D. Plexousakis (Eds.), *The Semantic Web - ISWC 2004: Third International Semantic Web Conference, Hiroshima, Japan. Proceedings (Lecture Notes in Computer Science, 3298).* (pp. 32–46). Germany: Springer-Verlag.

Guha, R., McCool, R., & Miller, E. (2003). *Semantic search*. Paper presented at the Twelfth International World Wide Web Conference, Budapest, Hungary.

Hägglund, M. (2009). Sharing is caring: Integrating health information systems to support patient-centred shared homecare. *International Journal of Integrated Care, 9*, e11.

Hayes, P. J. (2004). *RDF Semantics*, (W3C Recommendation 10 February 2004). World Wide Web Consortium (W3C).

Hazzard. (2008, October 28). UK - Another government IT scheme in trouble. *Telegraph*. Retrieved on June 27, 2010, from http://www.telegraph.co.uk/comment/telegraph-view/3563090/Another-Government-IT-scheme-introuble. html

Health Level Seven (HL7). (n. d.). Retrieved November 2013, from: http://www.hl7.org

HealthOne. Retrieved December 8, 2009 from http://www.openehr.org/114-OE.html

Heard, S. (2000). The Good electronic health record: Trial of a standard healthcare record in Australian general practice. *British Journal of Healthcare Computing and Information Management, 17*(1), 24–26.

Heiler, S. (1995). Semantic interoperability. *ACM Comput. Surv., 27*(2), 271–273. doi:http://doi.acm.org/10.1145/210376.210392

Hibernate. (2013). Relational Persistence for Java and. NET. Retrieved from http://www.hibernate.org/

Hitzler, P., Krötzsch, M., Parsia, B., Patel-Schneider, P. F., & Rudolph, S. (2009). *OWL 2 Web ontology language primer, (W3C Recommendation)*. World Wide Web Consortium.

HL7- EHR system functional model: A major development towards consensus on electronic health record system functionality. (2004). Retrieved December 8, 2009, from http://www.providersedge.com/ehdocs/ehr_articles/HL7_EHR_System_Functional_Model-White_Paper.pdf

HL7-clinical document architecture release 2.0. (n. d.). Retrieved December 8, 2009 from http://xml.coverpages.org/CDA-20040830v3.pdf

HL7V3 (2005). *HL7 version 3 message development framework*. Retrieved from http://www.hl7.org/ library/mdf99/mdf99.pdf

Hollingsworth, D. (1995). The workflow reference model. *Workflow Management Coalition*. Retrieved December 8, 2009, from http://www.e-workflow.org/standards/workflow_ref_model.pdf

Homola, M. (2007). Distributed Description Logics Revisited. In Calvanese et al. (Eds.), *Proceedings of the 20th International Workshop on Description Logics DL'07*. Brixen/Bressanone, Italy: Bolzano University Press.

Horridge, M. (2011). *A practical guide to building OWL ontologies using Protégé 4 and CO-ODE tools (Ed. 1.3)*. University Of Manchester. Retrieved December 20, 2013, from http://130.88.198.11/tutorials/protegeowltutorial/

Horridge, M., & Patel-Schneider, P. F. (2009). OWL 2 Web ontology language Manchester syntax (W3C Working Group Note 27 October 2009). World Wide Web Consortium (W3C).

Horrocks, I., Patel-Schneider, P. F., Bechhofer, S., & Tsarkov, D. (2005). OWL Rules: A Proposal and Prototype Implementation. *Journal of Web Semantics, 3*, 23–40. doi:10.1.1.65.9856

Horst, H. J. T. (2005a). Combining RDF and Part of OWL with rules: Semantics, decidability, complexity. In Gil et al., (Eds.), *The Semantic Web - ISWC 2005: 4th International Semantic Web Conference, Galway, Ireland, Proceedings (Lecture Notes in Computer Science 3729)* (pp. 668–684).Germany: Springer-Verlag.

Horst, H. J. T. (2005b). Completeness, decidability and complexity of entailment for RDF Schema and a semantic extension involving the OWL vocabulary. *Journal of Web Semantics*, *3*(2–3), 79–115. doi:10.1016/j.websem.2005.06.001

Hovenga, E. J. S. (2008). Importance of achieving semantic interoperability for national health information systems. *Texto Contexto Enferm. Florianópolis, 17*(1), 158–167.

Hsieh, S. H., Hsieh, S. L., Weng, Y. C., Yang, T. H., Feipei, L., Cheng, P. H., et al. (2007). *Middleware based inpatient healthcare information system*. Paper presented at the 7th IEEE International Conference in Bioinformatics and Bioengineering (BIBE 2007), Boston, MA.

Huang, Z., van Harmelen, F., & ten Teije, A. (2005). *Reasoning with inconsistent ontologies*. In L. P. Kaelbling & A. Saffiotti (Eds.), *IJCAI-05, Proceedings of the Nineteenth International Joint Conference on Artifical Intelligence, Edinburgh, Scotland*. (pp. 454–459). Professional Book Center.

Huizen, V. G., & Backman, A. J. (2005). *SOA: First principles. SONIC software*. Paper presented at the Conference of Oracle Global Business and Technology, Mumbai, India.

Hwang, S.-K., Gwak, H.-S., Paek, S.-H., Kim, D.-G., & Jung, H.-W. (2004). Guidelines for the Ligation of the sigmoid or transverse sinus during large petroclival meningioma surgery. *Skull Base*, *14*(1), 21–28. doi:10.1055/s-2004-821356 PMID:16145581

IBM EAS. (n. d.). Retrieved December 8, 2009 from http://www-01.ibm.com/software/data/ips/products/masterdata/eas/

IBM general parallel file system . (2013). Retrieved from: ftp://ftp.software.ibm.com/common/ssi/pm/fy/n/clf03001usen/CLF03001USEN.PDF

IBM network file system (NFS-IBM). (2013) Retrieved from: http://www03.ibm.com/servers/s390/os390/bkserv/r10pdf/nfs.html

IEEE. 1990. IEEE standard computer dictionary: A compilation of IEEE standard computer glossaries. New York: 1990.

IHTSDO. (n. d.). *International Health Terminology Standards Development Organization*. Retrieved December 8, 2009 from http://www.ihtsdo.org/

Indap, S. M., & Thakre, V. S. (2007). Weather monitoring system using JADE (Java Agent Development Environment), *Project Report*.

Innovative Medicine Initiative. (2009). *Innovative Medicines Joint Undertaking (IMI JU) 2009 Call for proposals*. Retrieved from http://www.imi.europa.eu.

Institute of Medicine. (1999). *To err is human: Building a safer health care system*. Washington, DC: National Academies Press.

Institute of Medicine. (2001). *Crossing the quality chasm: A new health system for the twenty-first century*. Washington, DC: National Academies Press.

International Organization for Standardization. (2008a). Health informatics — Electronic health record communication — Part 1: Reference model.

International Organization for Standardization. (2008b). Health Informatics-Electronic health record communication, Part II: Archetypes.

Isern, D., & Moreno, A. (2008). Computer-based execution of clinical guidelines: A review. *International Journal of Medical Informatics*, *77*(12), 787–808. doi:10.1016/j.ijmedinf.2008.05.010 PMID:18639485

ISO TR 20514:2005. (2005). *Health informatics - Electronic health record definition, scope and context standard.* International Organization for Standardization (ISO), Geneva, Switzerland.

ISO. (n. d.). *International Standard Organization.* Retrieved December 8, 2009 from http://www.iso.org/iso/home.htm

ISO/EN 13606 (ISO13606). (n. d.). Retrieved November 2013, from http://www.iso.org/iso/home.htm

ISO/TC 215. (2008). *CEN 12967 Health Informatics - Service Architecture*.

ITU. (n. d.). *International Telecommunication Union.* Retrieved December 8, 2009 from http://www.itu.int/net/home/index.aspx

Jahnke, J. H., Bychkov, Y., Dahlem, D., & Kawasme, L. (2005). Context-aware information services for health care. *Revue d'Intelligence Artificielle*, *19*(3), 459–478. doi:10.3166/ria.19.459-478

Japan medical engineering grid (MEGrid). (2013). Retrieved from: http://www.biogrid.jp

Java Agent DEvelopment Framework. (n.d.). Retrieved June, 2010, from http://jade.tilab.com.

Jiang, G., & Chute, C. G. (2009). Auditing the semantic completeness of SNOMED CT using formal concept analysis. *Journal of the American Medical Informatics Association*, *16*(1), 89–102. doi:10.1197/jamia.M2541 PMID:18952949

Jin, D., & Cordy, J. R. (2006). *Integrating reverse engineering tools using a service-sharing methodology*. Paper presented at 14th International Conference on Program Comprehension (ICPC 2006), Athens, Greece.

Jin, D., & Winter, A. (2005). *Working session on interoperable reengineering services*. Paper presented at the 13th International Workshop on Program Comprehension (IWPC 2005), St. Louis, USA.

Kalra, D. (2006). *Archetypes: The missing link*. Retrieved December 8, 2009 from http://www.eurorec.org/eurorec2006/programme.cfm?actief=programme

Kalra, D. (2008). Terminologies and EHR systems. In *Toward Semantic Interoperability of EHR systems: A joint effort for Europe. Expert Workshop*. Brussels.

Kalra, D. (2006). Electronic health record standards. *Yearbook of Medical Informatics*, *45*, 136–144. PMID:17051307

Kalra, D., Beale, T., & Heard, S. (2005). The openEHR Foundation. *Studies in Health Technology and Informatics*, *115*, 153–173. PMID:16160223

Kalra, D., Blobel, B., & Regensburg, G. (2007). Semantic interoperability of EHR systems. *Medical and Care Compunetics*, *4*, 231. PMID:17901615

Karla, D. (2009*). ISO EN 13606 electronic health communication (EHRCOM): The contribution of archetypes towards eHealth semantic interoperability*. Retrieved February, 2009, from http://www.kith.no/upload/5414/EHRCOM-Archetypes-DipakKalra-20091126.pdf

Kashyap, V., & Sheth, A. (1996). Semantic and schematic similarities between database objects: A context-based approach. *The Very Large Data Base Journal*, *5*, 276–304.

Kawamoto, K., Houlihan, C. A., Balas, E. A., & Lobach, D. F. (2005). Improving clinical practice using clinical decision support systems: A systematic review of trials to identify features critical to success. *BMJ (Clinical Research Ed.)*, *330*(7494), 765–772. doi:10.1136/bmj.38398.500764.8F PMID:15767266

Kifer, M., Lausen, G., & Wu, J. (1995). Logical foundations of object-oriented and frame-based languages. *Journal of the ACM*, *42*(4), 741–843. doi:10.1145/210332.210335

Kilic, O., Bicer, V., & Dogac, A. (2005). *Mapping archetypes to OWL* (Technical Report).

Kleer, J. D. (1986). An assumption-based TMS. *Artificial Intelligence*, *28*(2), 127–162. doi:10.1016/0004-3702(86)90080-9

Klyne, G. (2001). *Information modelling using RDF: Constructs for modular description of complex systems.* Retrieved from http:// xml.coverpages.org/Klyne-RDFInfoModelling.pdf

Knublauch, H. (2005). *User-defined datatypes in protégé-owl.* Retrieved from http://protege.stanford.edu/plugins/owl/xsp.html

Kolovski, V., Parsia, B., Katz, Y., & Hendler, J. A. (2005). Representing Web service policies in OWL-DL. In Gil et al., (Eds.), *The Semantic Web - ISWC 2005: 4th International Semantic Web Conference, Galway, Ireland, Proceedings (Lecture Notes in Computer Science 3729)* (pp461–475).Germany: Springer-Verlag.

Kraft, M. R., Desouza, K. C., & Androwich, I. (2002). Data mining in healthcare information systems: Case study of a Veterans' Administration spinal cord injury population. In *Proceedings of the 36th Hawaii International Conference on System Sciences*. Retrieved December 8, 2009 from http://csdl2.computer.org/comp/proceedings/hicss/2003/1874/06/187460159a.pdf

Krummenacher, R., Simperl, E., & Fensel, D. (2008). Scalability in semantic computing: Semantic middleware. In *Proceedings of the 2008 IEEE International Conference on Semantic Computing* (pp. 538-545). IEEE Computer Society.

Kuhn, I. M., Wiederhold, G., Rodnick, J. E., Ramsey-Klee, D. M., Benett, S., & Beck, D. D. (1982). *Automated ambulatory medical record systems in the US* (Report No. STAN-CS-82-928). Retrieved from ftp://reports.stanford.edu/pub/cstr/reports/cs/tr/82/928/CS-TR-82-928.pdf

Kutz, O., Lutz, C., Wolter, F., & Zakharyaschev, M. (2004). *E*-connections of abstract description systems. *Artificial Intelligence*, *156*(1), 1–73. doi:10.1016/j.artint.2004.02.002

Lau, F., Yang, J., & Brox, G. (2008). Initial experience in mapping minimum data set home care to SNOMED CT. *Electronic Healthcare*, online.

Lenat, D. B. (1995). CYC: A large-scale investment in knowledge infrastructure. *Communications of the ACM*, *38*(11), 33–38. doi:10.1145/219717.219745

Lenzerini, M. (2002). Data integration: A theoretical perspective. In *Proceedings of the Twenty-First ACM SIGMOD-SIGACT Symposium on Principles of Database Systems* (Vol. 4, pp. 233–246). doi:10.1145/543613.543644

Lenz, R., & Kuhn, K. A. (2004). Towards a continuous evolution and adaptation of information systems in healthcare. *International Journal of Medical Informatics*, *73*, 75–89. doi:10.1016/j.ijmedinf.2003.09.003 PMID:15036081

Lenz, R., & Reichert, M. (2007). IT support for healthcare processes – Premises, challenges, perspectives. *Data & Knowledge Engineering*, *61*(1), 39–58. doi:10.1016/j.datak.2006.04.007

Lezcano, L. (2009). A model for integrating disease and diagnosis semantics in clinical archetypes. In *Signs, symptoms and findings: Towards an ontology for clinical phenotypes (SSFW09)*. Milan, Italy. Retrieved from http://bimib.disco.unimib.it/index.php/SSFW09_Presentations

Lezcano, L., Sánchez-Alonso, S., & Sicilia, M. A. (2010). (in press). Associating clinical archetypes through UMLS metathesaurus term clusters. *Journal of Medical Systems*. doi: doi:10.1007/s10916-010-9586-9 PMID:20827566

Lezcano, L., & Sicilia, M. A. (2011). Connectivity and semantic patterns in automatically generated SNOMED-CT subsets. In *Metadata and semantic research* (pp. 117–125). Berlin, Heidelberg: Springer. doi:10.1007/978-3-642-24731-6_11

Lezcano, L., Sicilia, M. A., & Rodríguez-Solano, C. (2011). Integrating reasoning and clinical archetypes using OWL ontologies and SWRL rules. *Journal of Biomedical Informatics*, *44*(2), 343–353. doi:10.1016/j.jbi.2010.11.005 PMID:21118725

Lezcano, L., Sicilia, M. A., & Serrano-Balazote, P. (2008). Lecture Notes in Computer Science: Vol. 5288. *Combining OpenEHR archetype definitions with SWRL rules - A translation approach. Emerging Technologies and Information Systems for the Knowledge Society* (pp. 79–87). doi:10.1007/978-3-540-87781-3_9

Li-Fan Ko, E. A. (2006). *HL7 middleware framework for healthcare information system.* Paper presented at the 8th International Conference on e-Health Networking, Applications and Services (HEALTHCOM 2006), New Delhi, India.

Lindberg, D. A., Humphreys, B. L., & McCray, A. T. (1993). The unified medical language system. *Methods of Information in Medicine*, *32*(4), 281–291. PMID:8412823

Lindberg, D., Humphreys, B., & McCray, A. (1993). The unified medical language system (UMLS). *Methods of Information in Medicine*, *32*(4), 281–291. PMID:8412823

Linked Open Data . (n. d.). Retrieved from http://www.linkeddata.org/

LiU EHR GUI. (n. d.). Retrieved November 2013, from https://github.com/LiU-IMT/EEE

Liu, Y., Bacon, J., & Wilson-Hinds, R. (2007). On smart-care: Services studies of visually impaired users in living context. In *1st International Conference on the Digital Society* (pp. 32-40). French Caribbean: IEEE Press.

Lowe, H. J., & Barnett, G. O. (1994). Understanding and Using the Medical Subject Headings (MeSH) vocabulary to perform literature searches. *Journal of the American Medical Association*, *271*(14), 1103–1108. doi:10.1001/jama.1994.03510380059038 PMID:8151853

Loy, M., & Eckstein, R. (2002). *Java Swing*. Sebastopol, CA: O'Reilly Media, Inc.

Lustre file system . (2013). Retrieved from: http://www.sun.com/software/products/lustre

Lutz, C., & Sattler, U. (2000). Mary likes all cats. In F. Baader & U. Sattler (Eds.), *Proceedings of the 2000 International Workshop on Description Logics (DL2000), Aachen, Germany (CEUR Workshop Proceedings, 33)* (pp.213–226). Sun SITE Central Europe (CEUR).

Malamateniou, F., & Vassilacopoulos, G. (2003). Developing a virtual patient record using XML and Web-based workflow technologies. *International Journal of Medical Informatics*, *70*(2), 131–139. doi:10.1016/S1386-5056(03)00039-X PMID:12909164

Maldonado, J., Moner, D., Bosca, D., Angulo, C., Marco, L., Reig, E., & Robles, M. (2011). Concept-Based Exchange Of Healthcare Information: The LinkEHR approach. In *2011 IEEE First International Conference on Healthcare Informatics, Imaging and Systems Biology*, 150–157. doi:10.1109/HISB.2011.18

Maldonado, J., Moner, D., Boscá, D., Fernández-Breis, J. T., Angulo, C., & Robles, M. (2009). LinkEHR-Ed: A multi-reference model archetype editor based on formal semantics. *International Journal of Medical Informatics*, *78*(8), 559–570. doi:10.1016/j.ijmedinf.2009.03.006 PMID:19386540

Markwell, D., Sato, L., & Cheetham, E. (2007). Representing clinical information using SNOMED Clinical Terms with different structural information models. *KR-MED*, *2008*, 72.

Martínez-Costa, C., Menárguez-Tortosa, M., Fernández-Breis, J. T., & Maldonado, J. A. (2009). A model-driven approach for representing clinical archetypes for Semantic Web environments. *Journal of Biomedical Informatics*, *42*(1), 150–164. doi:10.1016/j.jbi.2008.05.005 PMID:18590985

Martin, J., & McClure, C. L. (1985). *Diagramming techniques for analysts and programmers*. Upper Saddle River, NJ: Prentice-Hall.

McCarthy, J. L. (1987). Generality in artificial intelligence. *Communications of the ACM*, *30*(12), 1029–1035. doi:10.1145/33447.33448

MEDCIN. (n. d.). Retrieved November 2013, from http://www.medicomp.com/

Mei, J., & Paslaru Bontas, E. (2005). Reasoning paradigms for SWRL-enabled ontologies. In *Proceedings of International Workshop on Protege with Rules*. Madrid, Spain.

Meilicke, C., Stuckenschmidt, H., & Tamilin, A. (2008). Supporting manual mapping revision using logical reasoning. In D. Fox & C. P. Gomes (Eds.), *Proceedings of the Twenty-Third AAAI Conference on Artificial Intelligence, AAAI 2008, Chicago, Illinois,* (pp. 1213–1218). AAAI Press.

Merriam-Webster Dictionary. (n.d.). Retrieved December 8, 2009 from http://www.merriam-webster.com/dictionary/health.

MOFScript. (n. d.). Retrieved November 2013, from http://www.eclipse.org/gmt/mofscript/

Moldovan, D. I., Clark, C., & Harabagiu, S. M. (2005). Temporal context representation and reasoning. In L. P. Kaelbling & A. Saffiotti (Eds.), *IJCAI-05, Proceedings of the Nineteenth International Joint Conference on Artifical Intelligence, Edinburgh, Scotland.* (pp. 1099–1104). Professional Book Center.

Moore, G. W. (2001). *What is a medical ontology?* Retrieved December 8, 2009 from http://www.netautopsy.org/whatonto.htm retrieved

Motik, B., Horrocks, I., & Sattler, U. (2007). Adding integrity constraints to OWL. In C. Golbreich, A. Kalyanpur, & B. Parsia, *Proceedings of the OWLED 2007 Workshop on OWL: Experiences and Directions, Innsbruck, Austria, (CEUR Workshop Proceedings 258).* Sun SITE Central Europe (CEUR).

Motik, B., Patel-Schneider, P. F., & Cuenca-Grau, B. (2009). *OWL 2 Web ontology language direct semantics* (W3C Recommendation 27 October 2009). World Wide Web Consortium (W3C).

Mulyar, N., van der Aalst, W. M. P., & Peleg, M. (2007). A pattern-based analysis of clinical computer-interpretable guideline modeling languages. *Journal of the American Medical Informatics Association, 14*(6), 781–787. doi:10.1197/jamia.M2389 PMID:17712087

Nardon, F. B., & Moura, L. A. (2004). Knowledge sharing and information integration in healthcare using ontologies and deductive databases. In *Medinfo 2004: Proceedings Of THe 11th World Congress On Medical Informatics* (p. 62).

National digital mammography archive (NDMA). (2013). Retrieved from: http://rt-image.com/0825digitalmammo

NCHS. (n. d.). *Nation Center of Health Statistics*. Retrieved December 8, 2009 from http://www.cdc.gov/nchs/icd9.htm

Nguyen, M. T., Fuhrer, P., & Pasquier-Rocha, J. (2009). Enhancing E-health information systems with agent technology. *International Journal of Telemedicine and Applications*, 2009. PMID:19096509

NHS. (n. d.). *NHS Connecting for Health*. Retrieved from http://www.connectingforhealth.nhs.uk/

NICTIZ. (n. d.). *AORTA*. Retrieved from http://www.nictiz.nl/

NLM. (n. d.). *National Library of Medicine.* Retrieved December 8, 2009 from http://www.nlm.nih.gov/healthit.html

O'Connor, M., Knublauch, H., Tu, S., Grosof, B., Dean, M., Grosso, W., & Musen, M. (2005). supporting rule system interoperability on the Semantic Web with SWRL. *The Semantic Web - ISWC 2005* (pp. 974–986). Retrieved fromhttp://dx.doi.org/10.1007/11574620_69

OASIS. (2005). *eXtensible Access Control Markup Language (XACML) version 2.0.* Retrieved July, 2009, from http://docs.oasis-open.org/xacml/2.0/access_control-xacml-2.0-core-spec-os.pdf.

Object Management Group (OMG). (n. d.). Retrieved November 2013, from http://www.omg.org/

Ocean OpenEHR Archetype Editor . (n. d.). Retrieved November 2013, from http://www.oceaninformatics.com/Solutions/ocean-products/Clinical-Modelling/ocean-archetype-editor.html

OMG. (2006) *Meta object facility (MOF) 2.0 core specification* (OMG Document Formal). Retrieved from: http://wwwomgorg/cgi-bin/doc?formal/2006-01-01. 2006

OMG. (n. d.). *Business process management with OMG specifications.* Retrieved December 8, 2009 from http://www.bpmroundtable.org/101807_BPM_Fact_Sheet.pdf

Online Mendelian Inheritance in Man. (n. d.). Retrieved from http://www.ncbi.nlm.nih.gov/omim/

OpenEHR architecture overview . (n. d.). Retrieved December 8, 2009 from http://svn.openehr.org/specification/BRANCHES/Release-1.0.1-candidate/publishing/architecture/overview.pdf

openEHR Community, (n.d.). *OpenEHR. Future proof and flexible EHR*. Retrieved June, 2010, from http://www.openehr. org.

OpenEHR repository. (n. d.). Retrieved November 2013, from https://github.com/openEHR

OpenEHR (OpenEHR). (n. d.). Retrieved November 2013, from http://www.openehr.org

O'Sullivan, D. M., Wilk, S. A., Michalowski, W. J., & Farion, K. J. (2010). Automatic indexing and retrieval of encounter-specific evidence for point-of-care support. *Journal of Biomedical Informatics*, *43*(4), 623–631. doi:10.1016/j.jbi.2010.03.003 PMID:20230908

OWL Web Ontology Language Reference (OWL). (2004). Retrieved November 2013, from http://www.w3.org/tr/owl-ref/

Pan, J. Z., & Horrocks, I. (2005). OWL-Eu: Adding customised datatypes into OWL. In The Semantic Web: Research and applications (pp. 153–166). Retrieved fromhttp://dx.doi.org/ doi:10.1007/11431053_11

Pan, J. Z. (2004). *Description logics: Reasoning support for the Semantic Web (PhD chapter)*. School of Computer Science, The University of Manchester.

Park, H. A., & Hardiker, N. (2009). Clinical terminologies: A Solution for Semantic Interoperability. *J Kor Soc Med Informatics*, *15*(1), 1–11. doi:10.4258/jksmi.2009.15.1.1

Paterson, G. I. (2004). Semantic interoperability for decision support using case formalism and controlled vocabulary. In *Proceedings of the e-Health 2004 Conference*.

Pathak, J., Solbrig, H. R., Buntrock, J. D., Johnson, T. M., & Chute, C. G. (2009). LexGrid: A framework for representing, storing, and querying biomedical terminologies from simple to sublime. *Journal of the American Medical Informatics Association*, *16*, 305–315. doi:10.1197/jamia.M3006 PMID:19261933

Patterson, N. L. (2004). *The mission of IT in health care: Creating a system that cares in healthcare information system management*. London: Springer. doi:10.1007/978-1-4757-4041-7_1

Pedersen, T. B., & Jensen, C. S. (1998). Research issues in clinical data warehousing. In *Proceedings of the 10th International Conference on Scientific and Statistical Database Management* (pp. 43–52).

Perkonigg, F. (2006). *Application of business process management in Web-based education* (Unpublished Master Thesis). Institute for Information Systems and Computer Media (IICM), Graz University of Technology, Austria.

PIPEDA. (2010). *Canada's Personal Information Protection and Electronic Documents Act*. Government of Canada. Retrieved on June 29, 2010, from http://www.priv.gc.ca/information/guide_e.cfm

Pirnejad, H., Niazkhani, Z., Berg, M., & Bal, R. (2008). Intra-organizational communication in healthcare. *Methods of Information in Medicine*, *47*(4), 336–345. PMID:18690367

Plsek, P., & Greenhalgh, T. (2001). The challenge of complexity in health care. *BMJ (Clinical Research Ed.)*, *323*, 625–628. doi:10.1136/bmj.323.7313.625 PMID:11557716

Poseacle repository. (n. d.). Retrieved November 2013, from http://miuras.inf.um.es/~researchehr/websvn/

PowerDesigner. (n. d.). *Sybase*. Retrieved December 8, 2009 from http://Sybase.com*/products/modelingdevelopment/powerdesigner*.

Preston, H. (2000). Information management and technology strategy in healthcare: Local timescales and national requirements. *Information Research, 5*(3).

Pulido, J. R. G., Ruiz, M. A. G., Herrera, R., Cabello, E., Legrand, S., & Elliman, D. (2006). Ontology languages for the Semantic Web: A never completely updated review. *Knowledge-Based Systems*, *19*(7), 489–497. doi:10.1016/j.knosys.2006.04.013

Qamar, R., & Rector, A. L. (2007). Semantic mapping of clinical model data to biomedical terminologies to facilitate data interoperability. In *Proceedings of Health Care Computing Conference*.

Qamar, R., Kola, J., & Rector, A. L. (2008). Interoperability of data models and terminology models: Issues with using the SNOMED CT terminology. *KR-MED*. Retrieved from http://ceur-ws.org/Vol-410/Paper09.pdf

Qamar, R. (2008). *Semantic mapping of clinical model data to biomedical terminologies to facilitate interoperability (PhD chapter)*. University of Manchester, Faculty of Engineering and Physical Sciences.

Qamar, R., Kola, J., & Rector, A. L. (2007). Unambiguous data modeling to ensure higher accuracy term binding to clinical terminologies. *AMIA ... Annual Symposium Proceedings / AMIA Symposium. AMIA Symposium, 2007*, 608–613. PMID:18693908

Raffio, A., Braga, D., Ceri, S., Papotti, P., & Hernandez, M. A. (2008). Clip: A visual language for explicit schema mappings. In *2008 IEEE 24th International Conference on Data Engineering*, 30–39. doi:10.1109/ICDE.2008.4497411

Rector, A. L. (1989). Helping with a humanly impossible task: Integrating knowledge based systems into clinical care. In J. Hanmu, L. Seppo (Eds.), *Proceedings of the Second Scandinavian Conference on Artificial Intelligence SCAI-89, 89*, 560–572.

Rector, A. L. (2007). *Barriers, approaches and research priorities for integrating biomedical ontologies* (No. D6.1). EC-supported FP6 SA. Retrieved from http://www.semantichealth.org/DELIVERABLES/SemanticHEALTH_D6_1.pdf

Rector, A. L., & Schreiber, G. (2005). *Qualified cardinality restrictions: Constraining the number of values of a particular type for a property*. Retrieved from http://www.w3.org/2001/sw/BestPractices/OEP/QCR/

Rector, A. L., Johnson, P., Tu, S., Wroe, C., & Rogers, J. (2001). Interface of Inference models with concept and medical record models. *Artificial Intelligence in Medicine* (pp. 314–323). Retrieved fromhttp://dx.doi.org/10.1007/3-540-48229-6_43

Rector, A. L., Qamar, R., & Marley, T. (2006). Binding ontologies & coding systems to electronic health records and messages. In O. Bodenreider (Ed.), *KR-MED 2006, Formal Biomedical Knowledge Representation, Proceedings of the Second International Workshop on Formal Biomedical Knowledge Representation: Biomedical Ontology in Action (KR-MED 2006)*. Sun SITE Central Europe (CEUR).

Rector, A. L., Rogers, J. E., Zanstra, P. E., & Van Der Haring, E. (2003). OpenGALEN: Open source medical terminology and tools. In *AMIA Annual Symposium Proceedings 2003* (Vol. 2003). Presented at the AMIA Annual Symposium.

Rector, A. L. (1999). Clinical terminology: Why is it so hard? *Methods of Information in Medicine, 38*(4/5), 239–252. PMID:10805008

Rector, A. L., & Brandt, S. (2008). Why do it the hard way? The case for an expressive description logic for SNOMED. *Journal of the American Medical Informatics Association, 15*(6), 744. doi:10.1197/jamia.M2797 PMID:18755993

Rector, A. L., Nowlan, W. A., & Consortium, G. (1994). The galen project. *Computer Methods and Programs in Biomedicine, 45*(1-2), 75–78. doi:10.1016/0169-2607(94)90020-5 PMID:7889770

Rector, A. L., Nowlan, W. A., Kay, S., Goble, C. A., & Howkins, T. J. (1993). A framework for modelling the electronic medical record. *Methods of Information in Medicine, 32*(2), 109–119. PMID:8321129

Rector, A. L., Qamar, R., & Marley, T. (2009). Binding ontologies and coding systems to electronic health records and messages. *Applied Ontology, 4*(1), 51–69.

Rogne, P. (1984). Use of electronic data processing in primary health care. Experiences and thoughts after 2 years' use of a record system for physicians. *Tidsskrift for Den Norske Lægeforening: Tidsskrift for Praktisk Medicin. Ny Række, 104*(14), 993–995.

Román, I., Roa, L. M., Reina-Tosina, J., & Madinabeitia, G. (2006). Demographic management in a federated healthcare environment. *International Journal of Medical Informatics, 75*(9), 671–682. doi:10.1016/j.ijmedinf.2006.04.006 PMID:16766223

Rose, J. S., Fisch, B. J., Hogan, W. R., Levy, B., Marshall, P., Thomas, D. R., & Kirkley, D. (2001). Common medical terminology comes of age, Part One: Standard language improves healthcare quality. *Journal of Healthcare Information Management*, *15*(3), 307–318. PMID:11642147

Ross Baker, G., Norton, P. G., & Flintoft, V. et al. (2004). The Canadian adverse events study: The incidence of adverse events among hospital patients in Canada. *Canadian Medical Association Journal*, *170*(11), 1678–1686. doi:10.1503/cmaj.1040498 PMID:15159366

Rossille, D., Laurent, J., & Burgun, A. (2005). Modelling a decision-support system for oncology using rule-based and case-based reasoning methodologies. *International Journal of Medical Informatics*, *74*(2-4), 299–306. doi:10.1016/j.ijmedinf.2004.06.005 PMID:15694636

Sackett, D. L., Rosenberg, W. M., Muir Gray, J. A., Haynes, B. R., & Richardson, W. S. (1996). Evidence based medicine: What it is and what it isn't. *BMJ (Clinical Research Ed.)*, *312*, 71–72. doi:10.1136/bmj.312.7023.71 PMID:8555924

Sahay, R., Akhtar, W., & Fox, R. (2008). PPEPR: Plug and play electronic patient records. In R. L. Wainwright & H. Haddad (Ed.), *Proceedings of the 2008 ACM Symposium on Applied Computing (SAC), Fortaleza, Ceara, Brazil,* (pp. 2298–2304). ACM Press.

Sahay, R., Fox, R., & Hauswirth, M. (2009). Semantic service-oriented design and development methodology for enterprise healthcare integration In J. Filipe & J. Cordeiro (Eds.), *WEBIST 2009 - Proceedings of the Fifth International Conference on Web Information Systems and Technologies, Lisbon, Portugal,* (pp. 159–166). INSTICC Press.

Samson, W. T., & Musen, M. A. (1996). The EON model of intervention protocols and guidelines. *EON Project at Stanford Medical Informatics*. Retrieved December 8, 2009 from http://www.smi.stanford.edu/projects/eon/96scamc/tu96scamc.html

Sánchez-Cuadrado, J., García-Molina, J., & Menárguez-Tortosa, M. (2006). RubyTL: A practical, extensible transformation language. *Proceedings of ECMDA-FA, 2006*, 158–172.

Sánchez-Macián, A., Pastor, E., Vergara, J. de L., & López, D. (2007). Extending SWRL to enhance mathematical support. In *Web Reasoning and Rule Systems* (pp. 358–360). Retrieved from. doi:10.1007/978-3-540-72982-2_30

Sartipi, K., & Mohammad, H. Y. (2008). Standard-based data and service interoperability in eHealth systems. *In Proceedings of the* International Conference on Software Maintenance (pp. 187 – 196). IEEE pres.

Schloeffel, P., Beale, T., Hayworth, G., Heard, S., & Leslie, H. (2006). The relationship between CEN 13606, HL7, and openEHR. In *Proceedings of HIC 2006 Bridging the Digital Divide: Clinician, consumer and computer.* Seattle, WA.

Schloeffel, P., Heard, S., Beale, T., & Rowed, D. (1999). *Overview of GEHR from an Australian perspective.* Retrieved December 8, 2009 from http://www.omg.org/docs/corbamed/00-01-17.txt

Schneider, M. (2009). *OWL 2 Web ontology language RDF-based semantics* (W3C Recommendation 27 October 2009). World Wide Web Consortium (W3C).

Schuler, T., Garde, S., Heard, S., & Beale, T. (2006). Towards automatically generating graphical user interfaces from openEHR archetypes. In MIE2006, 221-226.

Schulz, S., & Hahn, U. (2005). Part-whole representation and reasoning in formal biomedical ontologies. *Artificial Intelligence in Medicine*, *34*(3), 179–200. doi:10.1016/j.artmed.2004.11.005 PMID:15993045

Schulz, S., Suntisrivaraporn, B., Baader, F., & Boeker, M. (2009). SNOMED reaching its adolescence: Ontologists and logicians health check. *International Journal of Medical Informatics*, *78*, S86–S94. doi:10.1016/j.ijmedinf.2008.06.004 PMID:18789754

Seam . (n. d.). Retrieved November 2013, from http://www.seamframework.org/

Serafini, L., & Tamilin, A. (2005). DRAGO: Distributed reasoning architecture for the Semantic Web. In A. Gomez-Perez & J. Euzenat (Eds.), *The Semantic Web: Research and Applications, Second European Semantic Web Conference, ESWC 2005, Heraklion, Crete, Greece, Proceedings, (Lecture Notes in Computer Science 3532)* (pp. 361–376). Germany: Springer-Verlag.

Shabo, A. (2005). The implications of electronic health records for personalized medicine. *Personalized Medicine*. Retrieved on December 8, 2009 from http://www.haifa.ibm.com/projects/software/cgl7/papers/the_implications_of_ehrs_for_perso-nalized_medicine-shabo.pdf

Sheth, A. P. (1999). 0 changing focus on interoperability in information systems: From system, syntax, structure to semantics. In *Interoperating Geographic Information Systems* (pp. 5–29). Norwell, MA: Kluwer. doi:10.1007/978-1-4615-5189-8_2

Shortliffe, E. H., & Blois, M. A. (2006). The computer meets medicine and biology: Emergence of a discipline. In E. H. Shortliffe & J. J. Cimino (Eds.), *Medical informatics: Computer applications in healthcare and biomedicine (3rd Ed.),* Springer Press.

Shoshani, A., Kunszt, P., Stockinger, H., Stockinger, K., Laure, E., & Baud, J. P. ... Sim A. (2008). Storage resource management: Concepts, functionality and interface specification. In *International Conference on Computing in High Energy and Nuclear Physics*. Czech: IOP Publishing.

Shreeve, S. (n. d.). The Enabling technologies and reform initiatives for next generation health care. Retrieved December 8, 2009 from http://health20.org/wiki/Shreeve_Health_2.0_Whitepaper.

Sirin, E., Parsia, B., Grau, B. C., Kalyanpur, A., & Katz, Y. (2007). Pellet: A practical owl-dl reasoner. *Web Semantics: Science. Services and Agents on the World Wide Web*, *5*(2), 51–53. doi:10.1016/j.websem.2007.03.004

Smart Open Services for European Patients. (2009). *D.3.5.2. work package 3.5 - semantic services appendix G - CEN EN13606 technical specifications*. Retrieved from http://www.epsos.eu/uploads/tx_epsosfileshare/D3.5.2_Appendix_G_EN13606_Implementation_01.pdf

Smart Open Services for European Patients. (2012a). *D3.2.2 Final definition of functional service requirements- Patient summary*. Retrieved from http://www.epsos.eu/uploads/tx_epsosfileshare/D3.2.2_Final_Definition_Functional_Service_Req_Patient_Summary.pdf

Smart Open Services for European Patients. (2012b). *D.3.1.2 final definition of functional service requirements - ePrescription*. Retrieved from http://www.epsos.eu/uploads/tx_epsosfileshare/D3.1.2_Final_Definition_of_Functional_Service_Requirements_ePrescription_01.pdf

Smith, B. (2006). From concepts to clinical reality: An essay on the benchmarking of biomedical terminologies. *Journal of Biomedical Informatics*, *39*(3), 288–298. doi:10.1016/j.jbi.2005.09.005 PMID:16293444

Smith, B. et al. (2007). The OBO foundry: Coordinated evolution of ontologies to support biomedical data integration. *Nature Biotechnology*, *25*, 1251–1255. doi:10.1038/nbt1346 PMID:17989687

Smith, B., & Ceusters, W. (2005). An ontology-based methodology for the migration of biomedical terminologies to electronic health records. *AMIA ... Annual Symposium Proceedings / AMIA Symposium. AMIA Symposium*, *2005*, 704–708. PMID:16779131

Smith, C. (2003). *Open source meta-scheduling for virtual organizations with the community scheduler framework (CSF) (Technical Report)*. Platform Computing.

SNOMED CT style guide. Retrieved December 8, 2009 from http://www.ihtsdo.org/snomed-ct/snomed-ct-publications/

SNOMED-CT. (n. d.). Retrieved November 2013, from http://www.snomed.org

Sonnenberg, F. A., & Hagerty, C. G. (2006). Computer-interpretable clinical practice guidelines – Where we are and where we are going? *AMIA Yearbook*, *11*, 45–158.

Souder, T., & Mancoridis, S. (1999). *A tool for securely integrating legacy systems into a distributed environment*. Paper presented at the Sixth Working Conference on Reverse Engineering, Atlanta (WCRE '99), Georgia.

Spackman, K. A. (2008). *SNOMED CT style guide: Situations with explicit context. Style Guide 14 January 2008, Version 1.03*. SNOMED CT.

SPARQL. (n. d.). Retrieved November 2013, from http://www.w3.org/TR/rdf-sparql-query/.

Spetzler, R. F., Daspit, C. P., & Pappas, C. T. (1992). The combined supra- and infratentorial approach for lesions of the petrous and clival regions: Experience with 46 cases. *Journal of Neurosurgery*, *76*(4), 588–599. doi:10.3171/jns.1992.76.4.0588 PMID:1545251

Stahl, T. M. V. (2006). Model-driven software development. Hoboken, NJ: John Wiley and Sons.

Stearns, M. Q., Price, C., & Spackman, K. A. et al. (2001). SNOMED clinical terms: Overview of the development process and project status. *In Proc AMIA Symp, 2001*, 662–666. PMID:11825268

Stewart, G. A., Cowan, G. A., Dunne, B., Elwell, A., & Miller, A. P. (2008). Optimising LAN access to grid enabled storage elements. In *International Conference on Computing in High Energy and Nuclear Physics*. Pennsylvania: IOP Publishing.

Stoermer, H., Bouquet, P., Palmisano, I., & Redavid, D. (2007). A context-based architecture for RDF knowledge bases: Approach, implementation and preliminary results. In M. Marchiori, J. Z. Pan, & C. de Sainte Marie (Eds.), *Web Reasoning and Rule Systems, First International Conference, RR 2007, Innsbruck, Austria, Proceedings, (Lecture Notes in Computer Science, 4524)* (pp. 209–218). Germany: Springer-Verlag.

Strauss, A., & Corbin, J. (1994). Grounded theory methodology: An overview. In N. K. Denzin, & Y. S. Lincoln (Eds.), *Handbook of qualitative research* (pp. 273–285). Thousand Oaks, CA: Sage.

Stroetmann, V. N. (Ed.). Kalra, D., Lewalle, P., Rector, A., Rodrigues, J.M., Stroetmann, K.A., Surjan, G., Ustun, B., Virtanen, M., & Zanstra, P.E. (2009). Semantic interoperability for better health and safer healthcare. SemanticHEALTH Report. ISBN-13: 978-92-79-11139-6, DOI: doi:10.2759/38514

Stroetmann, V. N., Kalra, D., Lewalle, P., Rodrigues, J. M., Stroetmann, K. A., & Surjan, G. et al. (2009). *Semantic interoperability for better health and safer healthcare (Project report)*. Luxembourg: Office for Official Publications of the European Communities: European Commission.

Sutton, D. R., & Fox, J. (2003). The syntax and semantics of the PROforma guideline modeling language. *Journal of the American Medical Informatics Association*, *10*(5), 433. doi:10.1197/jamia.M1264 PMID:12807812

Syed, J., Ghanem, M., & Guo, Y. (2006). Supporting scientific discovery processes in discovery net. *Concurrency and Computation*, *19*, 167–179. doi:10.1002/cpe.1049

Szolovits, P. (1982). *Artificial intelligence in medicine*. Boulder, CO: Westview Press, Inc.

Taylor, P. (2006). *From patient data to medical knowledge*. London: BMJ. doi:10.1002/9780470994702

Tu, S. W., Bodenreider, O., Çelik, C., Chute, C. G., Heard, S., Jakob, R., et al. (2010). *A content model for the ICD-11 revision* (Technical Report BMIR-2010-1405). Stanford Center for Biomedical Informatics Research.

Tuecke, S., Czajkowski, K., Foster, I., Frey, J., Graham, S., Kesselman, C., et al. (2003). *Open grid services infrastructure (OGSI) version 1.0* (Technical report). Global Grid Forum.

Tzitzikas, Y. T. (2002, September). *Collaborative ontology-based information indexing and retrieval* (PhD chapter). Department of Computer Science, University of Crete.

UK E-Science eDiaMoND. (2013). Retrieved from: http://www.ediamond.ox.ac.uk

UMLS. (n. d.). Retrieved November 2013, from http://www.nlm.nih.gov/research/umls/

UniProt. (n. d.). Retrieved from http://www.uniprot.org/

United Kingdom. (2010). Retrieved on June 26, 2010, from http://www.connectingforhealth.nhs.uk/

United States. (2010). *Healthcare Information Technology Standards Panel*. Retrieved on June 26, 2010, from http://www.ansi.org/standards_activities/standards_boards_panels/hisb/hitsp.aspx?menuid=3

Vallecillo, A. (n. d.). RM-ODP: *The ISO reference model for open distributed processing*. Retrieved December 8, 2009 from http://www.enterprise-architecture.info/Images/Documents/RM-ODP.pdf

Van Bemmel, J. H., & Musen, M. (1997). *Handbook of medical informatics* (1st ed.). Houten, The Netherlands: Bohen Stafeu Van Loghum.

Van Donk, P. (2008). Challenges in relating supply chain management and information and communication technology. An introduction. *International Journal of Operations & Production Management*, *28*(4), 308–312. doi:10.1108/01443570810861534

Van Heijst, G., Schreiber, A. T., & Wielinga, B. J. (1997). Using explicit ontologies in KBS development. *International Journal of Human-Computer Studies*, *46*(2), 183–292. doi:10.1006/ijhc.1996.0090

W3C OWL Working Group. (2012). *OWL 2 Web ontology language document overview* (Second Ed.). Retrieved January 10, 2014, from http://www.w3.org/TR/owl2-overview/

W3C. (n. d.). Retrieved December 8, 2009 from http://www.w3.org

W3CGRDDL. (2007). *Gleaning resource descriptions from dialects of languages (GRDDL) working group*. World Wide Web Consortium (W3C).

W3CHCLSIG. (2005). *Semantic Web health care and life sciences (HCLS) interest group*. World Wide Web Consortium (W3C).

W3CRDB2RDF. (2009). *RDB2RDF working group*. World Wide Web Consortium (W3C).

Wagner, G. (2003). Web rules need two kinds of negation. In F. Bry, N. Henze, & J. Maluszynski (Eds.), *Principles and Practice of Semantic Web Reasoning, International Workshop, PPSWR 2003, Mumbai, India, Proceedings, (Lecture Notes in Computer Science 2901)* (pp. 33–50). Germany: Springer-Verlag.

Walker, J., Pan, E., Johnston, D., Adler-Milstein, J., Bates, D. W., & Middleton, B. (2005). The value of health care information exchange and interoperability. *Health Affairs*. doi:10.1377/hlthaff.w5.10 PMID:15659453

Wang, W., & Wang, M. (2005). *Healthcare information system integration: A service oriented approach*. Paper presented at the International Conference on Services Systems and Services Management, ICSSSM '05, 1475–1480.

Warren, R., Solomonides, T., Del Frate, C., Warsi, I., Ding, J., & Odeh, M. … Estrella, F. (2013). *Grid-enabled medical simulation services (EU GEMSS)*. Retrieved from: http://www.it.neclab.eu/gemss

Watkins, E. R., & Nicole, D. A. (2006). Named graphs as a mechanism for reasoning about provenance. In X. Zhou, J. Li, H. T. Shen, M. Kitsuregawa, & Y. Zhang (Eds.), *Frontiers of WWW Research and Development - APWeb 2006, 8th Asia-Pacific Web Conference, Harbin, China, Proceedings, (Lecture Notes in Computer Science 3841)* (pp. 943–948). Germany: Springer-Verlag.

Watry, P., & Larson, R. (2005). Cheshire 3 framework white paper: Implementing support for digital repositories in a data grid environment. In *IEEE International Symposium on Mass Storage Systems and Technology* (pp. 60-84). Sardinia: IEEE Press.

Westbrook, J. I., Gosling, A. S., & Coiera, E. (2005). Do online information retrieval systems help experienced clinicians answer clinical questions? *Journal of the American Medical Informatics Association*, *12*(3), 113–120. doi:10.1197/jamia.M1717 PMID:15561783

WfMC. (n. d.). *Workflow Management Coalition*. Retrieved December 8, 2009 from http://www.wfmc.org

WHO. (n. d.). *World Health Organization*. Retrieved December 8, 2009 from http://www.who.int/

Wiederhold, G. (1992). Mediators in the architecture of future information systems. *Computer*, *25*, 38–49. doi:10.1109/2.121508

Woolman, P. S. (2011). Challenges of managing interoperability in regional healthcare organisations. In *Proceedings of the First International Workshop on Managing Interoperability and Complexity in Health Systems (MIXHS '11)* (pp. 1-2). New York: ACM.

Wozak, F., Ammenwerth, E., Hoerbst, A., Soegner, P., Mair, R., & Schabetsberger, T. (2008). *IHE based interoperability – Benefits and challenges*. Paper presented at the 1st International Workshop on Describing Medical Web Resources (MIE 2008), Gotenburg, Sweden.

Wroe, C. (2006). Is Semantic Web technology ready for healthcare? In *3rd European Semantic Web Conference (ESWC'06)*. Budva, Montenegro. Retrieved from http://ftp.informatik.rwth-aachen.de/Publications/CEUR-WS/Vol-194/paper2.pdf

Wyckoff, P., McLaughry, S. W., Lehman, T. J., & Ford, D. A. (1998). T Spaces. *IBM Systems Journal*, *37*(3), 454–474. doi:10.1147/sj.373.0454

XForms. (n. d.). Retrieved November 2013, from http://www.w3.org/TR/xforms11/

Yang, E. A. T. H. (2006). *A scalable multi-tier architecture for the National Taiwan University Hospital Information System based on HL7 standard*. Paper presented at the 19th IEEE Symposium on Computer-Based Medical Systems (CBMS'06), Utah, USA.

Zhu, K., Kraemer, K., Xu, S., & Dedrick, J. (2004). Information technology payoff in e-business environments: An international perspective on value creation of e-business in the financial services industry. *Journal of Management Information Systems*, *21*(1), 17–54.

Zimmermann, A. (2007). Integrated distributed description logics. In Calvanese et al. *Proceedings of the 20th International Workshop on Description Logics DL'07, June 8 - 10, 2007, Brixen/Bressanone, Italy* (pp. 507-514). Bolzano University Press.

Zimmermann, A., & Duc, C. L. (2008). Reasoning on a network of aligned ontologies. In D. Calvanese & H. Lausen (Eds.), *Web Reasoning and Rule Systems, Second International Conference, RR 2008, Karlsruhe, Germany, Proceedings, (Lecture Notes in Computer Science 5341)* (pp. 43–57). Germany: Springer-Verlag.

Zimmermann, A., Sahay, R., Fox, R., & Polleres, A. (2009). Lecture Notes in Computer Science: Vol. 5871. *Heterogeneity and Context in Semantic-Web-enabled HCLS systems* (pp. 1165–1182). Germany: Springer-Verlag. doi:10.1007/978-3-642-05151-7_30

Zou, Y., & Kontogiannis, K. (2001). *Towards a Web-centric legacy system migration framework*. Paper presented at the 3rd International Workshop on Net-Centric Computing(NCC 2001), Toronto, Canada.

About the Contributors

Miguel-Ángel Sicilia was born in Madrid, Spain in 1973. He got a five-year degree in Computer Science from the Pontifical University of Salamanca (at the Madrid Campus) in 1996. He worked at the same university as lecturer for some time, and he also worked for several companies in the IT sector until he joined Carlos III University as assistant professor. He obtained a Ph.D. in Computer Science from Carlos III University in 2003. He then moved to the University of Alcalá, where he is currently associate professor. From 2001, he has been a virtual tutor of the Open University of Catalonia. In 2008, he obtained a postgraduate degree on Bioinformatics from the same university.

* * *

Diego Boscá received his M. Sc. in Computer Science from Universitat Politècnica de Valencia (UPV) and currently is a predoctoral research fellow at the ITACA Institute of UPV. He has been involved in the implementation and deployment of health information systems and use of health standards in the real world for over six years. His experience covers the analysis, design, implementation, and deployment of semantically interoperable health information systems using standards such as ISO 13606, HL7 CDA, and openEHR. He is a Certified Specialist in HL7 CDA. He has participated as external advisor at the European epSOS project and as an external expert in the SemanticHealthNet European project. He is part of the openEHR software committee. He has participated in several research projects and co-authored more than 30 papers about data integration and standardization of the EHR.

Alessio Carenini has been working since 2007 for CEFRIEL, both as researcher and consultant. After focusing his research activities on the application of Semantic Web and Semantic Web Services principles to business intelligence (in SUPER EU project), eHealth (in TRIPCOM EU project), and logistics (in NeP4B Italian project), he participated to the CHOReOS FP7 development of an ultra large scale application of service choreographies to a marketing scenario. His current research interests delve into distributed architectures for efficient collection and processing of continuous data.

Davide Cerri has extensive experience in information security as a researcher, consultant, trainer, and security manager. Before switching to industry, he worked for many years at the IT technology transfer centre of the Technical University of Milan, Italy and at the University of Innsbruck, Austria. He was involved in several national and European research projects as well as in consulting and technology transfer activities to industry and public bodies regarding information security topics. He now works as a security manager and change manager in the private sector.

Jesualdo Tomás Fernández-Breis obtained his PhD in Computer Science in 2003 and is currently serving as Associate Professor in the University of Murcia. His main research areas are Semantic Web technologies and their application in biomedical domains and education, including the development of semantic web solutions for semantic interoperability in healthcare, together with the transformation of clinical data and models between electronic healthcare records standards. He has been the PI of more than 10 research projects in the last ten years and participated in more than 20 projects related to his main research interests. He has published over 100 papers in international journals and conferences and has supervised 6 doctoral theses.

Ronan Fox is in software engineering Manager at Avaya specialising in the visualisation and management of real time streaming data. Before his current role Ronan was the Health Care and Life Science unit leader within DERI, Galway, Ireland. He holds a B.E in Engineering (1988) and a PhD (2011) in Informatics from NUIG. Ronan's research interests are in addressing interoperability and scalability issues which will arise within the society now facing us in the context of an ageing population and personalised medicine.

Manfred Hauswirth is the Vice-Director of the Digital Enterprise Research Institute (DERI), Galway, Ireland and a professor at the National University of Ireland, Galway. His research focus is on linked data streams, semantic sensor networks, sensor networks middleware, large-scale semantics-enabled distributed information systems and applications. Manfred has also worked extensively in peer-to-peer systems, Internet of things, self-organization and self-management, service-oriented architectures and distributed systems security. He has published over 160 papers in these domains, and has co-authored a book on distributed software architectures and several book chapters on data management and semantics. He is associate editor of IEEE Transactions on Services Computing and was program co-chair of IEEE P2P-2007, WISE-2011, and ODBASE-2011 and general chair of ESWC-2008.

Pedro Isaías is an associate professor at the Universidade Aberta (Portuguese Open University) in Lisbon, Portugal, responsible for several courses and director of the master degree program in Electronic Commerce and Internet since its start in 2003. He holds a PhD in Information Management (in the speciality of information and decision systems) from the New University of Lisbon. Author of several books, book chapters, papers and research reports, all in the information systems area, he has headed several conferences and workshops within the mentioned area. He has also been responsible for the scientific coordination of several EU funded research projects. He is also a member of the editorial board of several journals and program committee member of several conferences and workshops. At the moment he conducts research activities related to Information Systems in general, E-Learning, E-Commerce and WWW related areas.

Vassiliki Koufi is a postdoctoral researcher at the Department of Digital Systems at University of Piraeus, Greece. She received a B.Sc. in Informatics from the University of Piraeus, a M.Sc. in Data Communication Systems from Brunel University, UK and a Ph.D. from the Department of Digital Systems of the University of Piraeus. She has been working as a network engineer at the Network Management Center at the University of Piraeus and she has been a teaching/research fellow at the Department of Digital Systems of the same University. She has been involved in several projects concerning the development of web-based healthcare information systems as well as the development and management of network services and applications. She has published several research papers in internationally refereed journals, international conferences and books. Her research interests include ubiquitous and pervasive healthcare, context-aware healthcare information systems, healthcare information security and personal health records systems.

Reto Krummenacher, after concluding his engineering degree in communication systems at the Ecole Politechnique Federale de Lausanne (Switzerland), continued his academic career at the Semantic Technology Institute at the University of Innsbruck. Before concluding his doctoral studies in late 2010 with a dissertation on scalability in semantic web service middleware, he worked for many years on topics like semantic web services, middleware, service oriented architectures and as such served as principle investigator and project manager in various national and European research projects such as TripCom, LarKC or SOA4All.

Craig Kuziemsky, PhD, is an Associate Professor and director of the Master of Science in Health Systems Program in the Telfer School of Management at the University of Ottawa. He completed his PhD in Health Information Science from the University of Victoria in 2006. Craig's research focuses on developing new approaches for modeling collaborative healthcare delivery so we can better design information and communication technologies to support collaboration. His research is tackling this problem at two levels. The first level is the micro level where he is modeling healthcare delivery from the perspective of the micro level relationships between providers and teams. That research includes modeling how providers communicate and collaborate with each other as part synchronous and asynchronous healthcare delivery. For example he has developed models of awareness and common ground and looked at the role they play in collaboration and how they can inform HIS design. The second level is looking at collaboration from a meso or organizational level. Craig's research at this level makes a key distinction between data and process interoperability. To date his research has identified process interoperability needs such as workflow, knowledge, collaborative, and information management, and then applied those needs to different technical implementations.

Leonardo Lezcano obtained a degree in Computer Engineering from the University of Alcala (UAH) (2008) and a Ph.D. degree in Computer Science (2012) from the same university. He taught DDBB, Language Processing, and Algorithms Design at the Open University of Madrid (UDIMA) between 2008 and 2010, and Medical Informatics at the UAH during the subsequent two years. As a member of the Information Engineering Research Unit, he has collaborated in several Spanish health projects such as CISEP "Intelligent Clinical Records for Patient Safety." As a result, he joined the openEHR.org Java Project. In addition, he is an associated partner of the Patient-Project.eu and a collaborator of Emurgency.eu. Significant publications in the biomedical domain include "Integrating reasoning and clinical archetypes using OWL ontologies and SWRL rules" (2011, *Journal of Biomedical Informatics*) and "Associating Clinical Archetypes Through UMLS Metathesaurus Term Clusters" (2012, *Journal of Medical Systems*).

Mario Macedo, MSc, PhD **is an** Information Systems Architect with a deep knowledge of hospital and healthcare services management. He holds a PhD in Information Management, is a consultant on international healthcare information systems projects and a researcher on knowledge construction systems for healthcare and wellness domains. He is a member of the Working Group for Healthcare Normalization of Portuguese Institute of Quality and also a program committee member of several conferences and workshops. He is a professor in Portuguese and European universities.

Flora Malamateniou is Associate Professor at the Department of Digital Systems of the University of Piraeus, Greece. She has previously worked as a consultant and senior researcher in research centers and has published extensively in international scientific journals, conference proceedings and books on various subjects regarding digital healthcare services. She has been a referee in international scientific journals, conferences and books and has been involved in many Greek and EU-funded R&TD projects. She is a member of national and international scientific associations. Her current research interests include web-based digital healthcare services, pervasive healthcare systems, (personal) electronic health records, health information security and workflow systems.

Jose Alberto Maldonado received his B.Sc. in Computer Science from the John Moores University (UK) and his B.Sc. and Ph.D. degrees in Computer Science from Universitat Politècnica de Valencia (UPV). He is a postdoctoral research fellow at ITACA Institute of UPV. He was an expert of the Technical Committee 251 of CEN and the Spanish Association for Standardization and Certification (AENOR). Dr. Maldonado is a Certified Specialist in HL7 CDA and HL7 RIM. His research interest spans EHR information modeling, medical terminologies, data transformation, and web semantic technologies. He has been in charge of the technical coordination of several R&D projects and has co-authored several papers on medical informatics.

Catalina Martínez Costa obtained her PhD in Computer Science in 2011 at the University of Murcia. She is now a postdoctoral researcher at the Institute of Medical Informatics, Statistics and Documentation at the Medical University of Graz. Her main research area is medical informatics and more specifically the application of ontologies and semantic web technologies into this field. She has participated in several research projects and at this moment participates in the European network of excellence project SemanticHealthNet. She has published over 20 papers in international journals and conferences.

Marcos Menárguez-Tortosa is a Computer Engineer and is currently serving as Assistant Professor in the University of Murcia. His main research areas are the combination of Software Engineering, Model-Driven Engineering and Semantic Web technologies and their application for the semantic interoperability in healthcare. His doctoral research pursues the development of ontology-based models for the representation and exploitation of archetypes in health information systems. His research results show the possibilities of OWL technologies for supporting the validation and interoperability of archetypes. He has participated in more than 10 research projects related to his main research interests, and has published over 20 papers in international journals and conferences.

David Moner received his M. Sc. in Computer Science from Universitat Politècnica de Valencia (UPV) and currently is a predoctoral research fellow at the ITACA Institute of UPV. He is member of the Spanish Normalisation Organisation (AENOR) and Certified Specialist in HL7 CDA, HL7 v2.6, and HL7 RIM. He has participated as external advisor for the Semantic Interoperability Group of the Spanish Ministry of Health and is also member of the international Clinical Information Modelling Initiative (CIMI). David Moner has been involved in several projects on the development of semantically interoperable health information systems based on health information standards such as ISO EN 13606, HL7 v2.x, HL7 CDA, and openEHR. He is coauthor of more than 30 publications about data integration and standardization of the EHR and EHR systems.

Axel Polleres obtained his PhD in 2003 from Vienna University of Technology, Austria, and the habilitation in "Information System" in 2011 from the same university. He worked at universities in Austria, Spain and Ireland before joining Siemens Corporate Technology as senior key expert research scientist in 2011. His research interests include Knowledge Representation & Management (Querying and Reasoning about Ontologies, Linked Data/Semantic Web, Web Services) and applications. He is an active participant in international standardization activities in the World Wide Web consortium, such as the SPARQL1.1 working group which he co-chaired, and has published more than 100 scientific articles in journals and books as well as international conferences and workshops.

Nikolaos P. Preve received his BS, MS, and his PhD degree from the School of Electrical and Computer Engineering of the National Technical University of Athens (NTUA), Athens, Greece. He is currently working in the field of computer networks research in national, European and international projects while he is specialized in computer and telecommunication networks. He has been mainly involved as a project leader, and technical manager of several successfully integrated projects both in national and international level. He is also in parallel teaching in the School of Electrical and Computer Engineering at the National Technical University of Athens, Greece, and in the Department of Informatics at the Technological Educational Institute of Athens, Greece. His main research interests are in the fields of wireless networks, mobile and personal communications, healthcare computing, parallel and distributed computing, cloud and grid computing.

Eydel Rivero Ruíz graduated in Computer Science from the University of Havana in 2008. He has been a member of the Information Engineering Research Unit (IERU) of the University of Alcala since 2012. In this group, he has participated in the development of the tool ADL2OWL translator, a set of Java libraries to translate openEHR archetypes to OWL. Currently, he is involved in the Spanish project HEDECAMA, a semantic model and data mining algorithms applied to the treatment of breast cancer in specialized care centers. His research areas include interoperability in health information systems, integration of electronic health records, semantic web, and knowledge representation and reasoning.

Ratnesh Sahay is Research Associate at the Digital Enterprise Research Institute (DERI), Galway. He received his Bachelor's Degree in Information Technology from the University of Southern Queensland, Australia, in 2002. He received his M.Sc. with specialisation in Distributed Systems from the KTH Royal Institute of Technology, Sweden, in 2006. He received his PhD in Computer Science from the National University of Ireland, Galway, in 2012. His research interests include Knowledge Representation &

Integration, especially ontology building, alignment, and reasoning for the HCLS domain. He has been active in a number of European and National R&D projects with emphasis on e-health and Semantic Interoperability. He has published and served as reviewer in several international conferences. He is a member of the W3C OWL 2, W3C HCLS, and HL7 RIMBAA working groups. He previously served as member of the OASIS SEE Technical Committee.

Elena Simperl works as a senior lecturer at the Web and Internet Science (WAIS) group at the University of Southampton. Her research interests include knowledge engineering, Social Web technologies, and crowdsourcing. She has contributed and led more than 15 national and European research projects, has authored more than 75 scientific publications, and chaired the European Semantic Web Conference in 2011 and 2012. Elena initiated several activities targeted at the supervision and guidance of doctoral students and young researchers, including the ESWC summer school, the Asian Semantic Web School, and the IEEE Summer School on Semantic Computing. She is also co-founder of semsphere GmbH, a professional training company in the same area. She is actively involved in knowledge transfer and innovation management initiatives, including the European Data Forum, which she chaired in 2013.

George Vassilacopoulos has received his Ph.D. degree from the University of London, UK. He is currently a Professor at the Department of Digital Systems, Director of the Digital Health Services laboratory, Vice-Rector of Academic Affairs and Deputy President of the Council of the University of Piraeus, Greece. He has published extensively in peer-reviewed international journals and conference proceedings in various ICT fields, especially eHealth, has authored three books and several book chapters and has taken part as either a contributor or a committee member in many ICT conferences. He also has been an editor and associate editor in several conference proceedings and books. His current research interests include eHealth, business process management, service-oriented systems and cloud computing, and healthcare systems security. He is a member of the BCS and the IEEE.

Montserrat Robles Viejo, M.Sc. and PhD in Physical Science, is an Associate Professor of the Universitat Politècnica de Valencia (UPV), where she is involved in pre and postgraduate teaching in Biomedical informatics. She established and has led the Biomedical Informatics Group (IBIME, www.ibime.upv.es) since 1999. Currently, she is the Director of the Institute for the Applications of Advanced Information and Communication Technologies (ITACA) (ww.itaca.upv.es) of UPV. Her research areas span Electronic Health Records Normalization, Biomedical Data Mining, and Medical Image. She has been the principal investigator at UPV of several national and international research projects, including the EU projects E-Tumour on decision support for brain tumour diagnosis and prognosis and HealthAgents on the application of agent technology for decision support in health. She is co-author of more than 70 papers on biomedical informatics.

Antoine Zimmermann (MSc, PhD) is an associate professor at École des mines de Saint-Étienne. His research interests are in representing, reasoning, querying and managing contextual knowledge that are distributed and heterogeneous, in open environments. Antoine participated in several international research projets, conference committees and in the OWL 2 and RDF 1.1 W3C working groups. Between 2009 and 2012, Antoine has jointly chaired the working group on semantics in the COST Action Agreement Technologies.

Index

J

L

M

N

O

P

R

S

T

W

X

www.ingramcontent.com/pod-product-compliance
Lightning Source LLC
Chambersburg PA
CBHW082307051126
54379CB00060B/142
* 9 7 8 1 4 6 6 6 3 0 0 0 0 *